A HISTORY OF MEDICINE

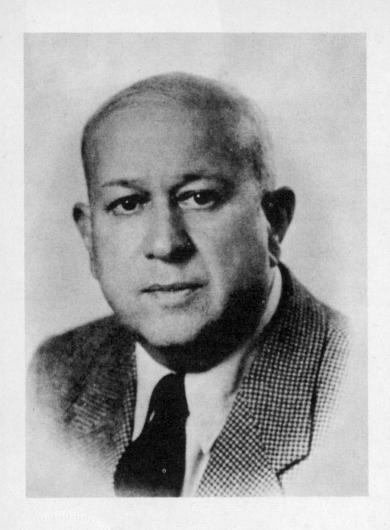

HENRY E. SIGERIST 1955

Photo House, H. Rüedi A.-G., Lugano

★

A HISTORY OF MEDICINE

HENRY E. SIGERIST

II

EARLY GREEK, HINDU, AND
PERSIAN MEDICINE

★ ★

OXFORD UNIVERSITY PRESS
New York   Oxford

Oxford University Press

Oxford   New York   Toronto
Delhi   Bombay   Calcutta   Madras   Karachi
Petaling Jaya   Singapore   Hong Kong   Tokyo
Nairobi   Dar es Salaam   Cape Town
Melbourne   Auckland

and associated companies in
Beirut   Berlin   Ibadan   Nicosia

First published in 1961 by Oxford University Press, Inc., 200 Madison Avenue,
New York, New York 10016

First issued as an Oxford University Press paperback, 1987

Oxford is a registered trademark of Oxford University Press

Publication No. 38
Department of the History of Medicine
Yale University

The Library of Congress has catalogued the
first printing of this title as follows:
Sigerist, Henry Ernest, 1891-1957.
A history of medicine. New York, Oxford University Press,
1951-61.
2 v. illus., ports., maps. 24 cm. (Publication / Historical Library, Yale
Medical Library ; no. 27) (v. 2: Publication / Department of the History of
Medicine, Yale University ; no. 38)
Includes bibliographies.
Contents: v. 1. Primitive and archaic medicine.—v. 2. Early Greek, Hindu,
and Persian medicine.
1. Medicine—History.   I. Title.   II. Series: Publication (Yale Medical Li-
brary, Historical Library) ; no. 27.   III. Series: Publication (Yale University.
Dept. of the History of Medicine) ; no. 38.
R131.S533   610.9   51-9041
Vol. 1 ISBN 0-19-500739-5(pbk.)
Vol. 2 ISBN 0-19-505079-7(pbk.)

2 4 6 8 10 9 7 5 3

Printed in the United States of America

Preface

The circumstances surrounding Dr. Sigerist's carefully laid plan to write a comprehensive eight-volume *History of Medicine,* which would place the subject in the broad framework of general history including all lands and cultures, were outlined in his Foreword to the first volume, and from another angle it was also touched upon briefly in the Preface which Professor Sigerist had invited me to contribute to that volume. Here he confessed to us that he had intended to begin drafting the book in 1941, when he would have been fifty years of age. World War II, however, precluded making a start at that time, and, when the conflict ended, he was obliged to face the difficult decision of giving up a post in which he had been happy in order to return to the land of his birth, where in the more isolated tranquility of the southern Alpine foothills of Ticino he could work with fewer interruptions. The first volume, *Primitive and Archaic Medicine,* made its appearance in 1951. It was accorded an enthusiastic reception by historians, being hailed as a new and highly original departure in medical historiography; the ensuing seven volumes were eagerly awaited, but his start was late, and circumstances quite unforeseen were to prevent completion of his great project.

The reasons for the slower progress during the five years prior to his death on 17 March 1957 were perhaps to some extent psychological, but failing health was primarily responsible. Henry Sigerist was stimulated by human contacts, especially of students old and young, and without these his old drive and extraordinary capacity for accomplishment noticeably slackened. In his beautiful Casa

Serena at Pura, he welcomed his friends in increasing numbers, and the obvious enjoyment which he derived from lecturing caused him to accept such assignments, the most notable being the Heath Clark series on *Landmarks in the History of Hygiene* given at The London School of Hygiene and Tropical Medicine in 1952.

Thus when an apoplectic stroke brought prematurely to an end the career of this many-sided man who had still so much to offer, only the second volume of the *History* had been drafted, and this was not complete. There were a few notes for Volume III and a topic outline for the remaining five volumes, but no drafted text could be found. Dr. Sigerist's titles for the remaining volumes were: III – Medieval Medicine; IV – Renaissance Medicine; V – The Seventeenth Century; VI – The Eighteenth Century; and VII and VIII – Medicine from the Industrial Revolution to the Second World War. As Dr. Sigerist's literary executor I therefore sought counsel from the Henry E. Sigerist Research Fund Committee* and on its advice decided to publish the present volume as Dr. Sigerist had left it, with his former associates, Professor Ludwig Edelstein acting as General Editor and Dr. Miriam Drabkin aiding in selection and arrangement of illustrative matter. Full consideration was given to the possibility of having the *History* carried on by other scholars along the lines originally envisaged by the author, but after thorough exploration, it was concluded that this would not only be difficult, but actually quite impossible.

His daughter, Mrs. Nora Sigerist Beeson of New York has now edited Dr. Sigerist's *Autobiography* which, when published, will throw further light on his original plan and the intended scope of his *History of Medicine*. The *Autobiography* is a human document

---

* This Committee, made up of Erwin Ackerknecht, Esther Lucille Brown, Leslie Falk, John F. Fulton, Iago Galdston, Alan Gregg, Robert Leslie, Genevieve Miller, Milton I. Roemer, George Rosen, George Silver, Ilza Veith, Gregory Zilboorg, was formed in 1953 to secure for administration by Yale University a subsidy for Dr. Sigerist and his projected *History,* one of his most pressing needs apart from his own stipend having been for a research secretary to work with him at Pura.

which will be invaluable to any future medical historian who is bold enough to undertake a history in such vast perspective. It will reveal much of the man who has inspired many, discouraged none— a scholar whose influence will long be felt as a living force by those who study the past to guide their future course of action, and who attempt to place the history of medicine and science in the broad cultural background of the general history of mankind.

JOHN F. FULTON M.D.

Department of the History of Medicine
Yale University
January 1960

★

Editor's Foreword

Shortly after Dr. Sigerist's death, Dr. Fulton and his Advisory Committee asked me to assume the responsibility of editing the second volume of Dr. Sigerist's *History of Medicine*. When I read the typed copy of the book, I found attached to the last page a note in Dr. Sigerist's handwriting, saying: 'Here my legacy ends.' These terse and moving words made it clear to me that he had hoped that the book would be published although he knew that he would be unable to finish it. I therefore undertook to carry out his wish as a token of my indebtedness to him as scholar and friend.

To all who have been eagerly awaiting this volume which was to deal with Greek, Indian, and Persian medicine as a whole, it will be disappointing that the analysis of only the early periods of the subject was completed. Also, unfortunately, there was no outline of the contents of the entire volume as Dr. Sigerist had planned it, nor were there any notes to give a hint of how he had intended to proceed. A few references here and there in the finished text point to topics he meant to discuss, but they are not detailed enough to permit any reconstruction of the sequel, which one might otherwise have attempted.

The problem of illustrations for the volume had occupied Dr. Sigerist's thoughts for a long time, and he had engaged in a far-flung correspondence to obtain material that was interesting and unhackneyed. At least in some instances he had succeeded. Dr. Howard Dittrick of Cleveland, Dr. P. M. Mehta of Jamagar (India), Dr. F. Merke of Basel and the Wellcome Museum at London had put photographs of little-known works at his disposal. However, for the bulk of the manuscript the question had been left in abeyance. I was sure that he would not have wished the book to appear without more illustrations than those he had already decided upon, and thus I have ventured to add what seemed most appropriate. It was difficult to act in his stead and not feel that he would have made a better selection.

As far as the text is concerned, I have left it as it stood even where I believed that Dr. Sigerist might have introduced changes or made additions after completing the work. Those concerned with the history of medicine are entitled to read this last writing of his in the form he gave it. I have merely tried to eliminate mistakes or inaccuracies that apparently escaped his notice, and I have throughout altered words or phrases, or tightened the style, wherever it seemed necessary. In short, I have read the text over as an author would read it once more before sending it to the press. Even in the notes, I have not inserted literature that might have been included by Dr. Sigerist, or that came out after his death and should now be referred to. The volume is not meant to be a bibliography; rather, what is important throughout is Dr. Sigerist's view of the development of medicine in antiquity.

In the stylistic revision of the text and in the choice of the pictures Mrs. Miriam Drabkin and I have collaborated. Without her help, given in the spirit of friendship and admiration for Dr. Sigerist, the publication of the book would have been delayed much longer, and I should have felt less hopeful of achieving at least part of my aim.

Had Dr. Sigerist been allowed to write the introduction to this volume he would, I know, have expressed his thanks to Yale University and to his friends who made it possible for him, even during his illness, to devote himself to writing. It is not for another person to speak on his behalf in this matter. But I think I may thank in his name those who provided him with illustrations. I should like to add my own thanks to all who have given permission to reproduce material in their possession, especially to the Archaeological Institute of America for the photographs from the Asclepi-

eion at Corinth, which to my knowledge have not yet been seen
except in the original publication, and to Professor O. Temkin for
the photographs of medical instruments deposited in the Institute
of the History of Medicine at The Johns Hopkins University and
hitherto unpublished.

Finally, I wish to express my gratitude to two friends who gave
me advice and assistance. Professor John Young of The Johns
Hopkins University made many valuable suggestions concerning the
illustrations for topics of Greek medicine. Mrs. W. E. Drake read
the proofs of the book and through her careful attention saved me
from many an error.

LUDWIG EDELSTEIN

August 1960
Baltimore, Maryland

Contents

IV. THE GOLDEN AGE OF GREEK MEDICINE

INDEX

★

List of Illustrations

ARCHAIC MEDICINE IN GREECE

HINDU MEDICINE

A HISTORY OF MEDICINE

To the Hippocratic Tradition in Medicine

———————

★

Introduction

A new epoch in the history of medicine began with the advent of the Indo-European peoples. Not all of them developed a high civilization. The Thracians, Illyrians, and Scythians remained barbarians. But in antiquity in Greece and in India cultures flowered such as the world had never seen before,[1] cultures created by the tribes that migrated from the Danube basin into the Balkan peninsula, and by the most Eastern branch of the Aryans that settled the Indus valley and gradually large sections of the Indian subcontinent. They too had their archaic period and archaic medicine, not so very different from that of the Ancient Near East and consisting of similar empirical, religious, and magical elements. But they went far beyond that. The separation of the various elements which in Mesopotamia never took place, and was only begun in Egypt, became here almost complete, at any rate in Greece. Both civilizations had forms of religious medicine, had magic, but on the basis of empiricism developed philosophical systems of medicine which looked beyond the sick man for universal laws.[2] And in both countries medicine became infinitely more effective than it had ever been in Egypt or Mesopotamia.[3] This occurred not only because of the element of time but also because the Greeks and Indians acquired a much more profound knowledge of nature and of man within nature, in health and in illness.

The parallelism in the development of Greek and Indian medicine is striking, both in chronology and in content. But there are also great differences determined to a certain extent by the fact that one culture unfolded in the temperate zone, the other in the tropics. The

Greek emphasis was on reason and logic; India also developed rational systems of medicine but had in addition another, a mystic approach to the problems of health and disease. The Greek method paved the way for modern Western science but Indian medicine was better prepared to handle mental and spiritual troubles, and in the various systems of meditation and Yoga created therapeutic methods unknown to the West in antiquity, or at least not as highly developed.

It may seem strange to discuss Graeco-Roman and Indian medicine in the same volume and to devote much space to Indian medical thought and achievements. As Western physicians living in the twentieth century, we are fully aware of the enormous progress made by medical science in the West, particularly during the last hundred years, advances which are reflected dramatically in the figures of our vital statistics. When we consult the history of medicine, we are inclined to do so from our present Western point of view, going backward, looking for precursors and ancestors. We trace the rise of science from the Renaissance and particularly from the seventeenth century on. The Middle Ages appear as dark ages or, at best, as a period good enough to produce cathedrals but not science. We glorify the Greeks, however, as our precursors and true ancestors who first developed the scientific method. Egypt and Mesopotamia may claim our attention only in so far as they were precursors of the Greeks and made a few contributions to our medicine through the channels of Greek literature and of the Old Testament.

It goes without saying that such an approach to history is utterly naïve and viciously wrong. We must study ancient medicine in the various countries as if it had never had any successors, and if we do this, we soon find that Western and Indian medicine were closely related and equally effective not only in antiquity but also in the Middle Ages. In the West, the turning point came in the Renaissance, and we shall have to discuss later why there was no similar movement in the East at that time. It may well be that India is today in the initial stages of a great renaissance, assimilating the technical knowledge of the West—without losing its soul—and blending it with the best traditions of its old culture. The future will tell whether this view is correct. In the meantime, there can be no doubt that whenever we approach the history of medicine not from the narrow Western, but from a universal, point of view, Indian medicine must be given full attention.

There was a time, probably around 3500 to 2500 B.C., when the Indo-European peoples who were to conquer Europe, the Near East, and India lived together.[4] There is no certainty as to their homeland but since their migrations took place from north to south, to southeast, to west and southwest, we are entitled to assume that they lived in the Russian plains, north of the Carpathian mountains, north of the Black Sea, north and east of the Caspian Sea. They were nomads, cattle breeders who in some regions must have settled down for a while to grow crops. At the time when Egypt and Sumer developed a pictographic script the Indo-Europeans were still barbarians, and it was not until two thousand years later that they adopted a foreign alphabet. What we know of their early history is derived entirely from linguistic studies. When we find the same word, or rather words, with the same root in Sanskrit, Greek, Latin, and other Indo-European languages, then we know that the concept existed before the tribes had scattered. Thus they had a common word for copper but not for iron, for which every language had its own word. From this fact we may deduce that the Indo-Europeans separated before the Iron Age but took the step from the Stone Age to the Copper Age while they were still together.

The language also tells us of their social organization, of the patriarchal family strictly ruled by the father, of the fraternities of warriors. The Indo-Europeans were divided into tribes which before 2500 B.C. were still in touch with one another. Their animals were cattle, sheep, goats, not yet pigs and geese. But they domesticated the horse and used it for riding and for pulling the cart. They worshiped Father-Sky and Mother-Earth and the sun that took its course through the sky as a horse or in a cart pulled by fiery horses. The gods of light were in constant struggle with the evil demons of darkness, and the thunderstorm was an eternally repeated picture of this fight. Much of this early mythology is reflected in that of the Greeks, Persians, Indians, and Germans.

Having no written records, we know nothing of the early history of the Indo-Europeans, of their battles among themselves or with neighbors, for better pastures or for revenge, or of their blood feuds. But then, toward the middle of the third millennium B.C., the great migrations began and the tribes were dispersed. We can only speculate about the causes of these migrations, but we may safely assume that here, as almost everywhere, it was economic pressure that set the people in motion and forced them to undergo all the dangers and hardships of a long journey into hostile territories, with women, children, domestic animals, and all household goods.

The Indo-Europeans were latecomers. In their wanderings into Asia Minor, India, Greece, and the Aegean Islands, they clashed with peoples who had been sedentary for a long time and had developed a much higher culture. Young, strong, uncorrupted, and very intelligent, they usually succeeded in defeating the peoples who opposed them; however, they could not but accept a great deal from the higher civilizations they met. The first to move south, the Hittites and Mitanni in the mountains of Asia Minor and on the upper Euphrates, came under the spell of Babylonia and adopted the cuneiform script. Their flourishing kingdoms were ultimately destroyed. The Aryans who migrated into the Indus valley through the mountain passes of Afghanistan also encountered an old civilization, and in order to adjust themselves to life in a tropical country were forced to change many habits, and to accept customs and views of the indigenous populations. The Greeks who settled the Balkan peninsula and the islands and shores of the Eastern Mediterranean basin came in contact with the civilization of Crete and thus indirectly with that of Egypt and Mesopotamia.

But however much the Indo-Europeans took over from the peoples they subjugated or otherwise came in contact with, they never gave up their individuality, and whatever they accepted they assimilated into their patrimony. Zeus might acquire attributes of a Cretan deity but he remained the old Indo-European Sky-Father. And thus great new cultures were born and new systems of medicine within them, showing a new approach to the problems of health and disease.

Our task in this volume is to study the development of Greek and Indian medicine in the West and East within the framework of the general culture of Greece and India. We begin with Greek medicine, although it is not older than that of India, merely because it is closer to a Western historian whose education was in the Greek humanistic tradition.

H. S.

NOTES

1. I am not forgetting China and will discuss Chinese medicine in Volume III; for I did not wish to burden this volume with a third civilization, especially since the uncertainties of the early chronology of China require detailed examination.
2. See W. Jaeger, *Paideia: The Ideals of Greek Culture,* New York, 1944, vol. 3, p. 5.
3. Philologists writing on Greek medicine, as a rule, are interested in theories only. To most of them medicine is merely one aspect of philosophy. And yet what counts in medicine is results. Was a treatment effective or not? Were the Greeks able to prevent illness and restore health, and if so, how? The value of medical theory is determined by the practical results it produces.
4. About the early history see E. Meyer, *Geschichte des Altertums,* 4th ed., Stuttgart and Berlin, 1921, p. 846ff.; J. H. Breasted, *Ancient Times, A History of the Early World,* 2nd ed., Boston, 1935, p. 237ff.; H. Hirt, *Die Indogermanen, ihre Verbreitung, ihre Urheimat und ihre Kultur,* Strassburg, 2 vols., 1905–7; O. Schrader, *Die Indogermanen,* Leipzig, 1911; V. G. Childe, *The Aryans,* New York, London, 1926.

I. ARCHAIC MEDICINE IN GREECE

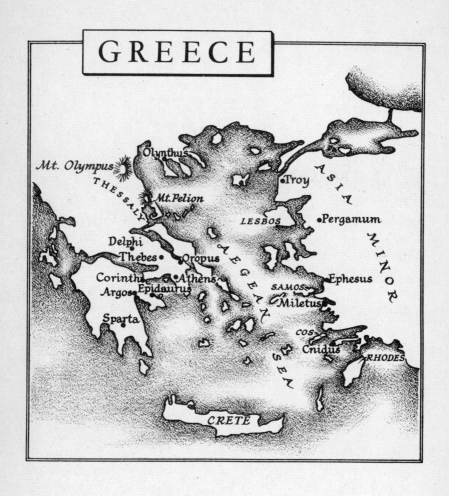

GREECE

Mt. Olympus

Olynthus

THESSALY

Mt.Pelion

Troy

ASIA

LESBOS

Pergamum

MINOR

Delphi

Thebes

Oropus

AEGEAN

Corinth

Athens

Argos

Epidaurus

SAMOS

Ephesus

Sparta

Miletus

SEA

COS

Cnidus

RHODES

CRETE

★

1. The Setting

The Greek tribes which in the course of time populated the Balkan peninsula, the islands of the Aegean Sea, and the coasts of Asia Minor, did not come all at once but in waves. The first invasion must have taken place around 2000 B.C. The Achaeans, as these early invaders were called, came from the north from the region of the Danube. Toward 1200 B.C., a second wave, the Dorian invasion, reached the Greek mainland, and Crete was conquered. The colonization of the Aegean Islands and of the Asiatic coast took place mainly in the centuries from 1300 to 1000 B.C. Different tribes, speaking different Greek dialects and differing also in social organization, shared in this task. Thus the northern part of the eastern Mediterranean basin was settled by Aeolians, whose language was immortalized by the poems of Sappho. The central part was Ionian and became the cradle of Greek science and medicine; Ionian is the language of the Hippocratic writings. The south was Dorian, and Dorian was the language of Sparta.

Our first impression when we travel in Greece today is that the country is extremely small. As in the case of Egypt, our imagination is inclined to magnify the land that has given the world such valuable gifts in every branch of culture. Yet from the Acropolis in Athens on a clear day we can see Corinth in the west. Attica is not larger than a small American county. Mount Olympus, seat of the gods, 9800 feet high, dominates large sections of the country. Wherever we are along the eastern coast we can see dozens of islands, and Crete is visible from the Peloponnesian Mountains. Indeed, the territory of continental Greece in antiquity covered an area of only approximately 25,000 square miles.[1]

The geography is very different from that of Egypt and Mesopotamia because four-fifths of the country is mountainous.[2] Two main ranges give it its profile: one, the continuation of the Central and Dinaric Alps reaching along the western sections to the Peloponnesus, including the Taygetus and ending up in Crete, the other, an extension of the Rhodope Mountains, including the elevations of Thrace, Macedonia, and Thessaly.

The mountains and the sea give the country its character. A peninsula, its fringes consist of a great many minor peninsulas and capes splitting up into islands. A multitude of valleys, with torrents large and small, discharge the water from the mountains into the sea, which through inlets and creeks reaches far into the land. Only 23 per cent of the soil is arable today; wheat, barley, and vegetables are grown. The grapevine and olive tree thrive on the slopes of the hills. Bread, wine, and olive oil have been the main food of the population for several thousand years. Twenty-three per cent of the soil is rocky and completely sterile, and 14 per cent is covered by forests today, but obviously that figure was greater in antiquity.

The climate in Thessaly and farther north is continental, with great changes in temperatures, short hot summers and long cold winters. It is continental-Mediterranean in the plains of the mainland, in the east and southeast, and on the Aegean Islands, with cool dry north winds and rain-carrying southwest winds. The sea acts as a regulator of the temperature, the yearly average ranging between 56° and 68° Fahrenheit. On the west coast and on the Ionian Islands the climate is even milder and more humid, and the vegetation, therefore, is more luxuriant.

Greece is a country that does not require irrigation. The summer is very dry and when you visit the land in autumn you find the hills turned brown. But then from October to March the rains fall; brooks and torrents swell, and from March on the pastures are green, flowers burst forth, and the crops begin to grow. An irrigation culture always requires co-operation of the population and centralized direction. Irrigation on a large scale cannot be carried out successfully unless there is a strong power to direct and enforce the work, and a disciplined population ready to obey orders. The need for irrigation united the people of Egypt and, to a certain extent, also the city-states of Mesopotamia. Greece was never united as long as it was independent. The city-states developed along individual lines. Athens and Sparta, so close geographically, were wide apart culturally, in their thought and entire mode of living. Only national emergencies, a common threat such as the Persian invasions, could unite the Greek states for a co-operative effort, and then only temporarily.

Most ancient Oriental cultural creations, buildings, statues, literary works, remained anonymous, while in Greece we almost always have a name attached to a work of art or to a poem or drama. And so great was the desire to grasp the individuality of an artist or writer that, even if the author of a literary work was not known, a name was attached to it, as was the case with the Homeric hymns or the Hippocratic writings. This extreme individualism so highly characteristic of ancient Greece was obviously not only the result of its geography. The civilization of western Europe, from the Renaissance on, was also individualistic, but showed strong collectivistic trends in the same area inhabited by the same people during the Middle Ages. The development of a man's personality as a desirable goal of education and of life in general is peculiarly Greek—Ionian in particular. But the geographic structure of the Greek land, the small plains, valleys, and islands where small groups could live individually, increased the general trend. And another geographic factor, the intimate connection with the sea,[3] played a still greater part in the formation of Greek culture.

Access to the sea always opens wide horizons, stirs the people's imagination, and makes them dream of foreign lands. Greece, however, not only has access to the sea, it is dipped into the sea. The sea is everywhere, a sea that is ἰοειδής, that has the deep, purple color of the violet, with white foam from which Aphrodite arose, and dolphins playing on the surface. Continental Greece was a small and not a rich country, with very limited arable area and pastures, most of which were good for sheep and goats but not for cattle. Its resources of lignites, iron pyrites, lead, silver, and a few other minerals were very limited also. But there was the sea, boundless and eternal, the sea that provided rich food for the poorest, that opened the doors to lands to be settled: the five hundred islands of the Aegean, bridge to Asia; Crete, bridge to Africa; and in the west, Sicily and southern Italy. Thanks to the sea, Greece did not remain a small peninsula but became a world.

To the Greek, sailing was not only a necessity but a passion, and long before the Venetian he could have said: *navigare necesse est, vivere non est.* Navigation is always a stimulus to science. The Aegean Sea is so crowded with islands that in the good season you may almost cross it to Asia in a rowboat. Today most navigation in the Levant is still coastal navigation, and you sail for days without ever losing sight of land. But once the Greeks reached out for the western shores of the Mediterranean and sailed by night, they needed more astronomical knowledge which, in turn, called for mathematics. A seafaring nation gets in touch with many foreign peoples and an exchange, not only of goods but also of technical knowledge and skills, takes place. Herodotus, although perhaps the most famous of the early Greek travelers, was only one of many who visited Egypt, Mesopotamia, and Asia Minor.

Greece, as a whole, is a healthy country. Since it is in the temperate zone, it does not have the diseases of the tropics. Nor does it have the violent changes of temperature and storms of Mesopotamia. And since it does not have the floods of Egypt, there are not as many water-carried diseases, or the infinity of ophthalmic maladies so frequent in the Nile valley. We shall discuss the main diseases of ancient Greece later when we analyze its medical literature. But for the sake of comparison, it may be worth while looking at health conditions in Greece as they existed in the years preceding the Second World War.[4]

In the period 1931-35 the average yearly birth rate per 1000 population was 29.5 and infant mortality was 122 per 1000 births, while the general annual average death rate per 1000 population was 16.6 for the period 1921-35. The death rate dropped to 13.3 in 1938 and to 13.0 in 1939.

In the year 1938 the main causes of death per 1000 deaths from all causes were the following:

Pneumonia   150.7
Tuberculosis of the respiratory system   70.3
Diarrhea and enteritis of children under two years of age   52.8
Influenza   36.1
Malaria   30.1
Dysentery   14.8
Typhoid and paratyphoid fevers   11.4
Acute and chronic nephritis   41.4
Senility   98.7
Ill-defined and unspecified causes   73.8

This is a very different picture from the one we find in economically advanced countries such as the United States or the United Kingdom, where the chronic diseases of maturity and old age represent the main causes of death. It is probably not so very different from that which prevailed in classical Greece. Pneumonia was then very frequent also and the incidence of malaria was extremely high. We also have many descriptions of gastro-intestinal diseases, and there is no doubt that tuberculosis of the lungs occurred, although it may not have been quite so frequent in antiquity. We shall come back to these problems in a later chapter.

NOTES

1. The territory of today's Greece reaches farther north. The area of the mainland is 41,328 square miles, that of the islands 8,819, a total of 50,147.
2. About the geography of Greece see C. Neuman and J. Partsch, *Physikalische Geographie von Griechenland mit besonderer Rücksicht auf das Altertum,* Breslau, 1885, 2nd ed., 1907; O. Maull, *Südosteuropäische Halbinsel* in O. Kende, *Enzyklopädie der Erdkunde,* Vienna, 1929; A. Philipson, *Das Mittelmeergebiet,* Leipzig and Berlin, 1922; *Beiträge zur Morphologie Griechenlands,* Stuttgart, 1930; G. A. Livadas and J. C. Sphangos, *Malaria in Greece (1930–1940),* Athens, 1941, vol. I, pp. 5–22.

3. See the beautiful book by A. Lesky, *Thalatta, der Weg der Griechen zum Meer,* Vienna, 1947.
4. The figures are from a mimeographed *Report on Public Health in Greece* prepared by the Milbank Memorial Fund in New York and kindly lent to me by the Library of the World Health Organization in Geneva.

★

2. Homeric Medicine

When the Greeks migrated from the north into the Balkan peninsula, they did not occupy an empty space. Mainland and islands were inhabited by tribes that were not Indo-European, but were composed of round-headed people who had emigrated from Asia Minor, and of long-headed Mediterraneans, the purest type of whom was to be found in Crete.

The first waves of Greeks subjugated the mainland and probably some of the northern islands but not Crete, whose high civilization was looked upon with admiration and awe. The Dorian migration, however, did not stop at Crete but caused serious dislocations in the Mediterranean basin. Displaced Cretans settled in Syria and are known to us from the Bible as Philistines.[1] Other displaced peoples who sought a home in the West were the Etruscans and Sardinians.

The Dorian migration was an invasion of barbarians; it destroyed the flourishing Cretan civilization which had been adopted by the early Greek settlers. The history of Crete ran a course closely parallel to that of Egypt and Mesopotamia, and here too culture reached its height soon after 2000 B.C. There was, however, a significant difference in that Crete did not share in the wars of the Asiatic and African mainland. It was a blessed island where people, protected by a strong fleet, could afford to live in cities that had no walls.[2] An aristocratic society, it was not geared to war but rather to hunting, games, and dances. The products of their craftsmen, pottery, jewelry, and seals, were much appreciated abroad, and had a market as far away as Sicily and Spain. Women were held in high esteem and seem to have had equal rights with men. They are frequently represented on wall paintings, dressing with the help of servants, or sharing the entertainments of men. The royal palace at Cnossus had bathrooms and a drainage system similar to those encountered in Egyptian and Mesopotamian palaces of the period. Plants and animals, particularly sea animals, fish, dolphins, and cuttlefish, are the frequent subject of wall paintings or appear on vases in designs of great beauty, which reveal not only a highly developed esthetic sense but also a keen power of observation.

Unlike their Oriental neighbors, the Cretans were not afraid of the dead, nor haunted by the fear of ghosts. All evil forces were relegated to an underworld which was far away and hence not threatening. The gods, immortal as they were, were the friends of man, and lived with him, moved by the same drives and passions, sharing the same urges and whims. It seems that the Cretan's attitude toward nature and life was outspokenly rational.

The Greek invaders who first came in contact with Cretan civilization were fascinated by it and did their best to imitate its ways, taking over artistic styles, giving their old Indo-European gods Cretan attributes and symbols, and worshiping them with music, songs, and dances learned from their neighbor. The culture that flourished in Greece from the sixteenth to the twelfth century, the Mycenaean Age, thus named after one of the main settlements, was apparently Cretan. The imitation, however, was not complete. No civilization has ever been taken over by a young foreign people without undergoing certain changes. The Greek barons, who with their subjects and slaves resided on the mainland, were warriors. Their residences, built on hilltops in Mycenae, Tiryns, Athens, Acrocorinth, and many other places, were castles rather than palaces, walled and well fortified. Men indulged in games and sports as did the Cretans, but from time to time they set out on war expeditions,

single-handed or in large groups, as they did when they sailed to
Asia and, after a long war, destroyed the flourishing city of Troy. This
and similar exploits were recorded in songs which itinerant bards
sang before the assembled noblemen in the *megaron,* the great hall
of the castle.

It was a patriarchal society in which men of the aristocracy were
expected to be strong and courageous, to live up to a well-defined
code of chivalry, while women who had a high social position were
expected to be beautiful and good housekeepers. Excavations have
shown that the arts and crafts flourished on the mainland as much
as in Crete, until the Dorian invasion brutally destroyed this entire
civilization.

A barbaric age followed, with centuries of stagnation, from about
1200 to 900 B.C. The greatest gain made during the period was that
the Greeks adopted the Phoenician alphabet and used it in writing.
This alphabet, derived from Egyptian hieroglyphs, had twenty-two
signs designating consonants. It was adopted by the Arameans who
carried it through western Asia as far as India, and by the Etruscans
who brought it to Italy. The Greeks learned the signs from Phoenician
merchants and used those signs which had no corresponding Greek
sound to designate the vowels. The Greeks thus had a complete
alphabet that did not require diacritical points or determinatives.
From the Phoenicians they also learned the use of pen, ink, and
papyrus. But it was a long time before writing was generally
accepted. For centuries poetry continued to be transmitted by word
of mouth; the nobility had no use for letters and handled the sword
rather than the pen, which seemed an appropriate instrument for
merchants only.

Now we would like to know from what diseases the Greeks suffered
in the Cretan-Mycenaean Age, who treated them in their illnesses,
and by what methods; and also the views they held of the nature of
life in health and disease. In other words, we would like to know
what were the beginnings of Greek medicine. Unfortunately, it is
almost impossible to answer these questions. We have no written
documents from the period, and archaeology merely tells us that the

palace of Mycenae like that of Cnossus had bathrooms, toilets, and a drainage system. We do have some indirect later sources which, however, must be consulted with caution, the *Iliad, Odyssey,* Homeric hymns, and, to a certain extent, Greek mythology as it is reflected in other literary documents.

This is obviously not the place to discuss the Homeric question, the part that Homer, the bard, played in the composition of the great epics. It is enough for us to remember that the *Iliad* and *Odyssey* in all probability took form in the ninth and eighth centuries B.C., and that parts of the poems were much older and had been passed on by word of mouth. We must also keep in mind that the world pictured in these epics is an artificial world, just as the language is an artificial language, a mixture of Aeolian and Ionian. The events described by the poet reflect memories of the glorious past, of the days before the Dorian invasion when the Greek barons resided in their castles and went on war expeditions from which they returned laden with booty. But these reminiscences were combined with the description of conditions as they prevailed in the days of Homer, in the impoverished world after the Dorian invasion, when the king's daughter did her own washing and lords ploughed their fields in person.[3]

The *Iliad* and *Odyssey,* of course, are not medical books but epic poems about the wrath of Achilles, the Trojan war, and the adventures of Odysseus. The *Iliad* is an epic of a world at war while the *Odyssey* has more the character of a novel, including miracle stories and fairy tales. In both poems medical matters are mentioned only incidentally, and we cannot possibly tell to what century a passage refers, whether it reflects a very old observation or view, or one that was current in the ninth century. And yet every single medical reference is important to us because the Homeric epics are the oldest Greek literature preserved. In interpreting medical passages, however, we must always keep in mind that they express a poet's, a layman's, view.[4]

Even greater caution is needed when we examine medical references in myths and legendary tales. There is no doubt that most of them are very old, that many are of Cretan origin or reflect events that took place in the early history of the Greeks. But we know of them from relatively late sources—Hesiod, Pindar, the tragic poets, or from even later sources, for example, Ovid—and while there can be no doubt that the poets made use of old traditions, it is equally certain that they let their imagination play and added episodes from their own experience or their own time.

The Homeric heroes endeavored to be healthy and fit. Their meals were frugal, as a rule, although large banquets were held on festive occasions. They drank wine, but it was mixed with water;[5] drunkenness was frowned upon.[6] They exercised in a variety of games and sports, and measured their strength and skill in various contests. They were clean, had bathrooms at home, and also bathed when at war. A passage in the *Iliad* tells us how Odysseus and Diomedes upon returning from a battle first went into the sea to wash off the sweat and to cool off, and then they had a regular bath in a tub and were anointed with oil.[7] The dress for men consisted of the χιτών, a tunic, worn as undergarment, and the χλαῖνα, a wrapper; women wore the πέπλος, a long garment made of linen or wool.

Health was highly desirable, disease a great evil, and death the worst lot of mankind. The soul of Achilles told Odysseus in Hades that he would prefer to be a laborer on earth slaving on a farm, with little food, rather than king in the realm of the dead.[8]

Disease [9] was inflicted by the gods. This view is not astonishing since here, as in other ancient civilizations, man's fate was believed to be entirely in the hands of the gods. Whatever good and whatever evil he experienced came from the gods, and in the *Iliad* we find the gods taking such an active part in battles that they even suffer wounds inflicted by mortal men.

Any god may cause illness. The Cyclops said to Polyphemus that no one could escape disease sent by the great Zeus.[10] But Apollo and Artemis were particularly known to send acute illness and sudden death by shooting their arrows at mortals, Apollo killing men and

Artemis women. Thus together they had killed Niobe and her
twelve children.[11] With his darts Apollo struck the helmsman of
Menelaus, Rhexenor, and many others, as they were nearing
Athens,[12] and Artemis killed Laodameia, daughter of Bellerophon,[13]
and the mother of Andromache.[14]

Arrows shot at a man symbolized sudden death not only in
Greece, but also in other civilizations.[15] More specifically, they were
symbols of the sudden death of pestilence, and the *Iliad* begins with
the description of a pestilence sent by Apollo to ravage the camp of
the Achaeans.[16] Agamemnon had offended Chryses, priest of Apollo,
by refusing to return his daughter to him, whereupon the god in
his wrath decided to punish the Greeks. He came down from the
peaks of Olympus and shot his arrows first at mules and dogs, then
at humans, and 'the pyres of the dead burnt continually in multitude.' The plague went on for nine days. Its cause was known:
none but Apollo could have sent it, but who had provoked the god,
what was the cause of his wrath? And what were the remedies to
placate him? Achilles suggested that they consult a soothsayer, a
priest, or an interpreter of dreams.[17] Calchas, the seer and augur,
was asked for advice; his answer was:

Neither by reason of a vow is he displeased, nor for any hecatomb,
but for his priest's sake to whom Agamemnon did despite, and set not
his daughter free and accepted not the ransom; therefore hath the
Far-darter brought woes upon us, yea, and will bring. Nor will he
ever remove the loathly pestilence from the Danaans till we have given
the bright-eyed damsel to her father, unbought, unransomed, and
carried a holy hecatomb to Chryse; then might we propitiate him to
our prayer.[18]

This was done, 'and Atreides bade the folk purify themselves. So
they purified themselves, and cast the defilements into the sea and
did sacrifice to Apollo, even unblemished hecatombs of bulls and
goats, along the shore of the unvintaged sea; and the sweet savour
arose to heaven eddying amid the smoke.' [19] Apollo was placated and
the plague ceased.

Here is a typical example of religious medicine. A god, provoked, sends illness in his wrath. The diviners find out what caused his anger and once he is placated by religious means, by reparation for the offense committed, by prayer, sacrifice, purification rites, he arrests the disease and relieves the people. These views are very similar to those we found in Babylonian medicine and in other civilizations, but in this instance the god acts directly and not through the intermediary of ghosts or evil spirits. The *Odyssey* mentions the case of a man who was attacked by a στυγερὸς δαίμων, a dreadful demon, fell sick, and suffered great pains until the gods relieved him of his illness.[20] 'Daimon' is not necessarily a spirit visualized anthropomorphically, but may simply designate divine power, or a man's fortune; but there can be no doubt that the Greeks believed in spirits who assailed man and punished him for evil deeds. The Erinyes, who avenged perjury, homicide, and other crimes, were such spirits.

The gods were responsible for other diseases mentioned in the Homeric poems. The melancholy of Bellerophon could have been amply explained by the fact that he had lost two children in a tragic way, but it is said in addition that he was hateful to the gods.[21] The gods caused illness and the gods healed. Reports of miracle cures are not rare. Diomedes, seriously wounded by an arrow and bleeding profusely, prayed to Pallas Athene, who immediately restored him to health so that he could return to the battle.[22] Aeneas, his hip crushed by a stone thrown by Diomedes, was rescued by Apollo, and nursed and cured by Artemis and Leto.[23] Apollo stopped a hemorrhage of Glaucus, who had been hit by an arrow and was suffering great pain.[24] Apollo and Artemis struck people not only with acute illness and violent death; they also had gentle darts which brought the death of old age.[25]

Illness is mentioned a number of times in the Homeric poems but, for obvious reasons, very few diseases are described. A man suffering from dysentery is not a heroic subject to be pictured in hexameters. But few as the passages are, they are numerous enough to allow us to conclude that there was religious medicine in early Greece, and we learn from Homer, in the words of Celsus, *morbos ... ad iram deorum immortalium relatos esse,* that diseases were attributed to the wrath of the immortal gods.[26] Celsus also points out that the Homeric physicians did not lend their services in the treatment of the plague or other internal diseases but treated wounds only, with surgery and drugs;[27] and Galen concluded that dietetics was unknown to these early doctors[28]—very correct remarks in view of the fact that internal diseases were a concern of religion rather than of medicine.

There is relatively little mention of magic in the Homeric epics although the ancient Greeks believed in magic and, like everyone else in antiquity, practiced some, as we shall discuss in a later chapter. The *Odyssey* is full of miraculous stories which must be accepted as fairy tales and are not to be interpreted rationally. Circe was a beautiful witch who could transform human beings into pigs,[29] and it is absurd to assume that Eurylochus who told the story had been the victim of hallucinations.[30] The drug given to Helen by the Egyptian lady, Polydamna,[31] had strongly euphoric properties, so that whoever took it forgot all unpleasant memories and would not shed a tear even if his closest relative died; this drug might be opium or hashish,[32] but it could just as well be the kind of miracle drug found in many fairy tales.

A truly magic rite, however, is mentioned in a passage of the *Odyssey.*[33] While hunting on Mount Parnassus Odysseus was wounded by a boar that caught him with its tusk and inflicted a flesh wound above the knee. Odysseus' companions, the sons of Autolycus, bound [34] his wound and staunched the dark blood, ἐπαοιδῇ, with a spell.[35] The stopping of a hemorrhage through the reciting of an incantation must be an old Indo-European rite, since it is found from Germany to India.[36]

It goes without saying that amulets and talismans were used in Greece as everywhere. The Gorgon on Agamemnon's shield [37] was not a mere decoration but a magic image which spread terror and caused panic. The Homeric heroes, moreover, believed in omens just as the Babylonians did. An eagle to the right signified that a wish would be fulfilled, one to the left, the contrary.[38] Sneezing at a critical moment was a good omen.[39] And we know well enough that the consultation of oracles played a great part throughout Greek history.[40]

Magic, nevertheless, plays a very minor part in the Homeric epics and although diseases were believed to be sent by the gods, we hear of many conditions resulting from what we consider natural causes, and for which the gods were responsible only indirectly. The wound of Philoctetes was caused by snake bite. He suffered excruciating pains and was left behind on the island of Lemnos.[41] Famine was considered an evil of the same category as disease, for it is said in the *Odyssey* of the island Syria that 'never does famine befall the people nor does any other terrible disease attack the poor mortals.' [42] A passage in the *Iliad* mentions that the hound of Orion, Sirius, is a sign of evil, since this constellation brings πολλὸν πυρετόν, much fiery heat to the people.[43] In the medical literature *pyreton* is the technical term for fever, but we have no evidence that this passage refers in any way to disease rather than to the traditional dog days.

The *Iliad* is the epic account of a bloody war in which the heroes fight with spear, sword, club, bow and arrow, and slingshot, wounding and killing one another. We hear of many wounds, some of which are deadly and some not. Some are merely mentioned while others are described in great detail. Much has been written on wounds and surgery in Homer,[44] and not all the comments are pertinent. In reading the poem, we should always keep in mind that it is not a medical book and that it was not written by an armysurgeon.[45] The fighting heroes were mortals, to be sure, but they enjoyed the special protection of the gods who themselves were deeply involved in the Trojan war. Their deeds were prodigious, and the wounds they inflicted were mighty and not always necessarily realistic. Thus Diomedes cut off Dolon's head which rolled into the dust still shouting.[46] In two passages of the *Iliad* a hero was hit in the face and the two eyeballs, 'all bloody, fell at his feet in the dust.' [47] Idomeneus hit the hero Alcathous in the heart with a spear, 'and he fell with a crash, and the lance fixed in his heart, that, still beating, shook the butt-end of the spear.' [48] Or we read that when Archelochus was struck by a spear 'at the meeting of the head and neck, on the last joint of the spine,' his head, mouth and nose 'reached the earth long before his legs and knees,' when he fell.[49] When Achilles cut off Deucalion's head the marrow spurted out of the vertebrae.[50] Or a hero dies immediately when a stone merely cuts the tendons and crushes the bone of one leg.[51]

It would be easy to give more examples of similar deadly wounds that are not described realistically but have sprung from the poet's imagination. The anatomical and physiological knowledge of the time was extremely limited. Yet we have many other descriptions which reveal a keen sense of observation and experience acquired on the battlefield. Phereclus was slain by Meriones who 'smote him in the right buttock, and right through passed the point straight to the bladder beneath the bone; and he fell to his knees with a cry, and death overshadowed him.' [52] Sarpedon was struck by a javelin 'where the midriff clasps the beating heart. And he fell as falls an oak,' whereupon Patroclus 'setting foot on his breast, drew the spear out of his flesh, and the midriff followed with the spear, so that he drew forth together the spear point, and the soul of Sarpedon.' [53] Erymas suffered a fatal wound at the base of the skull. Idomeneus wounded him 'on the mouth with the pitiless bronze, and the spear of bronze went clean through below, beneath the brain, and shattered his white bones, and his teeth were shaken out, and both his eyes were filled with blood, and he blew blood up through mouth and nostrils as he gaped, and the black cloud of death covered him about.' [54] This is a very graphic description which must have been based on some observation. Also realistic is the picture of Hector smitten 'on the breast, over the shield-rim, near the neck' by a stone that Ajax had thrown at him; 'it made him spin like a top with the blow, that he reeled round and round.' But he managed to escape and his companions 'lifted him from the chariot to the ground and poured water over him, and he gat back his breath, and looked up with his eyes, and sitting on his heels kneeling, he vomited forth black blood. Then again he sank back on the ground, and black night covered his eyes, the stroke still conquering his spirit.' [55]

The Homeric hero like every warrior and every hunter knew

which spots he must hit in order to kill an enemy or an animal. Nestor's horse was 'smitten with an arrow upon the top of the crest where the foremost hairs of horses grow upon the skull; and there is the most deadly spot.' [56] You struck a foe 'between navel and genitalia,' [57] and when shooting an arrow you aimed at the 'chest near the nipple of the breast.' [58]

Daremberg counted the number of wounds described with more or less detail in the *Iliad* and found that there were 141 affecting the following parts of the body: [59] skull 6, forehead 7, temples 3, region of the ears 8, eyes, nose, mouth 1 each, jaws 2, throat 6, neck 11, decapitation 1-2, region of the collar bone 4, chest 11, breast 10, heart 1, hypochondrium 1, abdomen 5, lower part of abdomen and flanks 10, navel 2, groin 1, liver 4, back 9, shoulder 12, ablation of shoulder 1, of arm 1, arm 2, forearm 5, hand 2, buttocks 2-3, hip 1, thigh 3, knee 2, calves 1, ankle 1, tarsus 1. Many more wounds are mentioned without being described and over two hundred heroes were killed, some of them dying from what would seem to us to be rather slight injuries. The wounded hero suffered pain, pain compared to the pain of labor.[60] He frequently fainted as people also did from strong emotions.[61] The 'knees gave way' [62] and the 'heart was loosened.' [63] Andromache beheld the body of her slain husband, 'then dark night came on her eyes and shrouded her, and she fell backward and gasped forth her spirit.' [64]

Not all wounds were fatal and the warrior could count on receiving some treatment. A hemorrhage sometimes ceased spontaneously.[65] If it did not, the wound was bandaged with wool: 'and the great-hearted Agenor drew the spear from his hand, and himself bound up the wound with a band of twisted sheep's-wool, a sling that a squire carried for him.' [66] Incantations against bleeding are not mentioned in the *Iliad*. If an arrow or other weapon stuck in the wound, it had to be removed and various methods were tried to this end. The dart was pulled out or pushed through the limb or, if necessary, was cut out of the body; these methods were later known as ἐξολκή, διωσμός, and ἐκτομή. When Menelaus was wounded Machaon treated him, 'anon drew forth the arrow from the clasped belt; and as it was drawn forth the keen barbs were broken backwards. Then he loosed the glistering belt . . . and when he saw the wound where the bitter arrow had lighted, he sucked out the blood and cunningly spread thereon soothing drugs, such as Chiron of his good will had imparted to his sire.' [67] Another good description of the treatment of a wound is given in Book XI of the *Iliad*. Eurypylus was struck by an arrow in the thigh. Dripping with sweat and bleeding heavily he limped out of the battle. When he saw Patroclus he said to him, 'but me do thou succour, and lead me to the black ship, and cut the arrow out of my thigh, and wash away the black blood from it with warm water, and sprinkle thereon kindly simples of healing power, whereof they say that thou hast learned from Achilles, whom Chiron taught, the most righteous of the Centaurs.' This was done, and Patroclus ended the treatment by casting upon the wound 'a bitter root rubbing it between his hands, a root that took pain away, and ended all his anguish, and the wound began to dry, and the blood ceased.' [68]

I think these two examples give a good idea of the treatment of wounds as it was practiced in early Greece. It consisted basically in the removal of foreign bodies, in the washing of the wound, and in the application of drugs. That the wound was bandaged is not reported in every case because it probably was taken for granted. Sutures are not mentioned nor do we hear of any surgical instruments. Of course we cannot compare the Homeric epics with a book such as Papyrus Edwin Smith, but if the early Greek treatment of wounds had been more elaborate we would in all probability have been told something about it, for the poet of the *Iliad* loved to describe details.

What were the drugs used in the treatment of wounds? The Greek word φάρμαχον *(pharmakon)*, usually translated 'drug,' has a much broader meaning. [69] *Pharmakon* originally designated a vegetable substance that had magic powers. It might be the power to turn humans into pigs, in which case we would call it a philter, or the power to kill when it acted as what we consider a poison, or finally, the power to cure. All these effects were the result of inherent qualities of the *pharmakon* which were originally considered to be magic here as in the ancient Orient. It is obvious that not all plants were *pharmaka* but only some, and their effects were very different, so that the witch, the physician, or whoever used them had to be skillful. Their general action was indicated by adjectives. Thus in the Homeric epics a *pharmakon* is designated as κακόν, evil,[70] or λυγρόν, baneful,[71] or οὐλόμενον, accursed,[72] or even stronger, ἀνδροφόνον, murderous,[73] or θυμοφθόρον, life-destroying.[74] Snakes were venomous not from some magic property but because they ate evil *pharmaka*.[75] Poisons were used not only by witches and criminals but also by warriors who poisoned their arrows with them. Thus Odysseus once went to the city of Ephyre in Epirus to get a murderous *pharmakon* with which he smeared his arrows.[76] What this poison was we do not know; Schmiedeberg, the great pharmacologist, thought that it must have been a substance that acted on the heart, such as could easily be extracted from *Helleborus orientalis Lam,* a plant frequently found in Greece.[77]

There were not only evil *pharmaka,* some were ἐσθλά, good,[78] or ἤπια, soothing,[79] or ὀδυνήφατα, killing, that is, stilling the pain.[80] These were the remedies used in the treatment of injuries and diseases, and the medicines applied to wounds. They were powders, as a rule, that had an astringent or styptic effect. Powders containing tannic acid could be prepared from gallnuts and a variety of plants. All we know of the Homeric wound powders is that they had a soothing effect, that they lessened the pain and dried out the wound, and this is just what an astringent would do. In one of the passages we quoted, Patroclus rubbed a bitter root between his hands and cast it upon the wound, whereupon the blood ceased, the wound began to dry, pain was removed, and the patient's anguish was ended. We can only speculate about the nature of such a root. Its effect was so spectacular that it might have been a magic remedy. On the other hand, it is possible that roots were actually applied in the treatment of wounds, and Schmiedeberg's guess [81] that onions could have been used for such a purpose is not unreasonable, particularly since we know that onions have not only an astringent but also a bactericidal effect.[82] We do not learn of any internal pharmacological medication but this does not mean that drugs may not have been given internally in early Greece. The epic was not the place for the discussion of such questions.

And now we must look at the medical personnel. Who treated the wounded heroes? First of all, we find that they treated themselves and one another. The Homeric hero was a versatile man prepared to play his part in very different situations. To be sure, not all the heroes were as resourceful as Odysseus, but they were all skillful in many trades. They knew how to cook: a scene in the *Iliad* depicts with great delight Achilles cooking a meal, carving and slicing the meat, piercing it through with spits, and roasting it over the embers.[83] And the hero was expected to be able to treat a wound. Diomedes himself removed an arrow that had perforated his foot, painful as the operation was.[84] On another occasion when he was shot in the shoulder, one of his comrades Sthenelus extracted the dart.[85] Patroclus attended to the wounded Eurypylus,[86] Nestor to Machaon;[87] Agenor dressed the hand of his friend Helenus.[88] Even the wounded gods helped one another when their physician Paeon was unavailable. Aphrodite wounded by Diomedes sought refuge with her mother Dione, who 'with both hands wiped the ichor [89] from the arm; her arm was comforted and the grievous pangs assuaged.' [90]

Among the heroes, however, some were particularly skilled in the treatment of wounds, and we know two of them by name, Machaon and Podalirius, the sons of Asclepius. To Homer, Asclepius was not a god but a mortal, a tribal chief like Agamemnon or Odysseus but one generation older, because not he but his sons took part in the expedition against Troy. They came from Thessaly; and the Catalogue of Ships in the *Iliad* says of them: 'And of them that possessed Trikke and terraced Ithome and that possessed Oichalia city of Eurytos the Oichalian, of these again Asklepios' two sons were leaders, the cunning leeches Podaleirios and Machaon. And with them were arrayed thirty hollow ships.' [91] The two brothers were warriors who, like other chiefs, had joined the expeditionary force with their troops, and who like the others fought valiantly in battles. But in addition to being heroes, they were also ἰητῆρ'ἀγαθώ, skilled healers, or leeches, or physicians, or whatever designation we may prefer.[92] Being the sons of Asclepius, they were Asclepiads just as the sons of Atreus, Agamemnon and Menelaus, were Atreids, and they had been instructed in leechcraft by their father who twice in the *Iliad* is called ἀμύμων ἰητήρ, 'blameless physician.'[93] He himself had been a pupil of the old Centaur Chiron who had given him 'soothing simples . . . with kindly thoughts,'[94] and who had also instructed Achilles.[95] But although Achilles had more knowledge of drugs than the rank and file warrior, he was never called a physician as were the sons of Asclepius, who were held in high esteem for their leechcraft. When Machaon was smitten 'on the right shoulder with a three-barbed arrow'[96] the Greeks were in great fear for him. Idomeneus delegated Nestor to get him out of the battle, back to the ships, and spoke the often quoted words:

ἰητρὸς γὰρ ἀνὴρ πολλῶν ἀντάξιος ἄλλων
ἰούς τ' ἐκτάμνειν ἐπί τ' ἤπια φάρμακα πάσσειν.

For a leech is of the worth of many other men
For the cutting out of arrows and the spreading of soothing simples.[97]

Podalirius, although a physician like his brother, never appears in the *Iliad* performing a medical function. He is mentioned only twice, in the Catalogue of Ships and in a passage where he is said to be in the thick of battle while Eurypylus was wounded.[98] Machaon, on the other hand, is mentioned more often and we have quoted the passage in which he is pictured as treating Menelaus.[99]

Later, when Asclepius had become the chief healing god, people wished to know more about his sons.[100] A scholion on Pindar[101] describes the treatment of Philoctetes who, 'washed clean by the oracles of Apollo, fell asleep; then Machaon, removing the gangrenous flesh from the festering ulcer and deluging it with wine, sprinkled over the wound an herb which Asclepius got from Chiron, and in this way the hero was cured.' Another tradition tells of Machaon's death and relates how he was killed 'in the Troad when ... he climbed out of the Horse and entered the city of Priam.' [102] In a similar way Podalirius is shown in action in the post-Homeric literature curing wounds by squeezing them out, stitching them with his hands, and spreading on them salves 'which his father once placed in his hands and by which even the unhealing wounds of men are quickly healed of their deadly evil on the very day,' [103] a description that combines rational and miraculous elements.

In the *Iliad*, Machaon appears as a surgeon treating wounds, and the fact that Podalirius is never seen performing any treatments had interesting consequences for the future. To the surgeons, Machaon was the obvious Father of Surgery, but when dietetics became the chief method of therapy, the physicians who treated their patients by prescribing diets needed an ancestor also. Might not Podalirius have been the Father of Dietetics? Nothing in Homer spoke against such an assumption although it must be admitted that we would look in vain for any prescription of diet. An old scholiast makes the very pertinent remark that it was not strange that Homer did not 'introduce someone being treated by diet,' and that he omitted such treatment 'because of its unseemliness.' [104] At any rate, Podalirius in various later texts appears as the physician who 'worked with the subject of diet,' [105] or who 'treated diseases by diet,' [106] or in a more general way, as the internist, compared to the surgeon Machaon. In the poem *The Sack of Troy*, this is expressed very clearly when Arctinus the poet says of the brothers: [107]

For their father himself, the glorious Earthshaker,[108] gave them both honors, but one he made more renowned than the other. To the one he gave more agile hands to draw the darts from the flesh and to heal all wounds; to the other he gave the power to know accurately in his heart all matters that are unseen, and to heal things incapable of healing. He first understood the eyes flashing forth like lightning and the depressed mind of the mad Ajax.

This differentiation between the brothers, however, was a later development. In the *Iliad* both are mentioned as fighting heroes and skilled leeches. And they are not the only physicians: Idomeneus turned a wounded comrade over 'to the physicians,' [109] men whose names are not given; and in a dramatic scene Patroclus in an endeavor to reconcile Achilles reminded him that Diomedes, Agamemnon, and Eurypylus were wounded, and were attended by ἰητροὶ πολυφάρμαχοι 'physicians skilled in many *pharmaka*,' [110] and this at a moment when Podalirius was fighting and Machaon was also wounded. There can be no doubt, therefore, that the Greek army had more than two men who possessed special skill in leechcraft. These other physicians were in all probability warriors also, and nothing entitles us to assume that the *Iliad* refers at all to professional doctors.

Different conditions are reflected in the *Odyssey* where we often find a picture of everyday life. In a very important passage Eumaeus, scolded for having brought in a beggar, answers: [111] 'Who would take it on himself to extend hospitality to a wandering stranger, unless he were one of the itinerant workers for the people,[112] a diviner, a physician, a carpenter, or a minstrel whose song makes you rejoice. Such people are welcome the world over.' The designation of the physician here as ἰητὴρ κακῶν, 'healer of evils,' points rather to the treatment of internal diseases than to surgery. This physician was not a warrior or a priest but a professional worker with the social status of a craftsman like the carpenter or the minstrel, the status that he still had in the classical period. The passage also reveals that physicians were few and practiced as itinerants, as was still the case in the days of Hippocrates.

And finally, in ancient Greece as everywhere else, women nursed the wounded and sick. Nestor's slave Hecamede washed the blood from Machaon's wound,[113] and restored the worn-out warriors with wine and food.[114] Or women knew of rare drugs, as we mentioned before.

Summing up, we may say that the Homeric heroes knew how to treat their own wounds and those of their comrades, and that some of them, such as the sons of Asclepius, were particularly skillful in this art. We saw, furthermore, that diseases were sent by the gods who relieved men from illness when they had been placated; but in the *Odyssey,* as we just noted, there is also evidence of a lay professional doctor. It remains for us to examine what theoretical views may be encountered in the Homeric poems. In this we can be very brief because the epic obviously was not the place for disquisitions on the nature of health and disease. And yet the poet who pictures the suffering and dying of people, whether he wishes to or not, always betrays his views on the nature of life and death.

In Greece, as in all ancient civilizations, the starting point of all physiological speculation was the elementary observation that life is bound to the presence of certain substances—substances of the outside world such as air and food, and juices of the human body such as blood. Physiology began when man tried to correlate these substances. The ancient Egyptians developed the theory of the *metu,* canals that connected all parts of the body and carried various substances to and from the organs. At the time of Homer a relation between food and blood was also assumed. The gods had no blood in their veins but another juice, ichor. Why? Because their food was different, consisting as it did of nectar and ambrosia, and not of bread and wine.[115] The necessity for air was recognized also. Life was an air-like substance which was exhaled and flew off at the moment of death.[116] The term *pneuma* that was to play such an important part in later Greek physiology was not yet in use. The spirit that was the principle of life was called θυμός, and this *thymos* resided in the whole body [117] and could escape from any wound. Sometimes, however, we find it localized in the φρένες, the diaphragm.[118] Man's soul, his *psyche,* was his bodiless double, similar somewhat to the Egyptian *ka,* the carrier of his self which after death 'flies around like a dream,' [119] and goes to the Lower World, where it leads a colorless dreary life.

Much has been said about anatomy in the Homeric poems. Daremberg claimed that 'the anatomical notions of Homer were hardly less advanced than those of Hippocrates,'[120] and Körner went even so far as to maintain that dissections of human cadavers were performed at the time of Homer.[121] Homeric anatomy actually was very much the same as that of other archaic civilizations, derived from observations in the kitchen, on the sacrificial altar, and on the battlefield. There is no evidence whatsoever, direct or indirect, of the dissection of human bodies. The main organs were known and had names, and the same was true of the main regions of the body. A warrior knew where to hit in order to kill, but we would look in vain for any detailed knowledge. Hippocratic anatomy was indeed primitive, but it was infinitely superior to that reflected in the epics.

One passage of the *Iliad* should be quoted because it has led to various interpretations. Antilochus attacked Thoon from behind and 'severed all the blood vessel that runs up the back till it reaches the neck; this he severed clean, and Thoon fell on his back in the dust.' [122] What was this blood vessel? Was it the aorta or the vena cava, or the aorta and carotis, or the cava and the jugularis? I am inclined to believe that it was an imaginary blood vessel, and I think that we should not expect accurate anatomical descriptions—no one had such knowledge at the time, and the poet was not bound by considerations of a rigid realism.

Although the chief organs were known and had names, the early Greeks obviously had little knowledge of their functions, with the exception of some elementary ones. Common observation had taught that the windpipe was needed for a man to 'make answer and speak unto his foe,' [123] that wine passed down the throat,[124] that the heart beat. Other similar elementary observations must have been made at an early date but many centuries were needed for man to gain a clearer view of the workings of his organs.

We know very little about the beginnings of Greek medicine, but scanty as our sources are, they tell us that archaic medicine, here as everywhere else, had religious, magic, and empirical elements, and that it is not by accident or merely because of the character of the sources that the empirical and rational component stood in the foreground. Religious medicine was soon to find its strongest expression in the cult of Asclepius. Magic practices were never abandoned but survived in uneducated groups of the population or assumed the character of superstitions—as in our present societies. The empirical

and rational component, however, was developed in the schools of
the early philosophers and physicians, and produced a system of
medicine such as the Mediterranean world had never before seen.

NOTES

1. Breasted, op. cit. p. 308ff.
2. About Crete and Mycenae see Sir A. J. Evans, *Palace of Minos*, London,
   3 vols., 1921–8; G. Glotz, *The Aegean Civilization*, London, New York,
   1925; D. Fimmen, *Die kretisch-mykenische Kultur*, Leipzig and Berlin,
   1921; T. Bossert, *Alt Kreta, Kunst und Kunstgewerbe im ägäischen Kul-
   turkreis*, 2nd ed., Berlin, 1923. About ancient Greek civilization in general
   see the highly original book of E. Howald, *Die Kultur der Antike*, 2nd ed.,
   Zurich, 1948.
3. See Howald, op. cit. p. 22f.
4. The literature on Homeric medicine is very large; from antiquity on the
   two epics have been read not only for their beauty but also for details of
   their content. According to a scholion on Oribasius (ed. Bussemaker and
   Daremberg II, 496, see also p. 897), Galen wrote a treatise on Homeric
   medicine, Περὶ τῆς καθ᾽ Ὅμηρον ἰατρικῆς, which is now lost. The most
   important literature of the last hundred years is the following: J. F.
   Malgaigne, 'Étude sur l'anatomie et la physiologie d'Homère,' Paris, 1842
   (from *Bull. Acad. Roy. Méd.*, 1841–2) ; C. Daremberg, 'Études d'archéolo-
   gie médicale sur Homère,' *Rev. Archéol.*, 1865, N.S., 12:95–111, 249–67,
   338–55, plate XXIII (also published separately as *La Médecine dans
   Homère*, Paris, 1865) ; O. Braumüller, 'Krankheit und Tod bei Homer,'
   Jahresber. K. Wilhelms Gymn., Berlin, 1879; H. Frölich, *Die Militär-
   medizin Homers*, Stuttgart, 1879; A. Floquet, *Homère médecin*, Thèse,
   Paris, 1912; O. Schmiedeberg, *Über die Pharmaka in der Ilias und
   Odyssee* (Schr. Wiss. Ges. Strassburg, 36), Strassburg, 1918; L. Lewin,
   'Heilmittel und Gifte bei Homer,' *Münch. med. Wschr.*, 1920, no. 33;
   B. Coglievina, *Die homerische Medizin*, Graz-Vienna-Leipzig, 1922; Q.
   Celli, *La Medicina greca nelle tradizioni mitologiche e Omeriche*, Rome,
   1923; O. Körner, 'Das Naturgefühl in der homerischen Dichtung,' *Das
   humanistische Gymnasium*, 1934, pp. 113–30; 'Die Empfindungen in Ilias
   und Odyssee,' *Jenaer medizin-hist. Beiträge*, 1932, Heft 15; 'Über Spuren
   des jonischen Forschungstriebs in Ilias und Odyssee und über die Ver-
   wertung homerischer Erkenntnisse im Corpus Hippocraticum und in der
   Tiergeschichte des Aristoteles,' *Arch. Gesch. Med.*, 1931, 24:185–201; *Die
   homerische Tierwelt*, Munich, 1929; *Die ärztlichen Kenntnisse in Ilias
   und Odyssee*, Munich, 1929; 'Wie entstanden die anatomischen Kenntnisse in Ilias und Odyssee?,' *Münch. med. Wschr.*, 1922, pp. 1484–7;
   *Das homerische Tiersystem und seine Bedeutung für die zoologische Syste-
   matik des Aristoteles*, Wiesbaden, 1917; *Wesen und Wert der homerischen*

Heilkunde, Wiesbaden, 1904; W. Artelt, *Studien zur Geschichte der Be-griffe 'Heilmittel' und 'Gift,'* Urzeit-Homer-Corpus Hippocraticum (Stud. Gesch. Med. 23), Leipzig, 1937; E. Fuld, 'Prähomerische Sektionen,' *Münch. med. Wschr.,* 1922, no. 50; 'Wissenschaft bei Homer und Kritik,' *Arch. Gesch. Med.,* 1930, 23:152–83; 'Bemerkungen zu der Abhandlung und Entgegnung O. Körners,' *Arch. Gesch. Med.,* 1931, 24:202–4; 'Quelques remarques sur les sciences naturelles et médicales dans Homère,' *Rev. des Études Homériques,* 1932, 2:10–17.

 5. In Greece throughout antiquity wine was mixed with water, probably not only because Greek wines are strong, but also because many of them are so sweet that one could not drink them in any quantity without feeling sick.

 6. The episodes of Polyphemus (*Odyssey,* IX, 371ff.) and Elpenor (ibid. X, 550ff.) illustrate the evil effects of drunkenness.

 7. *Iliad,* X, 572ff. Ἀσάμινθος was a bath tub in which one sat, the λουτήρ, a wash basin used later in the gymnasia. The ἀσάμινθος must be of Cretan origin. A specimen was found in the palace of Cnossus.

 8. *Odyssey,* XI, 489ff.

 9. The technical term for disease or illness is νοῦσος, but we find also other non-specific terms designating something evil, e. g. κακή (*Il.,* I, 10), κακότης (*Od.,* V, 397), ἀργαλέη (*Il.,* XIII, 667), στυγερή (*Il.,* XIII, 670; *Od.,* XV, 408).

10. *Od.,* IX, 411.

11. *Il.,* XXIV, 601ff.

12. *Od.,* III, 279ff.

13. *Il.,* VI, 205.

14. *Il.,* VI, 428.

15. Cf. Job, 6, 4.

16. *Il.,* I, 10ff. It is futile to speculate on the nature of this plague. An epic is not meant to be an epidemiological report.

17. The three categories are μάντις, ἱερεύς, ὀνειροπόλος, *Il.,* I, 62f.

18. Ibid. 93ff. All quotations from the *Iliad* are in the translation of A. Lang, W. Leaf, and E. Myers, London, 1891, unless otherwise indicated.

19. Ibid. 312ff.

20. *Od.,* V, 394ff.

21. *Il.,* V, 199ff.

22. *Il.,* V, 99ff.

23. *Il.,* V, 305ff., 447f.

24. *Il.,* XVI, 514ff.

25. *Od.,* XV, 411f.

26. Celsus, *De Medicina,* Prooem., 4.

27. Ibid. 3.

28. Galen, V, 869. All references to Galen are to the edition of C. G. Kühn, Leipzig, 1821–33.

29. *Od.,* X, 229ff.

30. Coglievina, op. cit. p. 27ff.
31. *Od.*, IV, 220ff.
32. See the discussion of Schmiedeberg, op. cit. p. 9ff.
33. *Od.*, XIX, 456ff.
34. The words ὠτειλήν ... δῆσαν usually interpreted as 'they bandaged the wound' mean, 'they bound the` wound,' namely with a magic spell. See *Pauly-Wissowa,* Supplement IV, col. 325, article *Epode* by Pfister.
35. 'Επαοιδή literally means, 'a song sung to' or 'over [the wound].'
36. See G. Ehrismann, *Geschichte der deutschen Literatur bis zum Ausgang des Mittelalters,* Munich, 1918, vol. I, p. 96ff.
37. *Il.*, XI, 36ff.
38. But see Hector's attitude (*Il.*, XII, 237ff.) when he said: 'One omen is best, to fight for one's country.'
39. *Od.*, XVII, 541ff.
40. See the classic book of A. Bouché-Leclercq, *Histoire de la divination dans l'antiquité,* Paris, 1879–82, 4 vols.
41. *Il.*, II, 721ff.
42. *Od.*, XV, 403ff., translated by H. E. Sigerist.
43. *Il.*, XXII, 31.
44. See note 4.
45. As Frölich quite seriously believed.
46. *Il.*, X, 455f. A similar scene occurs in *Od.*, XXII, 328f.
47. *Il.*, XIII, 615ff. The other passage is XVI, 739ff.
48. *Il.*, XIII, 442ff.
49. *Il.*, XIV, 467ff.
50. *Il.*, XX, 482f.
51. *Il.*, IV, 521ff.
52. *Il.*, V, 65ff.
53. *Il.*, XVI, 480f. and 503ff. The word for midriff, φρένες, designates the diaphragm which was considered the seat of ψυχή, the soul. Körner (*Die anatomischen Kenntnisse*) referring to this passage assumed that φρένες meant the pericardium, but I think that it is a mistake to try to make such distinctions. The anatomical concepts were vague.
54. *Il.*, XVI, 345ff.
55. *Il.*, XIV, 409ff., 433ff.
56. *Il.*, VIII, 83ff.
57. *Il.*, XIII, 568 (Sigerist).
58. *Il.*, VIII, 313 (Sigerist).
59. Daremberg, op. cit. p. 59ff.
60. *Il.*, XI, 267ff.
61. The passages are collected in Braumüller, op. cit. p. 12f.
62. *Od.*, XXIV, 345 (Sigerist).
63. Ibid. (Sigerist).
64. *Il.*, XXII, 466f.
65. *Il.*, XI, 267

66. *Il.*, XIII, 598ff.

67. *Il.*, IV, 210ff.

68. *Il.*, XI, 806ff. (slightly changed).

69. See the excellent discussion of this concept in W. Artelt, *Studien zur Geschichte der Begriffe 'Heilmittel' und 'Gift'*, Urzeit-Homer-Corpus Hippocraticum, Leipzig, 1937.

70. *Il.*, XXII, 94; *Od.*, X, 213.

71. *Od.*, IV, 230; X, 236.

72. *Od.*, X, 394.

73. *Od.*, I, 261.

74. *Od.*, II, 329.

75. *Il.*, XXII, 94.

76. *Od.*, I, 261. *Toxon* in Greek means 'bow', in the plural it also means 'bow and arrow'. *Toxicon pharmakon* is a poison for smearing arrows. We have forgotten the origin of the term when we speak of toxin, toxicology, intoxication, etc., words which no longer connote poisoned arrows.

77. Schmiedeberg, op. cit. p. 14ff.

78. *Od.*, IV, 227f., 230.

79. *Il.*, IV, 218; XI, 515, 830.

80. *Il.*, V, 401, 500.

81. Schmiedeberg, op. cit. p. 6.

82. See the experiments of B. Tokin and co-workers in *Am. Rev. Soviet Med.*, 1944, 1:236–50; also H. E. Sigerist, 'Ambroise Paré's Onion Treatment of Burns,' *Bull. Hist. Med.*, 1944, 15:143–9.

83. *Il.*, XI, 205ff.

84. *Il.*, XI, 397f.

85. *Il.*, V, 112.

86. *Il.*, XI, 822ff.

87. *Il.*, XI, 515ff.

88. *Il.*, XIII, 598ff.

89. The juice that flows in the veins of the gods corresponding to mortals' blood.

90. *Il.*, V, 416f.

91. *Il.*, II, 729–33.

92. In Homer, for the first time, we encounter the word ἰητήρ which in various dialectical variations, ἰητρός, ἰητώρ, ἰατρός, always designated the physician, and was to become part of our own nomenclature in such words as pediatrician, psychiatrist, etc.

93. *Il.*, IV, 194; XI, 518. See, however, U. von Wilamowitz-Möllendorf, *Isyllos von Epidauros*, Berlin, 1886, p. 46, note 3.

94. *Il.*, IV, 218f., translated by A. T. Murray, Homer, *The Iliad*, London, 1924–25, Loeb Classical Library.

95. *Il.*, XI, 831f.

96. *Il.*, XI, 504ff. (Murray).

97. Ibid. 514–5 (Murray). Quoting the first verse alone, as is frequently done, obviously alters the meaning.

98. *Il.*, XI, 836.

99. *Il.*, IV, 192ff.

100. See the testimonies collected by E. J. and L. Edelstein, *Asclepius, a Collection and Interpretation of the Testimonies,* Baltimore, 1945, vol. I, p. 60ff.

101. *Ad Pythias,* I, 109a. Trans. by Edelstein, op. cit. Test. 174.

102. Hippocrates, *Letters,* 27, Littré, IX, 426.

103. Quintus Smyrnaeus, *Posthomerica,* IV, 396ff.

104. *Scholia in Homerum, Ad Iliadem,* XI, 515. Trans. by Edelstein, op. cit. Test. 140.

105. Eustathius, *Commentarii ad Homeri Iliadem,* IV, 202. Trans. by Edelstein, op. cit. Test. 139.

106. *Scholia in Homerum, Ad Iliadem,* XI, 515.

107. Ibid. Edelstein, Test. 141.

108. Poseidon, who in this poem is the father of Podalirius and Machaon.

109. *Il.*, XIII, 213.

110. *Il.*, XVI, 28–9.

111. *Od.*, XVII, 382ff. (Sigerist).

112. This is the literal meaning of δημιοεργός; the term designates skilled laborers, craftsmen, artists.

113. *Il.*, XIV, 6.

114. *Il.*, XI, 624.

115. *Il.*, V, 340ff.

116. See *Il.*, IV, 524; θυμὸν ἀποπνείων, 'gasping out his life.'

117. E. g. in the white bones, *Od.*, XI, 224.

118. See *Il.*, XXII, 475.

119. *Od.*, XI, 222.

120. Daremberg, op. cit. p. 10.

121. Körner, op. cit. p. 1487.

122. *Il.*, XIII, 546ff. (slightly changed).

123. *Il.*, XXII, 328 (Murray).

124. *Il.*, XXIV, 641f.

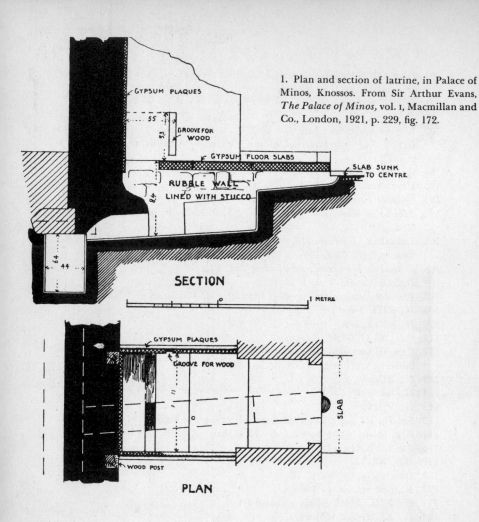

GYPSUM PLAQUES

55

GROOVE FOR
WOOD

53

GYPSUM FLOOR SLABS

SLAB SUNK
TO CENTRE

RUBBLE WALL
LINED WITH STUCCO

84

64

44

SECTION

1 METRE

GYPSUM PLAQUES

GROOVE FOR WOOD

SLAB

WOOD POST

PLAN

1. Plan and section of latrine, in Palace of Minos, Knossos. From Sir Arthur Evans, *The Palace of Minos,* vol. I, Macmillan and Co., London, 1921, p. 229, fig. 172.

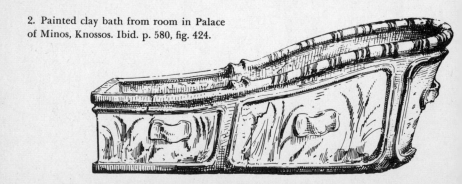

2. Painted clay bath from room in Palace of Minos, Knossos. Ibid. p. 580, fig. 424.

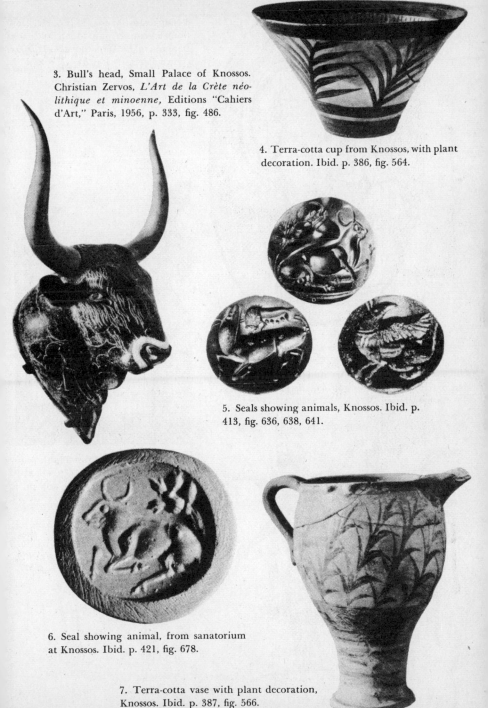

3. Bull's head, Small Palace of Knossos. Christian Zervos, *L'Art de la Crète néolithique et minoenne,* Editions "Cahiers d'Art," Paris, 1956, p. 333, fig. 486.

4. Terra-cotta cup from Knossos, with plant decoration. Ibid. p. 386, fig. 564.

5. Seals showing animals, Knossos. Ibid. p. 413, fig. 636, 638, 641.

6. Seal showing animal, from sanatorium at Knossos. Ibid. p. 421, fig. 678.

7. Terra-cotta vase with plant decoration, Knossos. Ibid. p. 387, fig. 566.

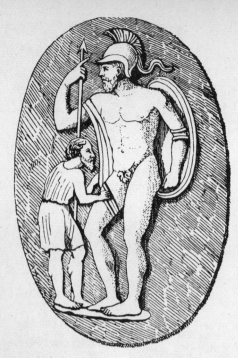

8. Menelaus bandaged by Machaon. From a manuscript in Milan, in Charles Daremberg, *La Médecine dans Homère*. Didier, Paris, 1865, p. 84 (cf. p. 83).

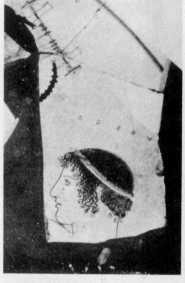

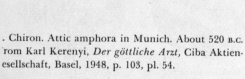

. Chiron. Attic amphora in Munich. About 520 B.C. rom Karl Kerenyi, *Der göttliche Arzt,* Ciba Aktien-esellschaft, Basel, 1948, p. 103, pl. 54.

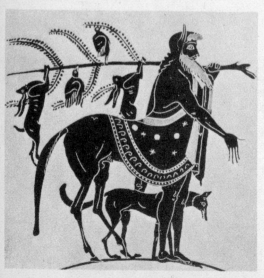

10. Orpheus. From Ernst Pfuhl, *Malerei und Zeichnung der Griechen,* F. Bruckman, München, 1923, vol. III, p. 135, pl. 416.

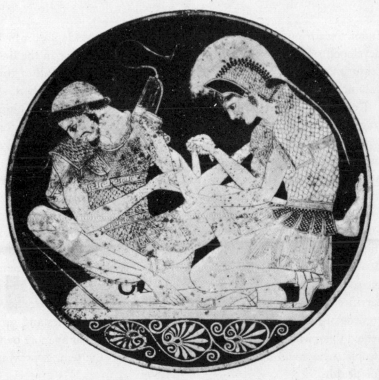

11. Patroclus bandaged by Achilles, Sosias vase. Ibid.
pl. 418.

★

3. Religious Medicine: Asclepius and His Cult

It may seem out of place to discuss the cult of Asclepius, which developed relatively late and exerted its greatest influence in the first centuries of our era, at the beginning rather than at the end of this volume. Yet, there are good reasons for placing this chapter here.

Religious medicine is timeless; we come upon it in the initial stages and throughout the course of every civilization, no matter what other forms of medicine may have been developed. It is always present because it satisfies an ever-existing need. In all civilizations, at all times, there have been religious individuals who in case of illness sought help from the priest rather than the physician. Temples and churches, furthermore, were the last resort of those patients who had been given up by their physicians and were hoping for a miracle. And finally, there was also an economic factor which must not be overlooked. Religious therapy was, as a rule, cheaper than diets, drugs, and operations. The god was satisfied with a small sacrifice while physicians had to be paid in hard cash. We have records of many rich people who sought healing in temples and presented them with opulent gifts, but we also know that many more poor people, who could not afford a doctor, went to the temple praying for health.

Greece was no exception to the rule. We found religious medicine in the Homeric poems, and there was no century without healing cults. The cult of Asclepius was by no means the only one, but, for reasons to be discussed later, it dominated the scene and set a pattern for the cults of other healing deities.

Another reason why we are justified in discussing the subject here is that religious medicine is always archaic in character and is, moreover, rather static. Pilgrimages to Lourdes and similar places, the

44

rites performed in such sanctuaries today, and the seemingly miraculous cures—which undoubtedly occur—are not expressions of modern but of archaic medicine with all its characteristic features; and the ritual changed very little in the course of the centuries. The Epidaurian pattern of the cult of Asclepius was followed in other Greek and Roman sanctuaries, and its ritual was even continued in Christian churches.

And finally, it seems opportune to present Asclepius and his cult now so that we may have a clear conception of the character of this medicine, because until not so long ago, it was generally assumed that the temples of Asclepius had been the cradle of Greek medicine. Egypt and Babylonia had priest-physicians and Greece had Asclepiads, priests of Asclepius, who, it seemed, must have been physicians also. The temples then appeared as sanatoria, centers of research and training, where medical experience accumulated and was passed on to younger generations. Was Hippocrates not an Asclepiad also? Was Cos, his birthplace, not the seat of a famous temple? With Hippocrates, it was said, medicine stepped out of the temples and emancipated itself from religious bonds. This seemed a logical development, but the excavations of Epidaurus and Cos destroyed this theory completely, and today we know that rational and religious medicine did not develop one from the other but took parallel courses. We also know that the roots of Greek medical science and practice are to be sought not in temple lore but in the observations and thoughts of the early philosophers, and in the experience gained by trainers in the gymnasia.

Asclepius became the chief healing god, and religious medicine centered in his cult;[1] but he was by no means the only deity with healing functions. In Greek, as in all ancient civilizations, all gods had the faculty to protect against evil and cure sick people.[2]

The early healing god was probably Paeon, who in the Homeric epics appears as physician of the gods. Doctors were *Paeonii*, members of his family,[3] and his name became an attribute of other gods, designating their healing function—or rather he was identified with them. Thus Zeus, whose oracle was consulted at Dodona, was worshiped as

Zeus Paian, Zeus the healer, on the island of Rhodes;[4] he was also invoked as Soter, the savior, in an ode of Pindar.[5] Like other gods, he was *apotropaios,* an averter of evil who protected mortal men. But Apollo, more than any of the older gods, became the deity of medicine and was recognized as such throughout antiquity. The rise of Asclepius was possible only because the legend made him the son of Apollo. In Delphi, Apollo had his famous oracle. He was seer but also physician, ἰατρομάντις, as Aeschylus calls him.[6] He is the first deity invoked in the Hippocratic Oath, where he appears as Apollo the physician.[7] A coin from Apollonia Pontice of about 300 B.C. represents him with a branch of laurel, the tree sacred to him, and the bow with which he inflicts pestilence upon the people. The inscription is to Apollo the physician.[8] A statue of Apollo Alexicacos made by the sculptor Calamis could be seen in Athens, and Pausanias tells us that he was named Alexicacos, the averter of evil, because through an oracle from Delphi he stayed the plague that afflicted the Athenians at the time of the Peloponnesian War.[9] Another epithet of Apollo has given rise to some speculation. In several texts he is called Smintheus,[10] which may mean the mouse-killer. On a late coin from Alexandria Troas he is pictured with bow and arrow and a mouse at his feet.[11] Since it was believed that Apollo sent the plague and relieved from it, and since we know that rodents play a part in the spreading of the plague, the possibility was considered that the Greeks might have connected the disease with rodents and that Apollo by killing mice would have stopped epidemics.[12] Such an interpretation, however, is too naïvely rationalistic, quite apart from the fact that the etymology is not at all certain.[13] Connection with mice as totem animals, moreover, would not be astonishing in a mantic deity whose chthonian character is easily apparent.

Of other gods who had healing functions, Hephaestus, the god of fire, was worshiped particularly on the island of Lemnos, and the earth upon which he fell when Zeus threw him from the heavens had medicinal properties. It was *terra Lemnia,* a fine clay used in the treatment of wounds, ulcers, and similar ailments; it was sold sealed, and hence also called *terra sigillata.* When Galen visited the island in the second century A.D., he was presented with a book that indicated the properties and uses of this famous medicament.[14]

The goddesses were the protectresses of women in all phases of their sexual life. Hera, the blameless consort of Zeus, was the patroness of matrimony, and assisted women in childbirth. Eileithyia, the divine midwife, was sometimes identified with her or considered one of her manifestations. Artemis, the virgin sister of Apollo, like him sent sudden death, shooting her darts at mortals. She was worshiped as the goddess of women in Athens, and protected young girls; in Sparta blood sacrifices were brought to her as Artemis Orthia.[15] Athena, the daughter of Zeus, had many healing functions. In Athens, in one of the porticoes on the way to the Cerameicus, stood the statue of Athena Paeonia, Athena the Healer.[16] On the Acropolis, Pausanias saw next to a statue of Hygieia, daughter of Asclepius, one of Athena 'whom they also name Hygieia.'[17] Athena Paeonia was worshiped in Oropus, in the temple of Amphiaraus, next to Panacea, Iaso, and Hygieia—that is, in close connection with the family of Asclepius.[18] In Sparta a temple was dedicated to Athena Ophthalmitis—that is, to the goddess of the eye. Tradition had it that the temple was founded by Lycurgus, who, after his eye was struck out by Alcander, fled to this spot where he was protected by the Lacedaemonians and thus could save his remaining eye.[19]

In addition to the gods, Greece knew heroes and demigods skilled in the art of healing such as the seer Melampus, who, according to legend, founded the cult of Dionysus, and understood the language of birds, after two snakes he had raised had cleansed his ears.[20] He was a famous physician and cured people, who were raving with madness. Thus he cured the daughters of Proetus, King of Tiryns, who, followed by other women, roamed the Peloponnesian Mountains in Dionysiac madness. The treatment is interesting because the underlying principle was to play an important part in later scientific medicine; he increased the women's raving with shouting and orgiastic dances, bringing it to an acme, whereupon he purified them with cathartic remedies.[21] He is supposed to have used black hellebore which thereafter was named after him, Melampodium.[22] And the water into which he threw the substances used for the purification rites had from then on a bad taste.[23] A sanctuary was erected to him at Aegosthena, in Attica, and an annual festival was held in his honor.[24] His descendants were seers and physicians also;[25] and later a divination book, composed probably at the time of the Ptolemies, a book in which muscular spasms were interpreted as omens, went under his name.[26]

By far the most famous of his descendants was Amphiaraus, in all probability a local chthonian demon whose oracle was consulted in the neighborhood of Thebes. A later legend explained why he had a subterranean residence in that locality. He had taken part in the ill-fated campaign against Thebes and when he was persecuted by the enemy and on the verge of being hit, Zeus saved him by opening the earth that engulfed him, his chariot, and horses, thus making him immortal.[27] His chief places of worship were Thebes, Oropus, and Athens. He was a seer and a divine physician; in his sanctuaries he cured through oracles by giving advice during the incubation to the people who slept on the earth in which 'he resided. A late source [28] tells us that supplicants who came seeking help and healing had to abstain from drinking wine for three days, and from taking any food for one day, whereupon they sacrificed a ram, on whose skin they went to sleep awaiting enlightenment in a dream. Pausanias, who gives a good description of the Amphiareion at Oropus, tells us that it was the custom for a patient who had been cured of a disease through an oracle to throw silver and gold coins into a spring near the temple, the water of which was never used for any other purpose.[29]

Related in many ways to Amphiaraus was another chthonian demon, Trophonius, a seer-physician too. The legends [30] tell that he was once an architect, a mortal man, who, to escape his enemies, entered the earth near Lebadeia. There he resided in a cave deep in the earth, giving oracles, appearing at times to supplicants in person, or giving responses through his serpents. The sight of him was frightening and no one entered the cave lightheartedly. Whoever saw him lost the power of laughter for some time. The ritual of his cult was described in detail by Pausanias.[31] It was similar to that of other mantic and healing cults, consisting in preparatory purifications and sacrifices, and reaching its climax in the descent into the cave.

The power of music and poetry over man's soul, and through the soul over his body, healthy or sick, found illustration in the lives of Orpheus and Musaeus. An inspired bard and seer, Orpheus was said to have wandered over Greece, and the power of his words sung to the strains of his lyre was such that it bewitched men, beasts, and plants, and moved even the rocks; the rivers halted their course to listen to him.[32] He was worshiped as the founder of a religious sect,[33] as a purification priest, and as a physician who with incantations and magic formulas appeased the wrath of the gods and cleansed the patient of impurity. His followers, the Orphics, were pledged to lead pure lives, and it seems that at one time, like the Pythagoreans, they abstained from eating meat. Many poems were attributed to Orpheus, including one on the magic virtue of precious stones.[34]

Musaeus is usually mentioned in close connection with Orpheus as his disciple, friend, or at least contemporary.[35] Like Orpheus he lived in the people's memory as a bard, seer, and physician, as one who, in the words of Aristophanes, taught oracles and the healing of disease.[36]

The Dioscuri, Castor and Pollux, the twin sons of Zeus and Leda, may also be mentioned here, although their function as healing gods seems to have been a later development. They were man's saviors; riding white horses, they came to the rescue of him who was in great danger on the battlefield, on the high seas, or on account of illness. Their cult was widespread, particularly in the Roman period, and patients came to sleep in their temples, to be cured in the incubation or to have dreams that the priests would interpret for them. Their healing activities did not end with the downfall of paganism; they continued to help people in distress as Christian saints. As Cosmas and Damian, they became the patron saints of physicians and pharmacists, and of medicine at large.[37]

There is one more demigod to discuss here, one who played a very important part in the mythology of medicine as healer and also as teacher of healers, the Centaur Chiron.[38] 'Half like a horse, half like a god,' [39] he dwelt in a cave on Mount Pelion, in Thessaly, like the other centaurs; but unlike that rough and savage breed, he was gentle, the most righteous of all centaurs, deeply skilled in the arts of hunting, music, and medicine. In the history of the mythologic founders of medicine, he was considered the discoverer of the medicinal properties of many herbs, who mastered the 'soft-handed lore of drugs' [40] and passed it on to his pupils. His name became part of the pharmaco-botanical nomenclature; we still have the genus *Centaurea*. According to Pliny,[41] the panacea *Centaurion* [42] was discovered by Chiron, as was another panacea, *Chironium*.[43] A further discovery attributed to him was that of Pliny's *ampelos Chironia*,[44] our white bryony. He and Asclepius were supposed to have revealed to Apuleius Platonicus the herbal that became so popular in the early Middle Ages.[45] He gave the plants, Artemisiae, their name and introduced them into the materia medica, after Diana had taught him their properties.[46] Until very recently Chiron's name was also attached to a certain type of chronic ulcer,[47] and Paul of Aegina explained that these old ulcers which were difficult to get cicatrized were called chironian, 'as if requiring Chiron himself to cure them.' [48] It may be, however, that the name was rather reminiscent of the wound that Heracles inflicted on him by accident with a poisoned arrow, and of which he ultimately died; because he longed for death, he was released of his immortality by Zeus who gave it to Prometheus.[49] Chiron was transported to the skies where he took his place in the zodiac as Sagittarius or Centaur, and we shall see in some other connection that in astrological medicine he was believed to rule over hips, buttocks, and thighs. Meanwhile he was worshiped on earth as one of the founders of the healing art.

Like the mythical Chinese emperor Shên Nung, Chiron was remembered primarily as the discoverer of drugs, and his treatments were said to have consisted mostly in the prescription of medicinal herbs. He was also a musician and knew songs; and songs have magic power. Pindar tells us that he taught his disciples to treat patients

with soothing incantations, with potions, with drugs applied externally, and with the knife, that is, with surgery.[50] And Chiron, like other
gods and demigods, also performed miracle cures. When Phoenix,
son of Amyntor, was blinded for having seduced his father's concu-
bine, he was brought to the cave of the Centaur, who restored his
eyesight.[51]

Chiron was not only a great seer, musician, and physician, he was
equally famous as the preceptor of heroes. He educated his own
daughter, Ocyrrhoë, in the art of prophecy; Melampus was his
pupil, as was Aristaeus, son of Apollo, and Jason, hero of the
Argonauts. But his most famous disciples were, undoubtedly, Achilles and Asclepius. We mentioned in the previous chapter that in the
Iliad Achilles appears as a hero who was more deeply skilled in the
use of drugs than other heroes, with the exception, of course, of
Podalirius and Machaon. This he owed to his education on Mount
Pelion. Achilles, however, was never called *iatros,* a physician, by
Homer, as was Asclepius.

The Greek patient who sought healing in religion rather than
medicine could invoke a wide range of gods, demigods, and heroes,
but in this multitude of divine healers one gradually stood out; one
became the leading healing deity, eclipsing Apollo himself; one came
to be worshiped universally on the mainland, the Aegean Islands,
and Asia Minor, and from 291 B.C. on, in Italy and as far as
Graeco-Roman civilization extended; one healing god became so
powerful that when Christianity entered the world as a religion that
promised healing and redemption, he, of all pagan gods, was the only
serious competitor of Christ. This was Asclepius. Who was he? What
gave him this unique position in the Greek pantheon? Why
did he, and not Amphiaraus or Trophonius, become the universal
healing god?

Asclepius presents many problems, and there is no agreement
among the historians of Greek religion about his origin. In order to
form an opinion, we must first look at the basic early texts that

mention Asclepius. The earliest such text is the *Iliad,* and in this epic, as we said before, he appears as a local chieftain, father of Podalirius and Machaon, the skilled leeches who held Tricca, Ithome, and Oechalia. Asclepius himself is called a blameless physician [52] who received soothing simples from old Chiron. [53]

Hesiod, probably around 700 B.C., is the first to tell a legend. [54] In the Boebian lake, the lake of Phoebus, the beautiful maiden Coronis, daughter of the Lapith Phlegyas, was bathing her feet when Apollo saw her and desired her. She became pregnant with the god's child but her father had promised her to her cousin Ischys. The day of the wedding came—what else could she do but obey her father's wishes? All preparations had been made for the wedding when the raven, a white bird until then, brought the evil news to Delphi, Apollo's seat. The god in his wrath first punished the messenger of evil tidings, who from then on exhibited the black color of mourning and was feared as the herald of disaster. He then killed Ischys, shooting his darts at him, while his sister Artemis hit Coronis and her innocent companions. But when the god saw the body of his beloved on the pyre, he felt pity for the unborn child, removed him from the mother's womb, and brought him to the cave of Chiron on Mount Pelion. There Asclepius grew up, instructed by the Centaur in the treatment of diseases with incantations, herbs, and the knife. He became a famous physician, sought by many from far and wide, and became so self-assured that he even resuscitated the dead, whereupon Zeus slew him with his thunderbolt. [55]

This is, in all probability, an old Thessalian legend. Pindar, who, in the early fifth century B.C. in one of his most beautiful odes addressed to Hieron of Syracuse, [56] told the story of Asclepius, made some significant changes. His sense of justice was offended by some elements of the old legend, and he changed the motivation for various actions. Thus Coronis was not the innocent maiden who, seduced by Apollo, married her cousin at her father's order. No, 'in the errors of her heart, bearing within her the pure seed of the god, yet without her father's knowledge she consented to be wedded to another,' and without waiting for the wedding, she 'slept in the couch of a stranger who came from Arcadia.' Thus she loaded guilt upon her head and deserved her dire fate. Pindar also did not mention the raven; the gods, he felt, did not require messengers to tell them what was happening on earth. And—a most significant change—he made Asclepius resuscitate a dead man for money!

Alas! even the lore of leechcraft is enthralled by the love of gain; even he was seduced, by a splendid fee of gold displayed upon the palm, to bring back from death one who was already its lawful prey. Therefore the son of Cronus with his hands hurled his shaft through both of them, and swiftly reft the breath from out their breasts, for they were stricken with sudden doom by the gleaming thunderbolt.[57]

We must reflect here for a moment on the meaning of the legend. There is no doubt that in it Asclepius does not appear as a god. He is the son of a god and of a mortal woman, a hero, to be sure, but also mortal. The fact that Zeus slew him for reviving the dead expresses graphically that the physician's interfering with the laws of nature, his keeping people alive whom fate had doomed, is not a self-evident right and may not be taken for granted. It is ὕβρις, wantonness. Society tolerates the physician in its midst and allows him to wield much power, but this puts great moral obligations upon him. Pindar's assumption that Asclepius overstepped the boundaries of his competence for venal motives is not only a further justification for the punishment inflicted upon him by Zeus, but at the same time a strong indictment of the greed that Pindar may well have observed in certain physicians of his time.

The legend made Asclepius the son of Apollo, perhaps for political reasons. The rising fame of Asclepius, the healer, was in competition with the Delphian Apollo, the old healing god. As Apollo's son, Asclepius was no longer a competitor but a co-worker to whom Apollo had delegated some of his main functions. And when temples were erected to Asclepius, Apollo, the father, was worshiped at the same time.

The later legends sound very different and picture the miraculous birth of a god. To give but one example, in the Epidaurian legend as Pausanias relates it,[58] Phlegyas, a great warrior, went on a military mission to the Peloponnesus accompanied by his daughter Coronis, who was with child by Apollo. In the land of the Epidaurians, she gave birth to the child and exposed him on the Myrtle Mountain, which thereafter was named Titthion, or the Nipple. A goat gave milk to the child and the herd's dog guarded him. And when the herdsman, Aresthanas, searched for the missing animals, he found the child. He wished to pick him up, but as he came near he saw lightning flash from the child and, thinking it was something divine, as it was, he turned away. Immediately the news was spread over every land and sea that the child could cure every disease and revive the dead.[59]

This sounds very different from the earlier legends; here Asclepius is a god, miraculously born, and performing miracles without being punished by Zeus. He was born not somewhere in the north but in the land where his most famous sanctuary for many centuries attracted sick people from far and wide. What was the process through which the Homeric chieftain, the hero of Hesiod and Pindar, became the most popular healing deity of Greece and later of Rome?

The traditional view is that Asclepius was originally an old local chthonian deity of Thessaly, a demon who dwelt in the earth, comparable to Amphiaraus and Trophonius. The sky is open for all to see but the earth is full of mysteries, full of hidden life. The snake sacred to Asclepius lives in the clefts of the earth, in the fissures of rocks.[60] People would lie down on the earth praying to Asclepius for help, and he appeared to them in their sleep or sent his snake or his dog who cured wounds and ulcers by licking them. When the Thessalians migrated into Greece they found this local demon, adopted him, and carried his cult to the Peloponnesus whence it spread to other places.[61]

This theory was taken up and developed recently in a very interesting way by Henri Grégoire.[62] His starting point was the etymology of the name Asclepius, which he thought derived from *skalops, aspalax,* or *spalax,* terms that designate the mole rat, or blind rat (*spalax typhlus*). The mole, indeed, is an animal that lives in the earth, was made blind, and cursed by the gods, just as Asclepius was destroyed by Zeus; it is an animal, moreover, that played a very important part in magic and popular medicine. According to Pliny, the Magi believed that whoever ate the fresh, still-palpitating heart of a mole, acquired the power of divination.[63] Liver, blood, head, teeth, legs, and other parts of the animal or the ashes therefrom were used in the treatment of a variety of diseases— and not only in antiquity. In the folklore of many peoples, and for centuries, the mole played a prominent part, and the belief was widespread that if a mole died in your hand, the hand acquired healing properties.[64] But not only the animal itself, the molehill, curse of our gardens, the earth thrown up by the mole building its lair, was also believed to have curative virtues. And this very lair is taken to explain a strange structure in the holy precincts of Epidaurus, the so-called Tholos, a round building, the foundations of which are still preserved, and to show that it consisted of a central chamber surrounded by communicating galleries similar in construction to the mole's lair. This then, according to Grégoire, would have been the tomb of Asclepius, the place where he lived in the earth. From time immemorial, the Asclepiads must have looked at such structures as the secret center of their cult where they sacrificed φαρμακοί, scapegoats, animals which carried evil disease into the molehill.

An analogous case is presented by another hero, Phineus, who opened the Bosporus to the Argonauts, thus violating the secrets of the gods, for which they punished him by transforming him into a mole.[65] And there may be a connection between the two heroes, as Asclepius appears on an Augustan coin from Nicopolis, in Epirus, as *Asklepios Phinaios*. But still more striking is the analogy to the Indian god Rudra, a Vedic deity, a bold archer who struck men and beasts but was also a healer.[66] An annual sacrifice was brought to him; it consisted of as many cakes as the family counted members, with an additional one which was buried in a mole's lair. 'This is thy share, O Rudra,' were the words spoken, 'the mole is thy animal ... Thou art remedy, remedy for the horned cattle, remedy

for horse and man, prosperity for the ram and the lamb.' [67] This is
not the place to go into further details and to discuss Grégoire's and
his co-workers' thesis of the relation between Apollo Smintheus and
the mole god Asclepius on one hand, and the Indian deities, Rudra
and Ganesha, on the other. Grégoire's theory cannot be proved by
texts but is based on considerations of etymology and folklore, both
somewhat shaky foundations. However, one cannot expect texts to
illustrate the exact origin of extremely old magic rites,[68] and people
were apt to forget the origin of a god who had been transformed into
an accursed animal. The mole was replaced by the serpent, and the
women sacrificing at Cos quietly put a cake into the serpent's hole.[69]
It has happened frequently in the history of religions that origins were
recorded merely in words and in certain rites the meaning of which
was later forgotten.

A totally different view of the origin of Asclepius and his cult was
taken recently by E. J. and L. Edelstein.[70] They collected and
published in the original languages with an English translation 861
testimonies, literary Greek and Roman references expressing the
beliefs of the upper classes, and a selection of inscriptions that to a
large extent reflect the views of the common man. They grouped the
collected materials so that they would illustrate the various aspects
of the problem: legend, descendants, the hero's deification and divine
nature, medicine, the cult, and finally the god's images and sanctuaries. Analyzing this wealth of material, the Edelsteins came to rather
novel and bold conclusions. No one had answered the question why
Asclepius became the universal healing deity. Why was it not an
Olympian god? Why not Apollo? Why did Paeon lose his personality? Why was not another hero deified, Amphiaraus or Trophonius
or Chiron himself? So many gods and demigods exercised healing
functions, why was Asclepius chosen?

The Edelsteins reject the common assumption that Asclepius was
an old local Thessalian deity who degenerated into a hero and was
incidentally restored to godhead. They look upon him as a culture
hero. He was the blameless physician of old, praised by Homer, and
as such became the patron of the physicians. For many centuries

doctors practiced as itinerant craftsmen. What united them and gave them standing was that they belonged to a guild based on the fictitious assumption that physicians were descendants of Asclepius the hero; they were Asclepiads just as minstrels were Homerids. Hippocrates was an Asclepiad, not a priest of the god but a fictitious descendant of the hero. Asclepius the hero did not cure people; he protected the physicians, and they treated patients rationally. Medicine was a secular craft. Wherever physicians went they carried the name of their patron hero, who more and more was identified with medicine and healing until he became the chief healer, competing with the physicians and supplementing their work. His deification took place, in the Edelsteins' opinion, toward the end of the sixth century B.C. At that time there existed a strong need for a personal god whom people in distress could freely approach, who would appear to them and would relieve their sufferings. Asclepius was predestined to become this god. He was the son of Apollo, and in the sixth century B.C. it seemed to fit into the policy of Delphi to relieve Apollo of some of his functions. As Apollo Maleatas he continued to be worshiped as the god of medicine in a number of places, but his son, the god Asclepius, became his coadjutor and finally eclipsed him as healing deity.

Historians of religion also disagree as to the place where Asclepius' deification occurred. If one assumes that he was an old indigenous Thessalian demon, Tricca would seem the logical place. Strabo says that the earliest and most famous temple of Asclepius was in Tricca,[71] and according to the Coan tradition the cult had been brought to the island from Tricca.[72] The temple, however, has not yet been excavated so that we have no archaeological evidence. A good case, on the other hand, can also be made for Epidaurus, in the Argolid,[73] where a flourishing sanctuary with an aggressive missionary policy developed early; and from this sanctuary the Asclepius religion spread to other sections of Greece, Asia Minor, and Rome. At the end of the sixth century B.C. an altar and a sacred building were erected at Epidaurus, and this was the beginning of a development which in the course of the centuries was to make Epidaurus one of the most famous and sumptuous holy places of the ancient world.

In the fifth century B.C. the new religion began its triumphant course.[74] By that time it had reached Sicyon in the Argolid, Mantinea in Arcadia, Corinth, Aegina, and a number of other places. In 420 B.C.—that is, ten years after the great plague—Asclepius took up his abode in Athens. He came from Epidaurus and, as he arrived 'at the time of the great mysteries, he took up his residence in the Eleusinium, and having summoned from his home the snake he brought it hither in the chariot of Telemachus. ... At the same time came Hygieia.' [75] A beautiful temple was built to him on the southern slope of the Acropolis, which even in ruins is still impressive; [76] a few years later in 408, a second sanctuary was built in Athens' port, the Piraeus.[77] The fact that the cult was firmly established in Athens early, undoubtedly contributed to its rapid expansion.

Asclepius reached the island of Cos relatively late.[78] At the time of Hippocrates there was no temple, no cult, and the island was famous for its secular school of medicine which flourished in the fifth and early fourth centuries B.C. The Coan Asclepiads were not priests but physicians who worshiped Asclepius as their patron, as their ancestral hero. It is easy to understand, however, that the Coan doctors took to the god Asclepius and joyfully adopted him when his cult spread to the Aegean Islands and to Asia Minor. However, the famous Coan medical school was not derived from temple medicine; on the contrary, the god and his temple benefited from the reputation of the secular school.

The cult of Asclepius was launched at Cos when an altar was erected to him in a cypress grove dedicated to Apollo Cyparissius. This occurred in the middle of the fourth century B.C. In the beginning of the third century, a small temple was built in front of the altar and a structure was erected around the spring that is always present in such places of worship. This first sanctuary was very modest compared to the rich temple and colonnades that followed in the second century B.C., but it contained great works of art. We have a charming description of them in a mime, a dramatic sketch of the poet Herondas written between 280 and 260 B.C.[79] Two women, natives

of Cos, at sunrise walk to the temple to sacrifice to the god in gratitude for having been cured of an illness. Standing before the altar
one of them, Cynno, invokes the god and the members of his family,
whose statues made by the sons of Praxiteles adorn the altar:

Hail Lord Paieon,[80] who rulest over Tricca and who dwellest in
our beloved Cos and in Epidaurus. And Coronis also who bore thee,
and Apollo. Hail to them both. And hail to her, Hygieia whom thou
touchest with thy right hand. Hail also to those who are honored at
these altars, Panacea and Epio and Iaso. Hail to them all. And
Podalirius and Machaon who destroyed the house and the great wall
of Laomedeon, both healers of sickness, them I salute also, with all the
other gods and goddesses that dwell about thy hearth, oh Father
Paieon. Come graciously and receive this cock, the herald of our walls
at home whom I offer to you as a slight addition to your meal. For
at home our well gives us not much water and that not all the time.
If it did, I would surely have offered you an ox or a pig heavy with
fat, instead of a cock, in thanksgiving for the sickness which thou hast
wiped away. Coccale, put up our little tablet to the right of Hygieia.

The tablet was a modest votive offering probably with the name
of the patient, and perhaps with a reference to the organ that had
been affected. It stood next to great works of art, offerings of wealthy
patients: a girl looking at an apple, an old man, a boy strangling a
goose. 'If the marble did not stand there lifeless before our eyes, you
would say that the goose was just about to cry out.' The women enter
the inner temple and admire a painting by Apelles, representing a
religious procession with sacrificial animals so realistically that 'if it
did not seem unbecoming for a woman, I could scream aloud, for
fear the ox would hurt me; he is looking so sideways at me, dear
Cynno, with one eye.' The sacristan, in the meantime, has killed the
cock and comes back with the report that the sacrifice has been well
received.

The cult of Asclepius thrived in Cos. Panhellenic festivals were
held every four years and attracted large crowds. The sanctuary was
enlarged considerably and survived the medical school by several
centuries.

The cult was established at Pergamum in the middle of the fourth century B.C., and the sanctuary soon became as famous as that of Cos.[81] Five hundred years later, in A.D. 129, Galen was born in Pergamum, and he tells of a new temple that was built to Zeus Asclepius while he was a student in that city.[82] Throughout his life he remained attached to the god who once saved him from a fatal illness.[83]

Epidaurus, Cos, and Pergamum were, without doubt, the chief centers of the Asclepius cult which, however, spread far beyond Greece and Asia Minor. In 291 B.C. Asclepius entered Rome. Livy,[84] Valerius Maximus,[85] Ovid,[86] and others[87] relate the dramatic story. For three continuous years the city had suffered from a pestilence. The Sibylline Books were consulted and revealed that no improvement might be expected unless Asclepius were summoned from Epidaurus. A legation was dispatched and was well received by the Epidaurians, who were always eager to see new branches established. The god was willing to help and appeared to the ambassadors in the form of a huge serpent which wound its way along the ground and took its place on the ship. Wreathed with flowers, the ship set sail, reached Italy on the sixth day, sailed along the shore and up the Tiber until it came to Rome. There the god-serpent disembarked, swam to the island of the Tiber, and, resuming his heavenly form, set an end to the people's woes and brought health to the city. A temple was erected to him on the island shaped like a ship. An obelisk took the place of a mast and a relief of Asclepius adorned one of the walls, parts of which can still be seen today.[88]

The cult spread to Africa. In Egypt Asclepius was identified with Imhotep and was worshiped as Asclepius Imouthes. Sarapis, the god introduced by the Ptolemies, became a fierce competitor of Asclepius as a healing deity, assuming many of his characteristic traits and taking over elements of his cult.[89] In Carthage, as in Phoenicia,[90] the Greek god was identified with the main local deity, and we shall see later the part Asclepius played in the struggle between Christianity and paganism.

All over the ancient western world more than four hundred

temples and shrines were dedicated to the son of Apollo and Coronis,[91] sanctuaries in which he was worshiped either alone or together with other gods and to which people came from far and wide in search of health, physical as well as spiritual health. The cult of Asclepius was one of the last to die and some of his temples were still functioning in the sixth century A.D.

We have seen that many points in the early history of Asclepius are highly controversial. We had to mention the various theories about his origins since they all have some bearing on medicine, but we could not go into any detail, and I think we need not take sides in the controversy since in this study we are interested primarily in health and disease, in the means to preserve or to restore health. The history of religion is probably more conjectural and more subject to changing ideas than any other branch of history. Every one of the theories proffered has some very convincing points but also some highly speculative links. We must be satisfied with the undeniable fact that from the sixth century B.C. on, Asclepius became the Panhellenic healing god, and that Greek religious medicine crystallized around his cult. Our task now is to find out what kind of patients sought help in the temples, and how they were cured. To this end we must again look at Epidaurus because it was the center of the cult for many centuries, because its site has long been excavated, because the testimonies found here, literary and epigraphic, are particularly revealing, and also because we have in Pausanias an unusually eloquent guide.[92]

Driving today from Nauplia through vineyards to Epidaurus, we enter a quiet valley surrounded by lofty hills. It is filled with ruins of mighty buildings: some, like the theater, are well preserved and very impressive; of others only the foundations can be seen, but the ground plan of the holy place may easily be discerned, and with the help of Pausanias we are able to reconstruct and revive this great sanctuary which for such a long time was teeming with life.[93] When Pausanias visited it in the second century A.D., the Asclepieion of Epidaurus was close to seven hundred years old. It was as active as ever and more magnificent even than before, because it showed the accumulated wealth of the centuries, and because a Roman senator, Antoninus, had restored the dilapidated buildings and constructed new ones.

The Asclepieion was not only a temple but an entire holy district. Like other holy places, it had its rules of purity. No child was to be born within the enclosure and no one was permitted to die there. This meant great hardship to many pilgrims until Antoninus had a special building erected outside the precinct in which a man could die and a woman be delivered without sin. The center of the place in the midst of the sacred grove was the temple in which stood the statue of the god, made by Thrasymedes of ivory and gold. The god was seated on a throne grasping his staff with one hand while he held the other over the head of the serpent. A dog was lying by his side. Thus we find him represented on Epidaurian coins and also on votive offerings. Stepping out of the golden-roofed temple, over its marble pavement, the visitor saw the Tholos or Rotunda that we mentioned before, built by Polycletus [94] of white marble, with graceful columns and famous paintings by Pausias.[95] One represented Methe, or Drunkenness, drinking from a glass cup through which her face could be seen, and the other Eros, who had thrown away bow and arrow and had taken up a lyre instead. There is no doubt that such paintings had a symbolic meaning, and Meier's interpretation that Methe stood for Dionysiac raving and Eros playing the lyre for its cure, may well be correct.[96] Close to the Tholos was the *Abaton,* the incubation hall, and temples of other deities, Artemis, Aphrodite, and Themis. All buildings were adorned with statues, and it goes without saying that the whole family of the god was represented, his wife Epione, his favorite daughter Hygieia with whom he is most closely associated and with whom he so frequently appears on reliefs, he, the Healer, and she, Health. His other daughters, Aceso, Iaso, and Panacea, personified healing functions as the names indicate; and the boy Telesphorus, 'he who brings the end,' namely, of the illness, was probably the god of convalescence and recovery.[97]

Water was to be found not only in the Tholos but also in a fountain 'worth seeing for its roof and general beauty.' Many other structures were erected in the course of time for the entertainment of patients and their families, and also for the mental preparation of those who were to partake in the mystery of healing: a theater, work of Polycletus, famous for its symmetry and beauty, today one of the best-preserved ancient theaters with astounding acoustics,[98] an odeon or concert hall, a stadium, a gymnasium, baths. And it is obvious that buildings were needed for housing people who had come from distant lands and wished to be close to the sanctuary, close to the god from whom they expected so much.

Asclepius was primarily a healing god. Physicians worshiped him as their patron, and healthy people prayed to him and sacrificed to him, seeking his blessings for the preservation of their health. Cities such as Athens, Syracuse, and Pergamum implored his protection.[99] But he was first of all the god of the sick who came to his temples from far and wide in the hope of having their health restored. He was the divine physician who succeeded where human doctors had failed.

People came to the temple, walking, or riding on a donkey, or on horseback, or in carts, accompanied by family members or friends, with slaves carrying gifts.[100] In Athens and Rome the Asclepieion was in the city, but in many other places, in Epidaurus, Cos, and Pergamum, the temple was in the country, in a valley or on a hill. Ancient authors speculated on the reasons for having the temples outside the cities. Was it because many sanctuaries were branches of that of Epidaurus which happened to be in the country, or should such shrines be in places which are both clean and high? [101] Or was it because the water is purer in the country, as Vitruvius thought? In his work on architecture, he recommended that healthy sites with suitable springs of water be chosen for all temples and particularly for those of Asclepius, 'for when sick persons are moved from a pestilent to a healthy place and the water supply is from wholesome fountains, they will more quickly recover. So will it happen that the divinity from the nature of the site will gain a greater and higher reputation and authority.' [102] I think no naïvely rational explanation is needed for the fact that Asclepieia were built in the country. We know today that they were not anything like sanatoria but were shrines where miracles took place. Like the temples of other gods in which people communed with the deity, they were built in quiet spots, far from the noise of city traffic.

When the patient arrived he first underwent purification rites as in the cult of other gods. Only the pure were admitted to the temple. But it was mainly a spiritual purity that was required. At the entrance of the temple at Epidaurus the suppliant could read: 'Pure must be he who enters the fragrant temple; purity means to think nothing but holy thoughts.'[103] This spiritual purity, however, was expressed also by certain rites as in other cults. The suppliant bathed and put on a white chiton. He then offered sacrifices to the god, according to his means, honey cakes, fruit, or a rooster. There was much to be seen in the holy precinct that struck the patient's imagination—statues and paintings, votive reliefs—and what probably impressed him most, case histories written on marble tablets, the stories of other patients who had come with seemingly hopeless diseases and yet had been cured by the god. If they had been helped, why should he not find healing also? Whoever has visited Lourdes at the time of a pilgrimage, or has read Zola's novel *Lourdes,* can well imagine in what frame of mind the Greek patient was when the great moment, long anticipated with hope and awe, had arrived, when he was going to face his living god. In such moments of greatest nervous tension miracles do occur, or at least happenings which are difficult to explain.[104]

The healing act took place in what the Greeks called ἐγκοίμησις, the Romans *incubatio*. When the sun had set and night had come, the patient was brought to the *Abaton,* the holiest part of the sanctuary, where he was instructed to lie down on a couch. There he waited for the god to come. The hours went by—and suddenly the god appeared looking like his statue in the temple, a bearded god somewhat like Zeus, with a kind face. He came alone or accompanied by his daughter Hygieia or another of his children, or the snake or the dog. He approached the patient, touched him, gave him medicine, or operated on him, or his dog licked the wounds. And when the glow of morning appeared on the hills, the blind would open their eyes and see the world in all its beauty. The deaf would hear the singing of the birds. Those who had been lame would find themselves able to walk without a limp. Old pains had vanished and sores were healed—sometimes, not always, of course; the god could not be forced. His epiphany, in a dream or vision, was a mystery in which not everybody participated. There can be no doubt, however, that patients were actually cured, just as true healings do occur today at Lourdes.[105]

When Pausanias visited Epidaurus he saw six tablets on which were engraved 'the names of men and women who were healed by Asclepius, together with the disease from which each suffered and how he was cured,' and he was told that there had been more such tablets in the past.[106] Similar steles could be seen at Cos and Tricca[107] and probably in other sanctuaries of Asclepius as well. The excavation of Epidaurus brought forth three of the tablets that Pausanias saw, and fragments of a fourth, with altogether seventy case histories. They were written in the fourth century B.C. and their general title is Ἰάματα τοῦ Ἀπόλλωνος καὶ τοῦ Ἀσκλαπιοῦ, 'Cures of Apollo and Asclepius.' [108] These tablets are a source of first-rate importance, for they give us information on the type of patient that sought healing in such a temple, and also on the kind of cure performed.

Every physician today who has had some experience with sick people apt to consult quacks or to seek healing in churches will immediately recognize the type. They are, to put it briefly, people suffering from certain chronic diseases—for instance old sores, or chronic ulcers such as the varicose ulcers—which resist treatment but may sometimes heal rather suddenly without apparent reason. They are, furthermore, the large group of patients showing symptoms due to hysteria, as described by Bleuler, whose concept of this mental disease is to me the most convincing.[109] Hysteria, according to

Bleuler, is a type of mental reaction to unpleasant situations that the individual refuses to face and from which he escapes by becoming ill. The normal individual has no choice but must bear such situations, must suffer, or overcome them, while the hysterical person escapes them by becoming blind, deaf, dumb, paralyzed, by developing pains, spasms, or other symptoms. He has a disease; the individual is sick, and as such benefits from all the privileges granted the sick man by society; and since his illness is the result of an unconscious desire, it is difficult to cure. But if one succeeds in influencing the patient's attitude toward life; if one can awaken in him the wish to recover and persuade him, for instance, to have recourse to Asclepius, it may very well happen that the blind man who saw the god in his dream will also see the world the following day, and that the paralytic will throw away his crutches. We know, however, that such seemingly miraculous but nonetheless real cures may not be permanent. The patient may relapse later or may develop other symptoms because his pathological disposition remains unchanged.

It is certainly not by accident that of the seventy cases listed on the Epidaurian tablets that have come down to us, eleven are cases of blindness, two of deafness, one patient had become voiceless, nine were paralyzed in some parts of their body, one had insomnia as a result of headaches. In other words, over one third of all cases listed may well fall into the category of hysteria, as we would expect. Bad sores are mentioned in a number of cases, and a type of suppliant that we usually find in religious medicine is not missing here either, namely, the barren woman seeking the god's help for offspring; four cases occur in our material. Some cases are frankly fantastic, like that of the woman who was with child for five years, and after having slept in the *Abaton*, 'bore a son who immediately after birth, washed himself at the fountain and walked about with his mother.' [110] I think it futile to try to explain such stories rationally. The cases engraved in these tablets and displayed so that they could be seen by every visitor were selected from thousands of cases. They related the most spectacular cures of the god, those most apt to inflame the patient's imagination, and we may readily believe that the priests who edited these stories added some of their own to the greater glory of their god.

The cures were miracle cures. The god healed the sick by appearing before him, by fondling him, or by giving him a verbal order, just as other ancient gods performed cures, or as Jesus Christ did. Or—and this is rather unusual in religious medicine—Asclepius acted like a mortal physician or surgeon in the patient's dreams, examining wounds and performing operations. In the people's mind Asclepius was not an ordinary god but a divine physician and hence acted as a doctor but not as an ordinary doctor. He performed miraculous operations. We must quote a few cases from the Epidaurian tablets in order to illustrate these various points.

In some cases we have no indications of the type of treatment performed. The patient went to sleep in the *Abaton* and woke up cured; the epiphany was apparently taken for granted. A barren woman from Troezen saw the god, who asked her whether she wanted a male or a female child. She answered she wanted a male and 'within a year a son was born to her.' [111] Another barren woman, Andromache of Epeirus, dreamt that a handsome boy uncovered her and that the god touched her, whereupon she too was blessed with a boy.[112] The sexual implications are obvious in the cases of sterility and diseases of the sexual organs; and we must forget Christian prudery when we read that Nicasibula of Messene saw the god approach her with his snake, and that she had intercourse with the snake, with the happy result that she gave birth to two sons within a year;[113] or when we hear that a man with a stone in his membrum dreamt that he was lying with a fair boy, 'and when he had a seminal discharge he ejected the stone.' [114]

A good example of magic transplantation of disease is found in the case of the Thessalian Pandarus, who had marks [115] on his forehead. The god bound the marks with a headband and 'enjoined him to remove the band when he left the *Abaton* and dedicate it as an offering to the temple.' This was done and the marks were gone. But then there was somebody else, Echedorus, who had marks also. He too went to the temple, with money that Pandarus had asked him to offer to the god in his name in gratitude for the cure. But he kept the money, and the god did not heal him, but bound the headband of Pandarus around his forehead. And when Echedorus awoke, he took off the headband, looked into the water, and saw his face with his own marks and those of Pandarus in addition.[116] The god was always anxious not to be cheated, and whoever attempted to deprive him of an offering due him was invariably punished. When the blind Hermon of Thasos was cured and did not bring the thank-offerings, the god made him blind again and he had to undergo another incubation.[117] Such cases were posted as a warning to all visitors, as were also cases in which lack of faith had met with punishment. Thus a certain Cephisias made the remark that if the god was able to heal lame people, why had he not cured Hephaestus? Whereupon he was hit by his horse so that his foot was crippled. He was cured by the god later, after he had repented and had entreated the god earnestly.[118] Another such case must be quoted literally—it is reported in such a delightfully naïve way:[119]

Ambrosia of Athens, blind of one eye. She came as a suppliant to the god. As she walked about in the Temple she laughed at some of the cures as incredible and impossible, that the lame and the blind should be healed by merely seeing a dream. In her sleep she had a vision. It seemed to her that the god stood by her and said that he would cure her, but that in payment he would ask her to dedicate to the Temple a silver pig as a memorial of her ignorance. After saying this, he cut the diseased eyeball and poured in some drug. When the day came she walked out sound.

In this case the god operated on the eye and treated it with a drug. Indeed, people knew that mortal physicians acted in such a way, and so they dreamt that the god was doing the same. We are of course not told what drugs he used; they were miracle drugs which, poured into the eye, restored the sight,[120] or rubbed on a bald head, made the hair grow.[121] The operations were similarly fantastic, such as a layman expected of a divine surgeon to whom nothing was impossible. A man had swallowed leeches, and 'the god cut open his chest with a knife and took out the leeches which he gave him into his hands, and then he stitched up his chest again.' [122] Still more miraculous was the case of Aristagora of Troezen who slept in the Asclepius temple of her home town because she had a tapeworm in her belly. The sons of the god cut off her head but were unable to put it back again. At daybreak the priest found her 'with her head cut off from the body.' But the following night Asclepius came from Epidaurus in person and 'fastened her head on to her neck. Then he cut open her belly, took the tapeworm out, and stitched her up again.' And after that she became well—a gruesome tale which illustrated the superiority of Epidaurus over Troezen, and of the father over his sons. [123] Like a mortal surgeon, Asclepius used assistants to grip the patient and hold him tightly while he was cutting his belly open to remove an abscess. [124] Touchingly naïve is the story of Cleinatas of Thebes who went to the temple because he was full of lice. His dream was that 'the god stripped him and made him stand upright, naked, and with a broom brushed the lice from off his body. When day came he left the Temple well.' [125]

These examples are sufficient to illustrate the general type of cures performed in the temples in the fifth and fourth centuries B.C. A few cases throw light on less common aspects of the god and his cult. We mentioned before that the healing act was sometimes not performed by the god himself but by his animals, the serpent and the dog. [126] Rather unusual was the case of Arata, a woman of Lacedaemon who suffered from dropsy. [127] She stayed at home, but her mother went to Epidaurus in her stead, slept in the temple and dreamt that the god cut off her daughter's head, hung her upside down and thus drained the water from her body, whereupon he fitted the head back to the neck. When she returned to her home, she found her daughter cured and heard that she had seen the same dream. This, in other words, was a case of vicarious incubation.

Asclepius sometimes also cured people outside of his temples.

Thus a woman who was suffering from worms had gone to sleep in Epidaurus but had had no distinct dream and had not been cured. Such failures must have been very frequent. However, the god appeared to her on her way home, and there on the road removed two washbasins full of worms from her belly. And he did not forget to enjoin her to send thank-offerings to Epidaurus.

The god restored miraculously not only human bodies but also objects, as he did the goblet of a man that was dropped on the way to the temple, to the great distress of the bearer. And finally we hear that the god was consulted not only in medical matters but also to find lost persons or objects. A father had lost his son who while swimming and diving had come to a place surrounded by rocks, whence he could not find his way out. Sleeping in the temple of Epidaurus, the father dreamt that the god was leading him to a certain place where, seven days later, he actually found his son.[128] Similarly, a widow was given an oracle in the incubation which told her where her deceased husband had buried his gold.[129]

We mentioned the sacrifices brought to the god as part of the preparatory ritual. They were plain and inexpensive, as a rule, but after the cure the god or rather the temple expected more, a fee in cash or kind, and a record of the case which could be a simple tablet relating name, illness, and cure, or might be an artistic representation of what had happened. Such votive offerings have been found in considerable number where temples of Asclepius have been excavated,[130] and we read about them in the ancient literature.[131] Particularly valuable and also beautiful is the large collection of reliefs found in the Asclepius temple of Athens and preserved today in the National Museum of Athens.[132]

These thank-offerings varied a great deal, and their choice was largely determined by the suppliant's means and generosity. 'After an illness men often in exchange for the god's beneficence picture Asclepius as the well-doer on an image. How great an expenditure would the picture have entailed? How large would have been the pay of the painter? Willingly would I have spent the money for such things,' we read in the *Declamationes*[133] of Libanius, a late sophist. On a number of such votive representations of the god, marble reliefs mostly, he appears standing or sitting, alone or with Hygieia, or with some other deity, who is a member of his family. In other cases the suppliant, who had been healed by the god's intervention, dedicated to the temple his own portrait or a reproduction of the organ from which he had suffered. Hausmann very justly pointed to the magic significance of having one's picture in the temple, that is, constantly within the sphere of the god's influence. And similarly, having an arm, a leg, bowels, a uterus, whatever the sick but now healthy organ had been, in the temple close to the god was not merely a gesture of gratitude but was originally meant to protect the organ against further illness.[134] Votive organs in terra-cotta have been found frequently in sanctuaries on Italian soil but rarely in Greece, and there chiefly at Corinth. It is very possible that the custom to dedicate such organs, which became so popular in the Christian church, came to Italy from Corinth.[135]

By far the most fascinating votive reliefs are those that tell a story. Looking at the Athenian reliefs, we see the very life of such a temple unfolding before our eyes. Suppliants come in endless succession, some singly, followed by a servant, others with their entire families, adults, children, and slaves, who carry boxes with gifts for the god. Some bring a sheep, a ram, or even a cow; they are the wealthy patients who will sacrifice more than a cake or incense or a cock. They stand before the god and his daughter, small as mortals are compared to deities. On other reliefs we find depicted the dreams that the patients had during the incubation, regular illustrations of the miraculous stories of the Epidaurian tablets. On one we see the patient lying on a couch; the god stands behind her and touches her shoulder gently. On another an assistant performs an operation on the patient's head while the god himself stands by leaning on his caduceus. On a third the serpent performs the healing act. On a relief in the Carlsberg Museum in Copenhagen, the patient is carried on a stretcher, probably on his way home after an unsuccessful incubation; but there in a tree is a huge snake— the god, who is now ready to perform the miracle. If we had to describe all these reliefs, we should be repeating the stories of Epidaurus. Word and picture presented the same type of religious medicine.

We know that the temples contained other offerings, in gold and silver. The silver pig of the Athenian woman Ambrosia was such a gift. Or they were works of art that pleased the god even though they had no direct connection with healing, paintings and sculptures such as the women described by Herondas admired at Cos. On the whole it may be said that Asclepius was not greedy as were some Olympian gods. He did not require hecatombs and was satisfied with modest gifts. This made him a physician not only of the rich but also of the poor people; the Edelsteins have very justly stressed this social and economic aspect of the cult.[136] The physicians, as we shall see in a later chapter, were craftsmen, and as such, men who worked for money and did not recognize an obligation to provide care for poor patients also. Society felt no responsibility for its indigent members, and illness in a poor family was a catastrophe far greater than it is today. In such an emergency the indigent sick man could always seek the god's help, hope for a miracle, or get some aid from the priests. And this leads us to the discussion of a relatively late development of the cult.

The cures that we have studied so far, particularly those of the Epidaurian tablets, were miracle cures that succeeded with a certain type of patient, whether rich or poor. Such miraculous cures the god continued to perform throughout antiquity, but it appears from the testimonies that in later centuries patients in the incubation received oracles rather than cures, oracles which told them what to do in order to recover their health, and which they reported to the priests. Around A.D. 100, at Pergamum, a certain Polemo who suffered from a disease of the joints was told in the incubation to abstain from drinking anything cold.[137] Another patient, also at Pergamum, was instructed to struggle hard which he did, and when perspiration resulted the disease was gone.[138] Particularly revealing are some inscriptions from Lebena in Crete. A certain Poplius Granius Rufus who suffered from chronic bronchitis was cured by a diet consisting of 'rocket to nibble on an empty stomach, then Italian wine flavored with pepper to drink, then again starch with hot water, then powder of the holy ashes and some holy water, then an egg and pine-resin, then again moist pitch, then iris with honey, then a quince and a wild purslane to be boiled together ...'[139] In the same temple a woman who had a malignant sore on her little finger was advised to make an ointment consisting of ground burned oyster shell with rose-ointment, mallow, and olive oil.[140]

The examples could be multiplied indefinitely but they are sufficient to illustrate what actually happened. This oracle medicine was decidedly a sign of decadence. One should not need a god to have an ointment or an enema prescribed, and it may well be that so many competitors of Asclepius arose because of the change in his treatment. Yet the change itself may have been due to strong social and economic pressure, to the fact that the proletarization of the ancient world and the loosening of family bonds called for some cheap pastoral medicine to serve poor people who could not count on a regular physician. It is possible that the hostels attached to the Asclepieia were the first Western hospitals and poorhouses where indigent sick people could stay for a while and be treated by the priests. The temples were rich. Wealthy patients continued to patronize them, made generous donations, and distributed alms among poor pilgrims. And where the community failed to give any help to the needy, the temple stepped in and filled the gap, at least to a certain extent. Asclepius was thus a forerunner and competitor of Christ in more than one respect.[141]

In the fourth century B.C. an anonymous poet sang:[142]

Welcome, and come thou propitious to my wide-spaced city,
     hail, Paean!
And grant we may see the sunlight in joy, acceptable with
    bright Hygieia, the glorious,
       hail, Paean!
Asclepius, most renowned of demigods,
       hail, Paean!

The centuries went by; Andromachus the Elder prepared an antidote, a treacle, for Nero, his Lord. He described it in verse and ended his poem with the prayer: [143]

Be gracious, blessed Paeon, you who fashioned this remedy, whether the Triccaean ridges hold you, O demigod, or Rhodes, or Cos and Epidaurus on the sea; be gracious, send your always gracious daughter, Panacea, to the emperor, who will propitiate you with pure sacrifices for the everlasting freedom from pain which you can grant.

And for centuries people in distress invoked him, Asclepius,

Healer of all, Lord Paean, softening the painful sufferings of men's diseases, giver of gentle gifts, mighty one, may you come bringing health and checking illnesses and the harsh fate of death ... come blessed one, savior, granting a good end to life.[144]

NOTES

1. On Asclepius in general, see Alice Walton, *The Cult of Asklepios,* Cornell Studies in Classical Philology, vol. III, Ithaca, N. Y., 1894; L. R. Farnell, *Greek Hero Cults and Ideas of Immortality,* Oxford, 1921; Karl Kerényi, *Der göttliche Arzt,* Basle, 1948; and especially Emma J. and Ludwig Edelstein, *Asclepius, A Collection and Interpretation of the Testimonies,* Baltimore, 1945, 2 vols. (referred to in this chapter as Edelstein).

2. On Greek religion in general, see E. Rohde, *Psyche, Seelencult und Unsterblichkeitsglaube der Griechen,* Tübingen, 7th and 8th ed., 1921, 2 vols.; O. Kern, *Die Religion der Griechen,* Berlin, 1926–38, 3 vols.; M. P. Nilsson, 'Griechische Religion,' *Handbuch der Altertumswissenschaft,* Munich, 1941; *Greek Popular Religion,* New York, 1940; W. H. Roscher, *Ausführliches Lexikon der griechischen und römischen Mythologie,* Leipzig, 1884–1937, 6 vols. On healing gods, see L. Hopf, *Die Heilgötter und Heilstätten des Altertums,* Tübingen, 1904; F. Kutsch, *Attische Heilgötter und Heilheroen,* Giessen, 1913; W. A. Jayne, *The Healing Gods of Ancient Civilizations,* New Haven, 1925.

3. This is probably the meaning of *Odyssey,* IV, 232, that in Egypt everybody is skilled in medicine, ἦ γὰρ Παιήονός εἰσι γενέθλης. See the discussion in Edelstein, vol. II, p. 56.

4. Hesychius, *Lexicon.*

5. Pindar, *Olymp.,* 5, 17.

6. *Suppliants,* 263.

7. Ὀμνύω Ἀπόλλωνα ἰητρόν . . .

8. A picture of this coin is in O. Bernhard, *Griechische und römische Münz-bilder in ihren Beziehungen zur Geschichte der Medizin*, Zurich, 1926, plate I, fig. 1.

9. Pausanias, I, 3, 4.

10. E. g. *Iliad*, I, 39.

11. Bernhard, op. cit. plate I, fig. 5.

12. Bernhard, op. cit. p. 2. See in this connection O. Neustatter, 'Mice in Plague Pictures,' *The Journal of the Walters Art Gallery*, 1941, 4:104–13.

13. Smintheus may also mean the god of Sminthos or Sminthe, a town in the Troad.

14. Galen, XII, 174.

15. Pausanias, III, 16, 7ff.

16. Ibid. I, 2, 5.

17. Ibid. I, 23, 4.

18. Ibid. I, 34, 3.

19. Ibid. III, 18, 2.

20. About him, see Herodotus, 2, 49; Diodorus, VI, 8; Apollodorus, II, 2, 2. See also the discussion in E. Rohde, *Psyche*, vol. II, p. 50ff.

21. Apollodorus, 2, 2, 2.

22. Theophrastus, *Hist. Plant.*, 9, 10, 4; Dioscorides, 4, 149; Pliny, *Nat. Hist.*, 25, 47.

23. Ovid, *Met.*, 15, 322ff.; Vitruvius, 0, 3, 21; Pausanias, VIII, 18, 7; Strabo, 8, 346.

24. Pausanias, I, 44, 5.

25. *Odyssey*, XV, 225.

26. See H. Diels, *Sitzungs-Berichte Akad.*, Berlin, 1908, 1ff.

27. Pindar, *Nemeae*, 9, 24ff.

28. Philostratus, *Vita Apollonii*, II, 37.

29. Pausanias, I, 34, 4.

30. The chief sources are listed in Rohde, *Psyche*, vol. I, p. 119ff.

31. Pausanias, IX, 39, 4–5.

32. Aeschylus, *Agamemnon*, 1629; Euripides, *Bacchae*, 304, *Iphigenia Aul.*, 1211, *Alcestis*, 966; Pausanias, IX, 30, 4.

33. See Rohde, *Psyche*, vol. II, p. 109ff.

34. *Lithica* in *Orphica*, ed. E. Abel, Berlin, 1885.

35. Plato, *Republic*, 2, 364E; *Protagoras*, 316D.

36. Aristophanes, *Frogs*, 1033.

37. See E. Bethe, *Pauly-Wissowa*, vol. 5, 1087ff.

38. The most recent study on Chiron is by Warren R. Dawson, 'Chiron the Centaur,' *J. Hist. Med.*, 1949, 4:267–75.

39. Apollonius Rhodius, *Argonautica*, II, 1241.

40. Pindar, *Nemeae*, III, 56.

41. Pliny, *Nat. Hist.*, XXV, 13–14.

42. Identified as *Centaurea salonitana* or *Centaurea centaurium L.*

43. *Inula Helenium* and also *Hypericum olympicum.* The name *Chironias* appears as synonym of *Centaurea maior* in Pseudo-Apuleius, *Herbarius,* XXXIV, 18.

44. *Nat. Hist.,* XXV, 16.

45. See the edition by E. Howald and H. E. Sigerist in *Corpus Med. Lat.,* vol. IV, Leipzig, 1927.

46. Ps.-Apuleius, op. cit. XII, 12.

47. See Galen, X, 1006: ὧν ἰδέαι τινές εἰσι τά τε χειρώνια καὶ τηλέφια καλούμενα.

48. Paulus Aegineta, IV, 46.

49. Apollodorus, II, 5, 4.

50. *Pythiae,* III, 51–3, where this is said of Chiron's most famous pupil, Asclepius.

51. Apollodorus, III, 13, 8.

52. *Il.,* XI, 518.

53. *Il.,* IV, 218–19.

54. In the *Ehoiai;* only fragments are preserved but von Wilamowitz-Möllendorf was able to reconstruct the legend, partly with the help of Pindar's Ode (*Pythiae,* III), in *Isyllos von Epidauros,* Berlin, 1886, p. 70ff. We follow his version.

55. The legend did not end with Asclepius' death but pictured the wrath of Apollo over the slaying of his son. See von Wilamowitz-Möllendorf, op. cit. p. 71f.

56. *Pythiae,* III.

57. Pindar, op. cit. 54–8; see Edelstein, vol. I, p. 4.

58. Pausanias, II, 26, 3–5.

59. Another Epidaurian legend is related by Isyllus, see von Wilamowitz-Möllendorf, op. cit. p. 13f.

60. E. Küster, *Die Schlange in der griechischen Kunst und Religion,* Giessen, 1913; E. S. Potter, *Serpents in Symbolism, Art and Medicine,* Santa Barbara, Calif., 1937; H. Scholz, *Der Hund in der griechisch-römischen Magie,* Thesis, Berlin, 1937.

61. Thus von Wilamowitz-Möllendorf, op. cit. p. 96ff.

62. Henri Grégoire avec la collaboration de R. Goossens et de M. Mathieu, *Asklèpios, Apollon Smintheus et Rudra; Études sur le dieu à la taupe et le dieu au rat dans la Grèce et dans l'Inde,* Ac. Roy. Belgique, Cl. Lettres Sc. Mor. Pol., Mémoires, tome XLV, fasc. 1, Brussels, 1950. An abstract was published in *Le Flambeau,* 1949, 32:22–54.

63. *Nat. Hist.,* XXX, 3.

64. Testimonies in Grégoire, op. cit. p. 59f.

65. Oppian, *Cynegetica,* II, 612ff.

66. Developed by Roger Goossens in Grégoire, op. cit. p. 127ff.

67. Ibid. p. 129.

68. The Indian analogy would be evidence of the antiquity of the rites.

69. Herondas, IV, 90–91.

70. See note 1.
71. Strabo, IX, 5, 17.
72. Herondas, II, 97.
73. Edelstein, vol. II, p. 97f.
74. About the spreading of the cult and the sanctuaries, see Edelstein, vol. II, p. 232ff.
75. *Inscriptiones Graecae,* II², no. 4960a; trans. by Edelstein, Test. 720.
76. W. Judeich, *Topographie von Athen,* 2nd ed., Munich, 1931; P. Gérard, *L'Asclépieion d'Athènes, d'après de récentes découvertes,* Paris, 1881.
77. F. Robert, 'Le Plutus d'Aristophane et l'Asclépieion du Pirée,' *Rev. Philol.,* 1931, p. 132–9.
78. R. Herzog, *Koische Forschungen und Funde,* Leipzig, 1899; *Kos, Ergebnisse der Deutschen Ausgrabungen und Forschungen,* Berlin, 1932; K. Sudhoff, *Kos und Knidos,* Munich, 1927.
79. Herondas, IV. English translation by J. R. Oliver in *Bull. Inst. Hist. Med.,* 1934, 2:504–11 (slightly changed).
80. Like Apollo, Asclepius was frequently addressed as Paieon.
81. O. Deubner, *Das Asklepieion von Pergamon,* Berlin, 1938.
82. Galen, II, 224f.
83. Galen, XIX, 19.
84. Livy, *Ab Urbe Condita,* XXIX, 1.
85. Valerius Maximus, *Facta et Dicta Memorabilia,* 1, 8, 2.
86. Ovid, *Met.,* XV, 622–744.
87. See Edelstein, vol. I, p. 431ff.
88. M. Besnier, *L'Ile Tibérine dans l'antiquité,* Paris, 1902.
89. Thus Sarapis is σύνναος with Isis as Asclepius is with Hygieia and is accompanied by a divine child, Harpocrates, as Asclepius is by Telesphorus. See C. A. Meier, *Antike Inkubation und moderne Psychotherapie,* Zurich, 1950, p. 53ff.
90. See Edelstein, vol. II, p. 252 and the corresponding testimonies.
91. Thrämer, in *Encyclopaedia of Religion and Ethics,* vol. VI, p. 550.
92. A. Defrasse and H. Lechat, *Epidaure,* Paris, 1895; P. Kavvadias, Τὸ ἱερὸν τοῦ 'Ασκληπιοῦ ἐν 'Επιδαύρῳ καὶ ἡ θεραπεία τῶν ἀσθενῶν, Athens, 1900; P. Maas, *Epidaurische Hymnen,* Schr. d. Königsberger Gel. Gesell., Geisteswiss. Kl. IX, 5, 1933.
93. Pausanias, II, 27.
94. Who lived in the middle of the fourth century B.C.
95. A painter who lived in the fourth century B.C.
96. C. A. Meier, op. cit. p. 78f.
97. About him, see Edelstein, op. cit. vol. II, p. 89; C. A. Meier, op. cit. p. 46ff.
98. A coin dropped on the *scene* can be heard from the top rows.
99. Edelstein, vol. II, p. 182ff.
100. We see them thus on votive reliefs of the National Museum in Athens.
101. Plutarch, *Aetia Romana,* 94, 286D.

102. Vitruvius, *De Architectura,* I, 2, 7. Trans. by Edelstein, vol. I, p. 370.

103. Clemens Alexandrinus, *Stromateis,* V, 1, 13. On the concept of purity, see T. Wächter, *Reinheitsvorschriften im griechischen Kult,* Berlin, 1910.

104. On ancient 'miracles' and miracle stories, see H. Reitzenstein, *Hellenistische Wundererzählungen,* Leipzig, 1906; O. Weinreich, *Antike Heilungswunder,* Giessen, 1909; P. Fiebig, *Antike Wundergeschichten,* Bonn, 1921.

105. On incubation, see G. Ritter von Rittershain, *Der medizinische Wunderglaube und die Incubation im Altertum,* Berlin, 1878; Mary Hamilton, *Incubation,* London, 1906; C. A. Meier, op. cit.

106. Pausanias, II, 27, 3.

107. Strabo, VIII, 374.

108. Edition by Hiller von Gaertringen, *Inscriptiones Epidauri, Inscr. Graec.* IV², 1, 1929, and R. Herzog, *Die Wunderheilungen von Epidauros,* Leipzig, 1931, with German translation. English translation of cases 1–43 by Edelstein, vol. I, p. 229ff.

109. E. Bleuler, *Lehrbuch der Psychiatrie,* Berlin, 1916, p. 388.

110. Case 1. All cases quoted in the following are in the translation of Edelstein, op. cit. vol. I, p. 229ff.

111. Case 34.

112. Case 31.

113. Case 42.

114. Case 14.

115. Στίγματα, whatever these may have been, possibly warts. Case 6.

116. Case 7.

117. Case 22.

118. Case 36.

119. Case 4.

120. Cases 4, 9, 10.

121. Case 19.

122. Case 13.

123. Case 23.

124. Case 27.

125. Case 28.

126. Such are the cases 17, 20, 26, 33.

127. Case 21.

128. Case 24.

129. Case 46.

130. About votive reliefs, see the recent monograph of Ulrich Hausmann, *Kunst und Heiltum, Untersuchungen zu den griechischen Asklepiosreliefs,* Potsdam, 1948.

131. See the testimonies collected by Edelstein, vol. I, p. 294ff.

132. Reproductions in the Catalogue of J. N. Svoronos, *Das Athener Nationalmuseum,* Athens, 1908–11. See also K. Sudhoff, 'Handanlegung des Heilgotts auf attischen Weihetafeln,' *Arch. Gesch. Med.,* 1926, 18:235-50.

133. XXXIV, 36, translation by Edelstein.

134. Hausmann, op. cit. p. 34.

135. G. Karo, *Weihgeschenke in Epidauros,* Stuttgart, 1937, p. 1 and note 3. On votive offerings in general, see W. H. D. Rouse, *Greek Votive Offerings,* Cambridge, 1902.

136. Op. cit. vol. II, p. 173f.

137. Philostratus, *Vitae Sophistarum,* I, 25, 4. These testimonies are all collected in Edelstein, vol. I, p. 240ff.

138. Aristides, *Oratio L,* 17.

139. *Inscript. Creticae,* I, xvii, no. 17.

140. Ibid. no. 19.

141. This thesis has been brilliantly defended by the Edelsteins who, however, are fully aware that the testimonies on hospital-like activities of the temples are very scanty.

142. Anonymus, 'Paean Erythraeus in Asclepium,' in Edelstein, vol. I, p. 327f.

143. Galen, XIV, 42. Translated by Edelstein, vol. I, p. 331.

144. *Orphei Hymni,* LXVII; Edelstein, vol. I, p. 335.

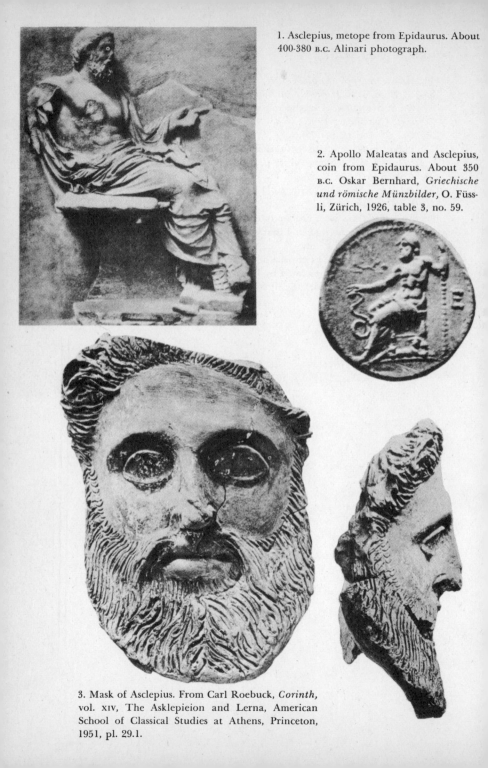

1. Asclepius, metope from Epidaurus. About 400-380 B.C. Alinari photograph.

2. Apollo Maleatas and Asclepius, coin from Epidaurus. About 350 B.C. Oskar Bernhard, *Griechische und römische Münzbilder*, O. Füssli, Zürich, 1926, table 3, no. 59.

3. Mask of Asclepius. From Carl Roebuck, *Corinth*, vol. XIV, The Asklepieion and Lerna, American School of Classical Studies at Athens, Princeton, 1951, pl. 29.1.

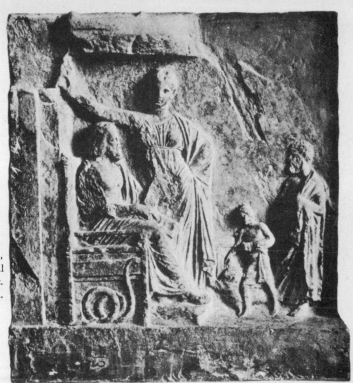

4. Asclepius and Hygieia, votive, Athens, National Museum. About 300 B.C. From Kerenyi, op. cit. pl. 46.

5. Asclepius and his family, from Thyrea in Argolis, Athens, National Museum. About 370-360 B.C. Ibid. pl. 47.

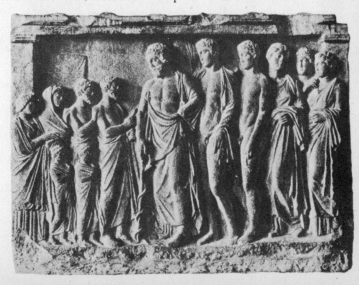

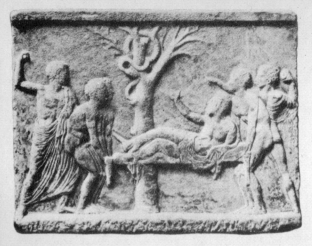

6. Asclepius Healing, in Kopenhagen Ny Carlsberg Glupt, fourth century B.C. From Ulrich Hausmann, *Kunst und Heiltum*, Stichnote, Potsdam, 1948, pl. 3.

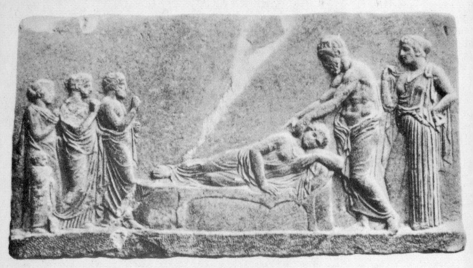

7. Asclepius Healing, in Piraeus Museum, fifth to fourth century B.C. Ibid. pl. 1.

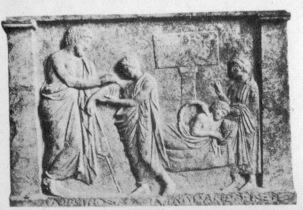

8. Asclepius Healing, in Athens, National Museum, fourth (?) century B.C. Ibid. pl. 2.

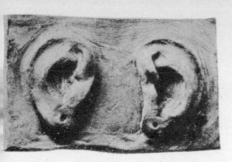

9. Ears, votives from Corinth. From Roebuck, op. cit. pl. 33, no. 9.

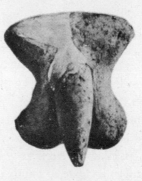

10. Genitals, votives from Corinth. Ibid. pl. 44.

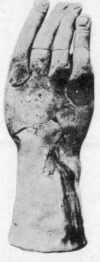

11. Hand, votive from Corinth. Ibid. pl. 66.

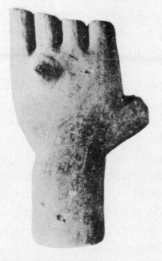

12. Hand, votive from Corinth. Ibid. pl. 40, no. 63.

13. Leg, votive from Corinth. Ibid. pl. 41.

Votive offerings from last quarter of the fifth to third quarter of fourth century B.C.

4. Pre-Socratic Philosophers and Early Medical Schools

We read Egyptian and Babylonian medical books and are impressed by the accuracy of some of the observations they relate, by the amount of accumulated empirical knowledge they reflect, or by the grandeur of some of their incantations. We search the Homeric epics and Greek religious texts for information on medical conditions, and are so captivated by the beauty of these poems that we almost forget that we are reading them with a purpose, and that our scrutiny is yielding very meager results. And then we turn to the Hippocratic writings, and suddenly we find ourselves in a totally different world. The *Corpus Hippocraticum* is a collection of medical books by different authors from different schools, most of them written in the fifth or fourth centuries B.C. It reveals an approach to the problems of health and disease and, in general, a type of medicine such as the world had never seen before. The overwhelming wealth of medical knowledge it conveys, the symptoms of disease observed and evaluated correctly, the illnesses traced throughout their course from the initial symptom to the happy or fatal end, the highly developed dietetic therapy reinforced by pharmacology, the very respectable surgery, and, last but not least, the theoretical studies on the nature of man in health and disease and on the mechanisms of illness—all this represents a state of medicine that must have been the result of a long development, the accumulated experience of many years.

Medicine had other great periods in the West when all forces seemed to be bursting forth at once, as in the Renaissance and in the nineteenth century, but their roots reached deep into the past. Such periods were culminating points in long developments. Pallas Athene was born spontaneously from the head of Zeus, but there is no spontaneous generation either in the crafts or in the sciences. We know the archaic statues that preceded the sculptures of Phidias; the art of decorating pottery developed step by step, and it is obvious that Hippocratic medicine, as we shall call it for brevity's sake, also had its antecedents. We would like to know what rational medicine was like between Homer and Hippocrates—that is, in the four hundred years from the ninth to the fifth century B.C. Unfortunately there is no medical literature earlier than the fifth century— not that it has been lost, it was never written. The writing of medical books in the fifth century was a new phenomenon.[1] This may seem strange because in other civilizations medical texts may be found, if not among the earliest, then certainly among the very early written records. In Greece, however, the physicians were itinerant craftsmen, *demiourgoi*, 'men who work for the people'; as such they first appear in the *Odyssey* and such they still were in the days of Hippocrates. The art and craft of medicine was transmitted by oral and practical instruction from father to son, from master to apprentice. This was entirely feasible, even without the help of books, so long as medicine was not too complicated, prescriptions not too long, and diets not too involved. It was also possible to acquire a vast store of knowledge in such a way as becomes evident when, for reasons to be discussed later, medical books began to be written. We have a similar development in medieval surgery which for many centuries was practiced and taught as a craft, with hardly any literature, and then suddenly in the thirteenth century was published in the splendid books of Italian surgeons who were university graduates and recorded in writing what they and other surgeons did, and what probably had been done for a long time.

The lack of any pre-Hippocratic medical literature, of any direct evidence of the status of medicine before the end of the sixth century B.C., has led some people to believe that there was no medicine at all, or in the words of Pliny 'that it was hidden in darkest night' from the time of the Trojan to that of the Peloponnesian War.[2] This obviously was not the case, and if we have no medical sources, we may hope to obtain some indirect evidence from non-medical books. The early Greek writers, however, were all poets, and we can hardly expect Sappho to sing of other pains than those of love. But before her, in the eighth century B.C., the peasant-poet Hesiod wrote a didactic poem known as *Works and Days* which might yield some information. The poem is a great human document, a passionate plea for justice, industry, and moral behavior. It is typically Western in its glorification of labor and desire for property. Written during hard times, when the poor farmer was becoming ever poorer and the rich nobleman ever richer, it does not complain about the hard work that was the farmer's lot, but extols it. Wealth is created by labor, and the man who works is dearer to the gods than he who is idle. Work is not a disgrace but idleness is.[3]

Reading the poem for its medical content we find relatively little: some common-sense hygiene, some views on religious medicine, some old taboos that must have been observed by peasants for a very long time, all elements of primitive medicine. We hear that mallow and asphodel were the poor man's fare.[4] The bulb of asphodel was probably roasted like an onion or pounded down with figs.[5] Of course, when the farmer could afford it he preferred other fare consisting of bread, goat milk, the tender meat of a heifer and of firstling kids, and bright wine, of which the gods received their share.[6] The advice given a man on his conduct was a mixture of common sense, religion, and magic. Get up early; do not postpone for tomorrow what you can do today;[7] drink your wine mixed with water, four parts of water to one part of wine;[8] wash your hands before you sacrifice or the gods will not listen to your prayers but will 'spit them back'; [9] do not make water standing upright and facing the sun, but in the early morning before sunrise and in the evening after sunset; do so sitting or against the wall of an enclosed court, and certainly not as you go along, on the road or off the road. And even at night, do not make water uncovered because the night too is sacred to the gods.[10] Do not make water or ease yourself in rivers that flow to the sea, nor in springs.[11] And do not expose your genital organs soiled with sperm by the fireside in your house.[12] Never wash yourself with water in which a woman has bathed.[13] Take a wife when you are about thirty years of age; let the bride be four years past puberty and marry her in the fifth.[14] Having an only son has the advantage that your property will not be divided. If you have two, may you live long enough to have time to increase your wealth; besides, more sons mean that more hands are at work and more wealth is produced.[15]

Hesiod obviously was a firm believer in divination, and the poem also has a whole section on hemerology, on 'the days which come from Zeus,' on the choice of lucky days and the avoidance of unlucky ones, particularly in reference to agriculture.[16] Not only the days come from Zeus but also famine and plague which may befall a city as a punishment for the sins and presumptuous deeds of a bad man.[17] And finally we may mention the saga of Pandora's box from which sprang all evils that befall man, countless plagues, diseases that come upon man continuously by day and by night, bringing evil to mortals and striking in silence because wise Zeus took speech away from them.[18]

This is folk medicine pure and simple, rules and views such as could be found not only in eighth-century Boeotia but among peasant populations all over the globe, yet it does not tell us anything about the practices of physicians. As a matter of fact, we cannot expect to find any data prior to the sixth century B.C. Life was primitive in Greece before that time, and we may safely assume that the kind of medicine that the itinerant *demiourgoi* practiced was also relatively simple and probably not so different from that of their Egyptian and Babylonian colleagues. The turning point was the sixth century, when the Greek spirit found its own expression not only in poetry but in all cultural fields, when rational systems of medicine, based on observation and reasoning, began to develop, and problems of health and disease were investigated by means of philosophy.

The language of the Hippocratic writings tells us where we have to look for the origin of this new approach to medicine. Most books of the Hippocratic collection were produced by the schools of Cos and Cnidus, and both the island of Cos and the peninsula of Cnidus were settled by the Dorians. Dorian was the language of these colonies, but all books of the Hippocratic collection were written in Ionian Greek. Why? Because Greek philosophy and science were born in the Ionian colonies, not on the mainland, not in Athens, but on the coast of Asia Minor in the flourishing cities where Greek and Oriental civilizations came in close touch.[19]

The earliest philosophers had no direct influence on medical thought. Their primary interest was not in man but in nature and in the universe at large. Yet we must mention them here because in their approach to the problems of nature, they developed a method that was to be used very profitably in the formation of medical theories. Unlike the naïve observer who saw the world and took it for granted, or if he sought an explanation for it had recourse to mythology, the philosopher did what the Greeks called θαυμάζειν—that is, he looked at the world in wonderment, in amazement. He took nothing for granted but reflected on the nature of things. What was their essence, what their origin? Everything has a cause and so the world must have a cause too. Endeavoring to find this cause, to explain the origin of the world with all it contained, animate and inanimate, he excluded mythology, excluded the transcendental. His explanation, although speculative, was rational in our sense of the word. His reasoning was based on careful observation of nature and on a wide range of personal experiences.

Miletus, in Caria on the coast of Asia Minor, was the cradle of Greek, and hence of European, philosophy; it was a flourishing city in the sixth century B.C. with an international population, rapidly developing industries, and far-reaching commercial relations with the outside world. Milesian ships carried the city's industrial products, textiles, leather goods, metal works, furniture, pottery, and also its wine and oil as far as the Black Sea, where Miletus had ninety-six trading stations, and whence the ships came back with raw materials, slaves, horses, cattle, salted fish, and amber. In Egypt, Miletus owned a whole section of Naucratis, the Greek settlement near today's Alexandria, and in Italy there were close relations with Sybaris on the Gulf of Tarentum.[20] All these cities on the coast of Asia Minor not only had an overseas trade but also maintained commercial relations with the hinterland, and we can easily visualize the international crowds in the streets of Miletus, speaking in many different tongues, as is still the case in the Levant today, exchanging goods, and also skills and ideas.

A flourishing port in which ships from all over the Mediterranean world were loaded and unloaded provided a strong stimulus to the people's imagination and raised many practical scientific problems connected with navigation. The skipper had to know about the stars, about winds and weather, and about the geography of the regions to which he was bound; the Milesian philosophers, Thales, Anaximander, and Anaximenes, provided answers to many of these questions. They were explorers of the world in which they lived and of the universe—geographers, astronomers, and cosmologists. In Miletus they enjoyed the freedom to engage in research instead of in business, to be different from their fellow citizens and yet popular with them.[21] We know little about them that is authentic, but enough to form an opinion. Thales, in all probability, wrote nothing, but a book which was said to be on nautical astronomy was attributed to him later. Anaximander and Anaximenes did write books but very few fragments are preserved. Later philosophers, however, from Plato on, discussed the views of these men and transmitted anecdotes about their lives which picture them sometimes as practical scientists, men of action taking part in politics, and sometimes as impractical dreamers.[22] They probably were both, and there is no doubt that they did not work in an ivory tower but were active members of the society in which they lived.

Thales flourished around 585 B.C. Aristotle considered him the first philosopher that Greece produced, and he was counted among the seven sages. He was a practical scientist who busied himself with the solution of technical problems. Plato praised his technical skill.[23] He was interested in problems of navigation and husbandry, of meteorology and physical geography, of astronomy and mathematics. According to tradition, he traveled to Egypt and Babylonia. In Egypt he acquired geometrical knowledge which made it possible for him to measure the height of a pyramid by its shadow, and the distance of a

ship at sea. In Babylonia he must have learned the use of astronomical tables because, according to Herodotus, he predicted the eclipse of
the sun that ended the war between the Lydians and the Medes. He is
said to have been active in politics, advising the Ionian cities to feder-
ate, and to have demonstrated that a philosopher can be a good busi-
nessman, cornering the oil presses when he expected a good crop of
olives.

All these practical scientific achievements, important as they were,
whether true or merely attributed to him by later generations, would
never have given him the position he holds in the intellectual history
of the West. The Egyptians and Babylonians could boast of greater
technical knowledge and were his teachers besides. What makes
Thales the first European philosopher is the fact that he was not
satisfied with the attempt to master nature but endeavored to interpret it—without the aid of mythology. He inquired into the reality
behind the phenomena, speculated about the origin of the world, and
came to the conclusion that water was the primary substance from
which all things were derived.

Thales had been in Egypt and had seen the fertilizing effect of the
waters of the Nile that flooded the land periodically. He even ventured an explanation of this natural phenomenon, as Herodotus tells
us.[24] Throughout the East he could see that life was bound to the
presence of water. Where water reached, vegetation was most
abundant, and where it ceased, the desert began. Whatever was
alive was moist, and Thales must have noticed that life-giving human
and animal sperm was moist. And so he came to believe that there
was a causal relationship between water and life. Did the rivers not
carve the profile of a landscape, cut valleys, create promontories and
deltas with alluvial soil? The earth they brought, could it not have
been generated from water? And when water evaporated, did it not
become air? Such observations and speculations must have guided
Thales in his assumption that water was the primary element. And
the earth, he thought, floated on water and was surrounded by a
vault of water whence came the rain.

Such a cosmological system marked the step from myth to science.

The earth and all that was on it and around it, the world at large, had not been created by an arbitrary act of the gods but had developed gradually from a primary element through natural processes which could be observed every day. No greater revolution in thought had ever occurred, and Thales is justly given the unique position he holds in the history of the Western world. Was there any place for gods in such a system? Indeed, there was. 'All things are full of gods,' Thales was reported by Aristotle to have said. Mythology, in other words, had been replaced by science and by a philosophic pantheism.

The assumption that water was the primary element from which all others were derived undoubtedly made a good working hypothesis, but Anaximander, another Milesian philosopher, who flourished around 560 B.C., apparently did not approve of the idea of having one element singled out in such a way. He thought that the elements commonly believed to constitute the world—water, earth, fire, and air, with their qualities, wet, dry, hot, and cold—were derived from one common indeterminate substance, τὸ ἄπειρον, as he called it.[25] From this infinite, inexhaustible primary substance which 'includes everything in itself, and guides everything,' two pairs of elements with opposite qualities were born, which seemed to be in ideal balance. In the beginning of the world these elements were separated with ·the earth in the center, and covered by a sphere of water, which was surrounded by air and ultimately by fire. Everyday experience taught what happens when fire acts on air, water, and earth. The earth became dry, water evaporated, pressure increased, and the ring of fire burst. Wheels of fire kept circling around the earth, each one encased in a tube of mist through the apertures of which we see the sun, the moon, and the stars. Thunder and lightning were not the work of Zeus but were caused in a perfectly natural way when air was compressed in a cloud and burst forth violently. All living creatures originated in the water, and some became land animals when the water evaporated. Man too arose from a fish-like creature.

Thus the world in which we live is part of a cosmos which is ruled by universal laws. Like Thales, Anaximander was not satisfied with speculating about the world but endeavored to improve it by using science in the service of man. He is said to have introduced the gnomon and sun-dial from Babylonia, and to have been the first Greek to use them. A true son of Miletus, he was keenly interested in geography and constructed the first map of the world known to the Greeks, a map later referred to as the 'Ionian map,' and revised and improved by another Milesian, Hecataeus. It revealed the same mathematical spirit that Anaximander had shown in his cosmology, and was a testimony to the discovery that not only the world at large but the earth, continents and waterways, mountains and plains, are constructed as a 'system which is orderly, not chaotic.'

Anaximander's 'non-limited' primary element was a hypothetical substance that did not satisfy his pupil and associate Anaximenes, who flourished around 546 B.C.; he looked upon air, one of the four elements, as the primary cause of all things. He wrote a book from which one sentence has survived: 'As our soul, being air, holds us together, so do breath and air surround the whole universe.' Air was unlimited also, surrounding as it did the whole universe, but it was a tangible element. Its vital importance in sustaining life was easily apparent, and no great effort was needed to identify it with the soul. Anaximenes' contribution is to be sought in the idea that quantitative changes may be responsible for changes in quality. Air was one of the four elements but it held a key position in so far as it was thought that the three others were born from it through changes of density, through rarefaction and condensation. Rarefied air became fire, and heat was generated in the process, while condensed air became water and finally earth, and produced cold. This was a logical explanation, and breath or air came to play an increasingly important part in biology.

Three generations of Milesians laid the foundation of Western philosophy and, at the same time, of Western science. They were investigators of nature. They observed phenomena, reasoned about them, and in doing so developed methods that could be applied also in the investigation of health and disease. Miletus took a leading part in the Ionian revolt against the Persians, and was conquered and destroyed in 494 B.C. The city was rebuilt in the course of the century, but its prosperity and intellectual leadership were lost for a long time. Other centers were active, however, and from the sixth century B.C. on, the exploration of nature never ended in Greece.

North of Miletus was Ephesus, a thriving commercial town, famous for the temple of the many-breasted Artemis, and like Miletus founded by Ionian colonists. One of her sons was Heraclitus, who flourished around 500 B.C.[26] Proud scion of a noble family he renounced all honors and retired to the temple of Artemis, if not to the wilderness, as one tradition has it. There, removed from the crowds to which he preferred the company of children, he reflected on the world and wrote a book that covered a wide range of subjects, scientific, metaphysical, and political—a book which in antiquity had the reputation of being difficult to understand, and of which many of the fragments preserved are dark to us also. Heraclitus was struck by the fact that everything changes constantly, a thought that was summarized in the sentence, πάντα ῥεῖ καὶ οὐδὲν μένει, everything flows, is in constant flux, and nothing remains unchanged. 'The sun is new every day.'[27] The world is not static but dynamic. And what makes things change? Like the Milesians, Heraclitus believed in the unity of the world, and to him the primary element was fire, not only because it was the most restless element but because fire was used in many technical processes where it caused great changes.[28] Hence it seemed not far-fetched to assume that fire had produced air, water, and earth. Heraclitus thought that change could be explained best through the concept of strife or of tension. War—that is, strife— is the father of all:[29] 'everything comes about by way of strife and necessity.'[30] All things are moved by an innate force, and from opposite tensions results harmony. 'That which is in opposition is in concert, and from things that differ comes the most beautiful harmony.'[31] It is through opposites that we become aware of things. Disease 'makes health pleasant; evil, good; hunger, plenty; weariness, rest.'[32] And everything in the world moves according to eternal laws. These very principles, unity of the world, eternal changing of all things caused by tension, and law and order ruling the world, were principles which proved to be strong stimulants to scientific research.

Of all early philosophical schools that of Pythagoras probably exerted the deepest influence upon medicine.[33] Pythagoras was a native of Samos, another great Ionian commercial center in the sixth century. The arts and luxury industries flourished at the court of the tyrant Polycrates where Anacreon wrote many of his poems. Pythagoras' father was a gem-cutter. We also hear of great technical feats performed at Samos, of a temple that was the largest of its time, of a mole around the harbor over three hundred yards long and twenty fathoms deep, and of a tunnel, cut through a mountain, which was seven stades or somewhat under a mile long, and which had a height and width of eight feet. At the bottom of the tunnel was a channel through which water was brought in pipes to the city. Modern excavations have shown that the tunnel was begun simultaneously at both ends and that there was a deviation of only a few yards when the two parties met—a remarkable engineering achievement at that time.

The life of Pythagoras is legendary in many ways. He is said to have traveled widely and to have visited Egypt,[34] which is possible although it cannot be proved. It is a fact, however, that he left Samos around 530 B.C. either because the pressure from Persia on the Ionian states was increasing and was making life unpleasant, or because he disliked the tyranny of Polycrates.[35] With a group of followers he sailed to the other end of the Greek periphery and settled in Croton in southern Italy. We are reminded of the early days of our medieval universities when professors and students moved to another city or another country when conditions became unfavorable at the place of their original residence. This was possible then as it was in antiquity, for the schools of learning were free associations of masters and disciples, not burdened by buildings, endowments, or other earthly goods which tie a school to a certain locality.

In Croton, Pythagoras oganized his followers into a well-disciplined school, and since a medical school developed at about the same time, Croton became the first and a very important Greek intellectual center on Italian soil. The school of Pythagoras was very different from the schools of the Milesian philosophers, and had much more the character of a religious order. The Milesians' object was the investigation of nature and this they pursued as rationalists and, to a certain extent also, as materialists, gaining experience from the observation of nature and the technology of their time. Pythagoras was carried along by the great religious movement that swept Greece in the second half of the sixth century. Many people were no longer satisfied with the naïve and primitive worship of the Homeric gods and felt shocked by the many scandals mythology reported about them. We saw that the cult of Asclepius developed in this atmosphere, as did a number of mystery religions under Asiatic influence. Pythagoras is one of the exponents of the great Orphic movement. He too, like the other pre-Socratic philosophers, investigated nature, and his school made great contributions to science, but his primary aim was religious, the redemption of man from the cycle of reincarnations. It was to be achieved through what Plato called 'the Pythagorean way of life,' about which much has been written from antiquity to our day.[36]

The Pythagorean order was aristocratic in character. Farrington very justly pointed out that at that time manual labor was more and more despised while slavery grew.[37] From now on occupation with intellectual matters was the privilege of a propertied elite, and we shall see that Hippocratic medicine was basically aristocratic also. The Pythagorean order accepted men and women without discrimination. Members were initiated after having absorbed the doctrine and proved their worth. There were several grades of membership, the inner circle, the μαθηματικοί or students, and the outer circle, the ἀκουσματικοί or hearers. Members were pledged to secrecy as in other mystery religions; thus it is impossible today to decide whether a thought or discovery belongs to Pythagoras personally or to one of his followers, particularly since loyalty to the master impelled his students to attribute every contribution of any importance to him. Αὐτὸς ἔφα, he himself said, were the words with which traditions were passed on from one generation to another, very much as the teachings of the Buddha were transmitted and ultimately collected. We know that Pythagoras did not write any book, and it was only after his death, in the middle of the fifth century, that books began to be written about his teachings and that of his school. Yet, however secret an organization may be, knowledge of its doings is bound to leak out through indiscretion or betrayal, and there is no doubt that Pythagorean views became known outside Croton in the first half of the fifth century.

The members of the school led an ascetic and pure life, endeavoring to maintain a perfect balance, physically and mentally.[38] To that end they followed a strict physical and mental diet. They observed many food taboos. According to some traditions they were not allowed to kill any animals, either for sacrifice or food. Once one believes in the transmigration of souls, as they did, the killing of animals appears as objectionable as the killing of human beings. They also abstained from eating beans, a strange and probably very old taboo.[39] They avoided all luxuries and learned to control their emotions. Meditation and mnemotechnics were employed to that end. One should not get up in the morning before having recalled the previous day's happenings in full detail, a method that is highly commendable today too, for it not only trains the memory but is at the same time an *examen de conscience* which makes one aware of shortcomings and failures. If in spite of careful living a man's equilibrium has been upset it must be restored, and this was done physically with medicine and mentally with music. This is why both medicine and music were greatly cultivated in the Pythagorean school.

The Milesians were interested in matter and speculated about the primary element of which all things were constituted. The Pythagoreans' chief concern was the soul, which after death seeks another body until it is redeemed from the cycle of reincarnations, a view reminiscent of Indian religious and philosophic ideas. Pythagoras and the Buddha were contemporaries, and the Orphic movement was undoubtedly inspired by the East.

If the school of Pythagoras had been a mystery religion and nothing else, there would be no reason for us to mention it in this book, just as we do not discuss Orphism or the mysteries of Eleusis.

The Pythagoreans, however, like the Ionians, investigated nature; many of them were scientists in addition to being mystics. And while the Ionians had been natural philosophers, the Pythagoreans became mathematicians and found that not only the world but also matters of the mind could be expressed in figures. Number appeared to them as the first principle: not water, not fire, not air, not the unlimited, but number. A tradition relates that Pythagoras while plucking a string discovered that the tone given was determined by the length of the string and that harmony was a mathematical proportion. Harmony, perfect equilibrium, perfect balance, were the goal of the Pythagorean life and also the key to health. Hence the desire to investigate numbers and to engage in mathematical studies. It was an approach that was at the same time scientific and religious. The famous theorem that the square of the hypotenuse of a right-angled triangle is equal to the sum of the squares of the other two sides may not be the discovery of the master himself, but it certainly originated in the early school, and many mathematical discoveries later systematized and developed by Euclid were the results of Pythagorean investigations, which also laid the foundation for the science of acoustics. But mathematics to the Pythagoreans was infinitely more than it was to Euclid; it was, in Farrington's words, 'a key to the riddle of the universe and an instrument for the purification of the soul.' [40]

Among the numbers, four played a particularly important part, for it seemed logical that two pairs of forces with opposite qualities would constitute an ideal balance, and we shall see that this view had a profound influence on medical theory, as had the Pythagorean doctrine of opposites in its dualistic form in general. These opposites were necessary to explain the harmony of the world. Aristotle tells that some Pythagoreans spoke of ten such pairs, namely, limited-unlimited, odd-even, one-many, right-left, male-female, rest-motion, straight-curved, light-darkness, good-bad, square-oblong,[41] a theory that may be of Babylonian origin.[42] The principle of the cosmos was harmony, achieved by the perfect balance of all elements—that is, of numbers. The earth was considered a star among other stars, all perfect spheres moving in circles around a central fire. The Ionians sought the substance that constituted the world, animate and inanimate, while the Pythagoreans emphasized the eternal mathematical laws that rule macrocosm and microcosm.

The school was very active politically and this activity resulted in its ultimate destruction. Upon Pythagoras' advice Croton went to war with Sybaris and defeated this city of proverbial luxury in 510 B.C., whereupon Pythagoras and his followers ruled supreme. Most Greek philosophers took an active part in the political life of their country or at least showed great interest in problems of state and statesmanship, because to them philosophy was not a mere subject for meditation but a very practical matter, a guide to action, which taught men how to understand the world and how to act in it intelligently. In the course of time opposition arose in Croton against the rule of the brotherhood. A conspiracy drove the master to Metapontum, where he died about 500 B.C. The school was almost entirely destroyed when political opponents around the middle of the fifth century B.C. stormed the assembly house and set fire to it. Many of the members perished in the conflagration.

The significance of Pythagorean doctrines for medicine is easily apparent. Health is a condition of perfect equilibrium, a view as true today as it was in antiquity. The Pythagorean way of life was meant to preserve this equilibrium, by practicing moderation in every respect and maintaining equanimity in every situation. There could be no better ideal set for a hygienic mode of living. If the balance of health has been upset it must be restored, and the psychosomatic approach of the Pythagoreans, the use of diet, as well as of music, was full of promise. Many pathological processes develop in ways which may be expressed in figures. Malaria is quotidian, tertian, or quartan—that is, the patient has an acute attack of fever every day, or every third or fourth day. Pneumonia and other diseases have crises after certain biologically determined periods. It is obvious that the Pythagorean theory of numbers played a part in the study of the critical days about which we shall have more to say in a later chapter. And, finally, Pythagorean ideals exerted a strong influence on medical ethics. Since Edelstein's epoch-making study there cannot be any doubt that the so-called Hippocratic Oath was a Pythagorean document.[43]

Medicine, like mathematics and music, was a field of investigation for the followers of Pythagoras. Philolaus of Tarentum, who lived in the latter half of the fifth century and who is supposed to have been the first to write about the teachings of the master, discussed matters of physiology; one of the fragments preserved reads as follows:

There are four vital organs in the rational living being: brain, heart, navel, genital organ. The brain is the seat of the mind, the heart of the soul and of sensation, the navel of the rooting and growth of the embryo, the genital organ of the emission of sperm and of procreation. The brain signifies the principal of man, the heart that of the animal, the navel that of the plant, the genital organ that of all of them, for they all sprout and grow from sperm.[44]

Philolaus in other words differentiated between nervous, animal, and vegetative functions. He was a late Pythagorean and long before his time a medical school had developed in Croton independently of the brotherhood. The man who first made it famous in the world was Democedes, the son of Calliphon.[45]

Herodotus has a great deal to say about Democedes[46] and, although he may have embroidered his stories, there is no reason to doubt their basic veracity. They are very interesting, particularly as they record several aspects of medical practice in the sixth century. Democedes left Croton because he could no longer stand his father's irascible temperament. He went to Aegina unequipped, without the tools of his craft, but his skill was such that within a year he surpassed the most famous physicians. In the second year the Aeginetans appointed him state physician and paid him an annual salary of one talent, about $1200. But then, in the third year, the Athenians lured him to their city by offering him a somewhat higher salary; as his fame grew Polycrates of Samos attracted him to his court by paying him two talents a year. Through him the school of Croton gained its great reputation, for at that time the

Crotonian physicians were considered the first in Greece, those of Cyrene were second.[47]

The downfall of Polycrates around 522 B.C. brought misery to his physician too. As a captive loaded with chains Democedes was brought to Persia, homesick, concealing his identity, because he knew well enough that the Persians would never let him go if they knew that he was the most famous physician of Greece. But a doctor cannot remain in hiding when an emergency occurs. Darius, the king, dislocated an ankle while getting off his horse at a hunting party. His court physicians were Egyptians, at that time considered the best doctors and surgeons. They tried to reduce the dislocated ankle by force but failed, and for seven days and seven nights the king was in such pain that he could not sleep. Then somebody recognized Democedes among the prisoners; he completely cured the king, who had begun to despair of ever being able to use his foot again. The Greek doctor was richly rewarded, lived from then on at the court in Susa, and ate at the king's table. His first action was to obtain pardon for the Egyptian physicians who were to be crucified for their failure. Medical practice at an Asiatic court in those days was not without perils. But Democedes was homesick, and he meditated on an opportunity to escape the golden bonds of the Persian court and return to Croton. His chance came when Atossa the queen, a daughter of Cyrus, had an abscess of the breast. She kept it hidden at first, for she was ashamed, but when it broke open and became worse she called Democedes, who cured her. Thereupon at the queen's intercession he was sent with a Persian delegation on a spying mission to Greece. Once they touched Italian soil he escaped to Croton, where he married the daughter of another famous Crotonian, the athlete Milo, who six times was victor in wrestling at the Olympian games, and six times at the Pythian.

This story teaches us a great deal. We learn from it that medical schools were developing in the last third of the sixth century in the periphery of the Greek world, in Croton, in Cyrene, and, as we shall see later, in Sicily, Rhodes, Cnidus, and Cos. They were not schools of philosophers but of physicians, free associations of teachers and students, of practitioners and their apprentices, many of whom worked as itinerants, as doctors had done for centuries, carrying with them the tools of their craft—instruments, appliances, drugs— and practicing internal medicine as well as surgery. Their number could not have been large but must have been increasing, for competition was becoming stiffer. In this story we also have the first record of a Greek salaried doctor being appointed by a community and paid from public funds, a custom that became universal in Greece and seemed the best way to secure for a community the permanent services of a competent doctor.[48] And finally the story relates the first clash between the old Egyptian and the young Greek medicine, a contest from which the Greek doctor emerged as the victor.

Democedes was a practitioner. We know that he performed successful cures on high personages, but we do not know by what means he effected them, nor do we know what he thought and according to what theories he acted. We are quite well informed, however, about another Crotonian physician who won fame not as a practitioner but as a philosopher and scientist, Alcmaeon.[49] He probably was a younger contemporary of Democedes and lived in the first half of the fifth century.[50] He wrote a book of which only six fragments are preserved, but we have in addition eighteen testimonies, some old, some very late but good enough to make it possible for us to form an opinion of his work. Although not a Pythagorean, he must have had relations with members of the school, because nobody could live in Croton at that time without being influenced by, or himself influencing, Pythagorean doctrine.

Like many philosophers, Alcmaeon was interested in problems of physiology, but, unlike other philosophers, he dissected animals [51] and performed some simple experiments. We are best informed about his studies on the physiology of the sense organs because Theophrastus in his treatise *On Sense Perception* discussed them, and also because Aristotle, who was in basic disagreement with Alcmaeon, attacked him. According to Chalcidius, a late commentator on Plato's *Timaeus,* Alcmaeon was the first to dare to remove

and dissect an eye.[52] He found it to be covered by several diaph-
anous membranes and to be connected with the brain by 'light-
bearing paths.' [53] These paths come together behind the forehead,
where they become one; this explains why both eyes always move
together. The eye contains water and fire. The water comes from
the brain and may easily be found when an eye is dissected, and
the fire you see when your eye is hit. Through the paths this fire
is transmitted to the brain. The ears are similarly connected with
the brain. They hear sounds because they are hollow; there is res-
onance like the echo we hear in a hollow vessel; air enters and
leaves them. Smell enters the nose with the air and is transmitted
to the brain. The tongue distinguishes flavors because being wet,
soft, and hot, it melts them and separates them according to their
looseness of texture and tenderness. All sense organs then are connected with the brain, the seat of sense perception. In the brain all
sensations come together and are somehow fitted together and stored
up, whence the brain is also the seat of memory and the organ of
thought. All animals have sensations but man alone συνίησι, fits
them together. The brain is the seat of the ἡγεμονικόν, the govern-
ing faculty. When a man has a concussion of the brain he is unconscious, his sense organs stop functioning and the brain is in-
capacitated: it has moved and shifted its position and by doing so
has obstructed the paths.

Today we know that Alcmaeon was right; that the brain is the
center of the nervous functions, and not the heart, as Aristotle and
so many ancient philosophers believed. Alcmaeon is therefore frequently considered the founder not only of physiology but of what
was later called experimental psychology. There is no doubt that
he deserves great credit, but we must keep in mind that his physiology was largely based on speculation, and that in those days
when so little was known about arteries, veins, and nerves, and their
function and significance, a strong case could be made for the
primacy of the heart. Alcmaeon was also interested in the blood
vessels and explained sleep, awakening, and death by the amount
of blood in the veins. Repletion with blood resulted in sleep, de-

pletion led to awakening, and maximal repletion caused death.[54]
Philosophers of the fifth century were much concerned also with
questions of embryology. What determines the sex of the child? Man
and woman produce semen, it was believed, and the semen that is in
larger quantity determines the sex. A puzzling practical problem
was presented by the sterility of mules, which Alcmaeon explained
speculatively by assuming that the female's womb did not open and
that the male's seed was too fine and cold. Like other naturalists
of the century he opened birds' eggs to watch the embryo, and he
thought that the head developed first, not the heart, the *punctum
saliens* of Aristotle, but he was not sure about it.

One of the few fragments preserved is extremely important, for
it reflects a theory of health and disease that we shall encounter
again in the Hippocratic writings. 'Health is maintained,' Alcmaeon
wrote, 'by the ἰσονομία, the equality of rights, of the qualities wet,
dry, cold, hot, bitter, sweet, and the rest; but the μοναρχία, the
single rule among them, causes disease, for the single rule of either
pair of opposites causes disease.' In other words, we recognize here the
Pythagorean theory of opposites, although we cannot tell who
initiated it, whether Alcmaeon or a Pythagorean, and who borrowed
from whom. Alcmaeon developed a physiological and pathological
theory, limiting himself to pairs of opposite qualities encountered
in the human body. The Pythagorean aim, to explain the cosmos,
was broader, and to this end ten pairs of opposites were needed.

Health then is a condition of perfect equilibrium and its material
substratum is to be sought in the δυνάμεις, the qualities or forces
that are active in the body. Illness results when this balance is upset.
But what causes a quality or a pair of opposites to dominate? The
answer is given in the same fragment: 'So far as cause is concerned
disease may be traced at times to an excess of heat or cold, it may be
occasioned by an excess or deficiency of food, and as to the affected
parts blood, marrow, or brain are involved, but these parts are
sometimes also affected by external causes such as certain waters,
or a particular locality, or fatigue, or constraint, or similar reasons.
But health is the harmonious mixture of the qualities.'[55]

As we shall see, Alcmaeon influenced Empedocles, Democritus, and several writers of the Hippocratic collection. At an early time he was a great philosopher and a great scientist, free from the mysticism of Pythagoras, and modest in his awareness of the limitations of science. By sheer accident the opening sentence of his book has been preserved. It says that only the gods have certainty about things unseen and things mortal, whereas all that man can do is to make conjectures.[56]

While in southern Italy there developed these intellectual centers where philosophy, science, and medicine were cultivated, another school, which was to have a profound influence on medical developments, sprang up elsewhere on the Greek periphery. It was the Sicilian school, dominated by the forceful personality of Empedocles, the most colorful of the early Greek philosopher-physicians.[57] We know little about Empedocles' life, not much more than what he tells us or lets us deduce from his works, but legends arose about him such as we usually find only in the biographies of religious leaders. Born at Agrigentum as the scion of a noble family, he took an active part in the political life of his country, and was offered the crown but refused it. He had democratic leanings, gave dowries to poor women, and dedicated one of his works to his fellow citizens:

> Ye friends, who in the mighty city dwell
> Along the yellow Acragas hard by
> The Acropolis, ye stewards of good works,
> The stranger's refuge venerable and kind,
> All hail, O friends.[58]

Philosopher, poet, statesman, scientist, physician, seer, and priest, he toured the island dressed in purple, with wreaths and garlands of flowers:

> But unto ye I walk
> As god immortal now, no more as man,
> On all sides honored fittingly and well,
> Crowned both with fillets and with flowering wreaths.
> When with my throngs of men and women I come

> To thriving cities, I am sought by prayers,
> And thousands follow me that they may ask
> The path to weal and vantage, craving some
> For oracles, whilst others seek to hear
> A healing word 'gainst many a foul disease
> That all too long hath pierced with grievous pains.[59]

Many stories were told about his miraculous cures, how he woke a woman from a long trance so that it looked as if he had resuscitated a corpse,[60] how he cured a maniac by music,[61] and also about other deeds. Thus he liberated the city of Selinus of an epidemic through an engineering feat by draining off its polluted water and giving it a better water supply.[62] He improved the climate of his home city by changing its physical geography.[63] These stories are intrinsically true in so far as they all illustrate one of Empedocles' chief contentions, namely that knowledge gives power over nature. His death was as miraculous as his life. It is possible that he died as the result of an accident, but legend had it that he jumped into the crater of Mount Etna or that he went to heaven in a trail of light. But he was not a quack. Renan called him a mixture of Newton and Cagliostro, but I think he was more Newton than Cagliostro; he was an outstanding representative of a period in which scholars and scientists were not specialized, when one individual could embrace all science and learning and be active in many fields.

Empedocles flourished in the middle of the fifth century B.C. He wrote at least two books, *On Nature* and *Purifications*. A book on medicine mentioned by several later writers was probably a part of the book on nature. Both books were written in verse, and while it does not seem strange to us to have religious and spiritual matters in general presented in poems, we are no longer accustomed to seeing scientific subjects discussed in verse. Yet this was done for thousands of years. The poem of the Roman Lucretius, *De Rerum Natura*, the medieval *Regimen Sanitatis Salernitanum*, and the Renaissance treatise on syphilis by Fracastoro, are outstanding examples of the genre. A scientific treatise in verse appealed to the esthetic sense of a reader who was not a narrow specialist, and it had the further advantage that it could be memorized more readily.

Over one hundred and fifty fragments of Empedocles' works are preserved, some of them short but some long; and we have in addition close to one hundred testimonies of unequal value about his life and work. Essentially his teachings represent a combination of Ionian science and Pythagorean mysticism. Science and religion are the pivots of his doctrine, the gaining of knowledge which gives power over nature, and purity which is the key to a happy and blissful life and death. Dominion over nature was the aim of his scientific thinking, and he turns to it over and over again. Thus in his book on nature, dedicated to a disciple, the physician Pausanias, he states explicitly:

> And thou shalt master every drug that e'er
> Was made defense 'gainst sickness and old age—
> For thee alone all this I will fulfil—
> And thou shalt calm the might of tireless winds
> That burst on earth and ruin seedlands; aye,
> And if thou wilt, shalt thou arouse the blasts,
> And watch them take their vengeance, wild and shrill,
> For that before thou cowedst them thou shalt change
> Black rain to drought at seasons good for men,
> And the long drought of summer shalt thou change
> To torrents, nourishing the mountain trees
> As down they stream from ether. And thou shalt
> From Hades beckon the might of perished men.[64]

It was such boastful passages that gave rise to the many legends about his life. More important for scientific and medical developments was his theory of nature. He declared that four elements constituted the world: earth, water, fire, and air; and he demonstrated that air although invisible was nevertheless a tangible reality, a corporeal substance able to exert power just like the other elements. Experimenting with a water-clock, he showed in truly scientific fashion that it was the pressure of air that made the water flow out or prevented it from entering the clock, depending on which opening was closed.[65] He compared this phenomenon with the flow of blood which he linked up with breathing through an endless number of tubes.[66]

Four elements then are at the root of all things. When they come together life is generated, and they separate at death. All objects of nature, animate and inanimate, are combinations of elements. They combine in different quantities and this determines the quality of an object. The driving forces, however, that impel elements to combine or separate are love and hate, attraction and repulsion.[67] Empedocles is frequently pictured as the founder of modern chemistry.[68] Indeed, his assumption that the world is constituted of a limited number of elements, that these elements combine in different quantities, and his concept of affinity and its contrary are strangely reminiscent of modern theories. We often find in the work of Greek thinkers views that seem to anticipate modern scientific discoveries, and we are naturally inclined to look at them as our ancestors and to admire them for having intuitively found what we today consider to be true. However, we should always keep in mind that from the speculations of Greek philosophers to the results of the modern laboratory there was still a long way to go. The Greeks did make scientific discoveries; they were keen observers and did perform experiments. Watching a little girl play with a water-clock, Empedocles discovered that the invisible air was corporeal. Most Greek theories, however, were the result of speculation, based on observations, to be sure, but even correct observations can be interpreted speculatively in many different ways. This is why we never find one generally accepted scientific theory at any given time in antiquity but always a plurality of contending theories.

Empedocles has also been praised as a precursor of Darwin,[69] and there is no doubt that he had the vision of an evolution from imperfect to perfect forms. In his poetical way he said that in the beginning of the world separate limbs were created. Love drove them together, hate separated them. Some beings thus generated were not able to reproduce while others were. In other words, there was a kind of survival of the fittest. But here again we must remember that these were purely speculative theories, and the fragments on this point, moreover, are by no means clear.

Love brings man and woman together and the result is the child, whose sex is determined by the part of the womb in which the seed falls, for the womb has two parts, 'the divided meadows of Aphrodite'; [70] on the right, the warmer part, males are generated, and on the left, the colder part, females are generated; also, the heart develops first, not the brain.

Like nurtures like, 'and Earth through Earth her figures magnifies, and Air through Air.' [71] This was the underlying principle not only of growth but also of sense perception. From all objects emanate efflorescences which reach the sense organs through paths. They are perceived through the like quality of the organs. The eye perceives light through its fire. *'Wär' nicht das Auge sonnenhaft, Die Sonne könnt' es nie erblicken,'* another poet-scientist, Goethe, was to say more than two thousand years later.

Chance plays an important part in the creations of nature, but behind it stands Ἀνάγκη, Necessity, the iron rule of Fate, just as behind and above the material world stands the realm of the spirit. Purity, asceticism, and the observation of taboos similar to those of the Pythagorean school were the paths leading to it.

Empedocles' theory of the four elements was to play a very important part in medical thought. Brought into relation with the theory of the four cardinal humors which constitute the human body, all endowed with elementary qualities, the theory proved to be a very workable instrument for the interpretation of the macrocosmos, the great world, universe and nature, and also of the microcosmos, the world of the animal body. It was able to explain both from the same principles just as our present chemical and physical theories do. We stand on firmer ground today because the scientific experience of two thousand years is available to us, but the Greeks worked in the same spirit.

A flourishing medical school developed in Sicily under the impulse given by Empedocles.[72] We mentioned Pausanias as the disciple

to whom the book *On Nature* was dedicated. Other outstanding physicians were Philistion—who lived at the court of Dionysius of Syracuse where he met and influenced Plato and Diocles of Carystus—
Akron, Euryodes, and others. They built on Empedocles' theory of
the four elements, considered the heart the center of the blood
vessels, the source of origin of the blood and seat of the soul. They
developed the theory of pneuma which permeates the whole world,
hence also the organism, and, like Empedocles, declared that respiration takes place not only through mouth and nose but also
through the pores of the entire organism. The school exerted a far-
reaching influence which can be traced not only in the works of
Plato and Diocles but also in some Hippocratic writings of Cnidian
origin.

When you divide gold or any such simple substance into ever
smaller particles you still get gold, not earth, water, fire, or air. Was
it not limiting nature too much to assume that it was constituted
of four and only four elements? Why not admit a plurality of elements, of seeds, as Anaxagoras of Clazomenae called them? [73] How
was it that a more complex substance such as bread, after it had
been eaten, became bone, flesh, and other parts of the body? Was
it not logical to assume that bread in the process of digestion was
split up into its constituent seeds which then were regrouped to
become flesh, bone, or whatever the part was? To this it could be
answered that the smallest particles of the four elements were invisible. But Anaxagoras knew well enough that an invisible substance
may well be corporeal; he himself had demonstrated the corporeality
of air by means of inflated skins.

Granted that the smallest particles of matter were invisible, was it
necessary to limit the elements to four? At this point Democritus
stepped into the picture with a theory that again had a far-reaching
influence on medical and scientific thought. [74]

Democritus was a native of Abdera in Thrace, a northern point
of the Greek periphery. He is said to have traveled widely all over
the Greek world, in Egypt and the Near East, before he settled
down in his native city. Flourishing in the second half of the fifth

century B.C., he was a mechanist and a philosophical materialist who explained religion as a result of the fear of man facing a hostile nature. He wrote books on many subjects including prognosis,[75] diet and regimen, and perhaps fevers. The fragments preserved are numerous but mostly very short. Some are priceless aphorisms: 'Poverty in a democracy is as much to be preferred to opulence under an autocracy as freedom to slavery.' [76] His endeavor to maintain equanimity or cheerfulness (εὐθυμίη) earned him the reputation of being a 'laughing philosopher' [77] which he certainly was not. We knew before Osler [78] how important equanimity and cheerfulness are in the maintenance of mental and physical health. 'Cheerfulness,' Democritus said, 'is created for men through moderation of enjoyment and harmoniousness of life. Want and abundance are apt to change and cause great disturbances in the soul. Souls which are stirred by great divergences are neither stable nor cheerful. Therefore one must keep one's thought on what is attainable and be content with what one has, paying little heed to things envied, and admired, and not dwelling on them in one's mind.' [79]

The world consists of an infinite empty space and of matter, and matter is built of atoms. We do not see the individual atoms just as we do not see air, but they are as real and as tangible as air. They are different in size, shape, position, and weight; since the heavier atoms have the tendency to fall in the empty space, motion is created. And in this motion atoms collide, become entangled, and combine in an infinite variety of combinations; this explains the variety of all objects of nature, animate and inanimate. Atomism was a very fruitful hypothesis which explained a great deal and inspired scientific research down to our day. Like Empedocles, Democritus is considered one of the great precursors of modern science, but again, it was a long way from his atomism to that of Dalton. Nevertheless, even in its speculative, philosophic rather than scientific form, atomism forged a very useful tool for the interpretation of the world (such as Lucretius gave in his great poem *De Rerum Natura*) as well as for the understanding of physiological and pathological processes and for the treatment of diseases. One of the most successful ancient schools of physicians, the Methodists, based their theories on atomism.

In later centuries Democritus acquired the reputation of having been a great magician, and all kinds of mystic treatises were attributed to him,[80] from those containing magical prescriptions for the treatment of diseases, or a magic sphere to ascertain whether a patient will live or die,[81] to mere *Jocular Prescriptions*.[82] The story was also told that he became mentally deranged, and that the citizens of Abdera, grieving over the illness of their first citizen, sent a delegation to Cos to invite the greatest physician of Greece, Hippocrates, to come and cure the philosopher. The story is developed in a very picturesque way in the *Letters of Hippocrates*, a forgery probably of the first century A.D.[83]

The relations between Democritus and Hippocrates are pure fiction, but, as often happens with fiction, the relationship has a deep symbolic significance: Democritus, the last link in the chain of pre-Socratic philosopher-scientists who from Thales on investigated the nature of the universe, is thus connected with Hippocrates, who symbolizes the Golden Age of Greek medicine. With Socrates, philosophy concentrated its attention on the nature of man, and Hippocrates investigated the ills and well-being of man.

We are now deep in the fifth century B.C. and have long overstepped the boundaries of the archaic period of Greek civilization. East and West had clashed in the long and bloody Persian Wars, from which the small Greek city-states had emerged victorious, young, strong, full of self-confidence, and with unexhausted creative forces. A period of cultural flowering, short but unbelievably rich, was to follow in which all arts and sciences had a share; an artistic and intellectual capital was amassed from which the Western world has been drawing for over two thousand years. Greek art and literature became a source of inspiration and happiness for generations to come, even to the present day. Greek science and medicine gave new insights into the workings of nature and of the human body in health and disease, and laid the solid foundations upon which our modern systems of medicine and science are erected.

NOTES

1. See Jaeger, *Paideia,* vol. III, p. 10.
2. *Nat. Hist.,* 29, 1, 2.
3. *Works and Days,* 308–11.
4. Ibid. 41.
5. See T. A. Sinclair's excellent commentary in his edition of the *Works and Days,* London, 1932.
6. *Works and Days,* 489ff.
7. Ibid. 410.
8. Ibid. 596.
9. Ibid. 724–6.
10. Ibid. 727–32. The idea of these taboos is that unseemly acts should not be performed in the sight of the gods. For further testimonies see Sinclair, op. cit. p. 74.
11. *Works and Days,* 757–9; rivers and springs were inhabited by nymphs.
12. Ibid. 733–4; in other words, purify yourself after sexual intercourse before you approach a holy place (the fireside).
13. Ibid. 753f., for it weakens a man.
14. Thirty years, the age for the man to marry, ibid. 695–8, also recommended by Plato (*Rep.,* V, 460E), is rather old and presupposes pre-marital intercourse with slave girls or with boys. As for the girl, assuming that she reaches puberty at about twelve, we would find her getting married at about sixteen or seventeen. Plato (loc. cit.) recommended the age of twenty.
15. *Works and Days,* 376–82.
16. Ibid. 765ff.
17. Ibid. 240–45.
18. Ibid. 102–5.
19. The fragments of the early Greek philosophers were collected by H. Diels, *Die Fragmente der Vorsokratiker,* 5th ed. by W. Kranz, Berlin, 1934–8. References are to this book (quoted here as Diels). Two recent books by Kathleen Freeman will be found very useful, *The Pre-Socratic Philosophers, A Companion to Diels, Fragmente der Vorsokratiker,* Oxford: Blackwell, 1946, and *Ancilla to the Pre-Socratic Philosophers,* Oxford: Blackwell, 1948; the latter is an English translation of the fragments. See also Aldo Mieli, *La Scienza greca, I. Prearistotelici,* Florence, 1916; P. Brunet and A. Mieli, *Histoire des sciences: Antiquité,* Paris, 1935; F. Enriques and G. de Santillana, *Histoire de la pensée scientifique, I. Les Ioniens et la nature des choses,* Paris, 1936; B. Farrington, *Greek Science, I. Thales to Aristotle,* Penguin Books, 1949; R. Baccou, *Histoire de la science grecque de Thalès à Socrate,* Paris, 1951.
20. See P.-M. Schuhl, *Essai sur la formation de la pensée grecque,* Paris, 1949, p. 165ff., where further literature is given.
21. See Jaeger, *Paideia,* I, 154.

22. Thus Thales was said to have fallen into a well while gazing at the stars and to have been jeered at by his maid for being so impractical, Plato, *Theaetetus,* 174A.
23. Plato, *Republic,* X, 600A, calls him εὐμήχανος εἰς τέχνας.
24. Herodotus, II, 20.
25. We are not giving references for every fragment since they are all easily available in Diels.
26. About Heraclitus see G. Burckhardt, *Heraklit, seine Gestalt und sein Künden,* Zurich and Leipzig, 1925; F. J. Brecht, *Heraklit, ein Versuch über den Ursprung der Philosophie,* Heidelberg, 1936.
27. Fragment 6.
28. See Farrington's discussion, op. cit. vol. I, p. 35.
29. Fragment 53.
30. Fragment 80.
31. Fragment 8, translated by K. Freeman, op. cit.
32. Fragment 111. See J. Burnet, *Early Greek Philosophy,* London, 1948 (4th ed.), fragment 104.
33. About the Pythagoreans in general see A. Delatte, *Étude sur la littérature pythagoricienne,* Paris, 1915; E. Frank, *Plato und die sogenannten Pythagoreer,* Halle, 1923; I. Lévy, *Recherche sur les sources de la légende de Pythagore,* Paris, 1926; L. Brunschwicg, *Le Rôle du pythagorisme dans l'évolution des idées,* Paris, 1937; K. Kerényi, *Pythagoras und Orpheus,* Amsterdam, 1940.
34. Herodotus, III, 60.
35. *Cambridge Ancient History,* vol. IV, p. 92f.
36. Chief ancient sources were the 'Pythagorean Maxims' of Aristoxenus (fourth century B.C.) mostly preserved in the 'Pythagorean Life' of Iamblichus (ca. A.D. 300).
37. Op. cit. vol. I, p. 45.
38. See the analysis of the 'Pythagorean Life' in Freeman, op. cit. p. 256ff.
39. See A. Delatte, *Faba Pythagorae cognata,* Serta Leodiensia, Liège, Paris, 1930.
40. Op. cit. p. 41.
41. Diels, 45, B5.
42. See T. Gomperz, *Griechische Denker,* 4th ed., Berlin and Leipzig, 1922, p. 90.
43. L. Edelstein, *The Hippocratic Oath.* Text, Translation and Interpretation (Bull. Hist. Med., Suppl. 1), Baltimore, 1943.
44. Diels, op. cit. 32, B13.
45. According to Suidas (Diels, op. cit. 9, 2) Calliphon was a priest of Asclepius who went from Cnidus to Croton where he had friendly contacts with Pythagoras. However, he cannot have been a priest of Asclepius for there was no cult of the god at Cnidus in the sixth century.
46. Herodotus, III, 125, 129–37. The Paris thesis of R. Houdry, *La Vie d'un médecin du VIe siècle avant J.-C., Démocèdes de Crotone,* Paris, 1921,

merely repeats the stories of Herodotus. C. Daremberg, *État de la médecine entre Homère et Hippocrate,* Paris, 1869, is a better study. The testimonies are in Diels, op. cit. 9.

47. Herodotus, III, 131.

48. R. Pohl, *De Graecorum Medicis Publicis,* Thesis, Berlin, 1905.

49. About him see A. Olivieri, 'Alcmeone di Crotona,' *Atti Acc. Arch. di Napoli,* 1919, 4:15ff.; L. A. Stella, 'Importanza di Alcmeone nella storia del pensiero greco,' *Acc. Naz. Lincei,* Ser. VI, vol. VIII, Fasc. IV, Rome, 1939, (see L. Edelstein's review in *Am. J. Philol.,* 1943, 63:3.); P. S. Codellas, 'Alcmaeon of Croton, His Life, Work and Fragments,' *Proc. Roy. Soc. Med.,* Sect. Hist. Med., 1932, 25:25–30; J. Ramón Beltrán, 'Alcmeon de Crótona y la psico-fisiologia,' *Rev. Asoc. Méd. Argentina,* 1940, vol. 54, no. 447–8, 4 p.; H. Erhard, 'Alkmaion, der erste Experimentalbiologe,' *Sudhoffs Arch. Gesch. Med.,* 1941, 34:77–89; and the histories of ancient philosophy and science; the fragments and testimonies are in Diels, op. cit. 14.

50. The assumption that he lived in the second half or last third of the sixth century is based on one short sentence in Aristotle's *Metaphysics* according to which he was supposed to have been young when Pythagoras was old. This sentence occurs only in inferior manuscripts and may be a later interpolation from Porphyrius' *Life of Pythagoras.* See W. H. Heidel's discussion in *Am. J. Philol.,* 1940, 61:3ff., and also in his *Hippocratic Medicine,* New York, 1941, p. 43f. Like K. Deichgräber (*Hippokrates, über Entstehung und Aufbau des menschlichen Körpers* [Περὶ σαρχῶν], 1935, p. 37), Heidel thinks that Alcmaeon flourished around 450 B.C. Quite apart from philological reasons, internal evidence makes it likely that Alcmaeon did his work in the fifth century and rather toward the middle than in the beginning.

51. There is no evidence that he dissected human cadavers or that he performed vivisections.

52. Diels, op. cit. 14, A10: 'primus exsectionem (oculi) adgredi est ausus.' It is futile to discuss whether by *exsectio* the author means 'excision' or a 'dissection.' The testimonies show unmistakably that Alcmaeon did dissect eyes, and in order to dissect them he had to cut them out of their sockets.

53. Πόροι or *luciferae semitae.* Since arteries and veins were designated as φλέβες, πόροι here undoubtedly mean nerves.

54. Diels, op. cit. 14, A18, a fragment from Aëtius.

55. Ibid. 14, B4, from Aëtius. The last sentence is particularly important: τὴν δὲ ὑγείαν τὴν σύμμετρον τῶν ποιῶν κρᾶσιν.

56. Ibid. 14, B1.

57. About him see the histories of Greek philosophy and science mentioned before; also, J. Schumacher, 'Der Physis-Begriff bei Empedokles,' *Sudhoffs Arch. Gesch. Med.,* 1941, 34:179–96. The fragments of his works are in Diels, op. cit.; English translation by K. Freeman, op. cit.; a beautiful translation in English verse by W. E. Leonard, *The Fragments of Empe-*

docles, Chicago, 1908. Our quotations are from this translation by courtesy of the Open Court Publishing Company, Chicago.

58. Fragment 112.

59. Ibid.

60. Diels, op. cit. 21, A1, § 61.

61. Iamblichus, *Vita Pythagorae,* 113.

62. Diels, op. cit. 21, A1, § 70.

63. Ibid. § 60.

64. Fragment 111.

65. Fragment 100.

66. Ibid.

67. Fragment 17.

68. So particularly by Gomperz, op. cit. p. 190.

69. Ibid. p. 201.

70. Fragment 66.

71. Fragment 37.

72. The chief study on the school is M. Wellmann, *Die Fragmente der sikelischen Aerzte, Akron, Philistion und des Diokles von Karystos,* Berlin, 1901.

73. In addition to the histories mentioned before see H. Erhard, 'Anaxagoras als Biologe,' *Sudhoffs Arch. Gesch. Med.,* 1942, 35:117–40; F. M. Cleve, *The Philosophy of Anaxagoras,* New York, 1949.

74. See Paul Tasch, 'Diogenes of Apollonia and Democritus,' *Isis,* 1941, 40:10–12; J. Ilberg, 'Hippokrates und Demokrit,' *Arch. Gesch. Med.,* 1913, 6:1–11.

75. Not to be confused with an apocryphal short *Prognostic* attributed sometimes to Democritus, sometimes to Hippocrates or Soranus. Literature on this subject is listed in W. Puhlmann, 'Die lateinische medizinische Literatur des frühen Mittelalters,' *Kyklos,* 1930, 3:407–8.

76. Fragment 251.

77. So in the pseudo-Hippocratic letters.

78. W. Osler, *Aequanimitas,* Philadelphia, 1889.

79. Fragment 191.

80. On the forged writings see K. Freeman, op. cit. p. 323ff., with references to Diels.

81. H. E. Sigerist, 'The Sphere of Life and Death in Early Mediaeval Manuscripts,' *Bull. Hist. Med.,* 1942, 11:292–303.

82. In a manuscript of the British Museum. See K. Freeman, op. cit. p. 325.

83. Littré, IX, 320ff.

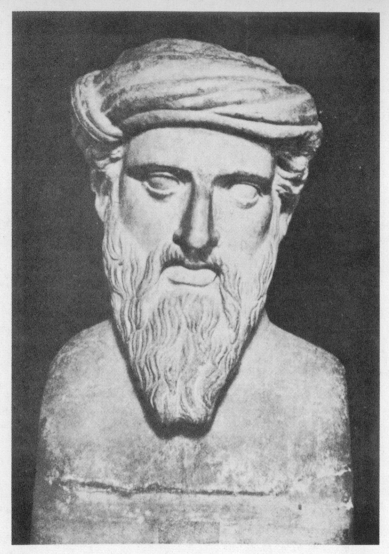

1. Pythagoras (?), Rome, Capitoline Museum. From Karl Schefold, *Die Bildnisse der antiken Dichter, Redner und Denker,* Benno Schwabe & Co., Basel, 1943, p. 161, no. 1.

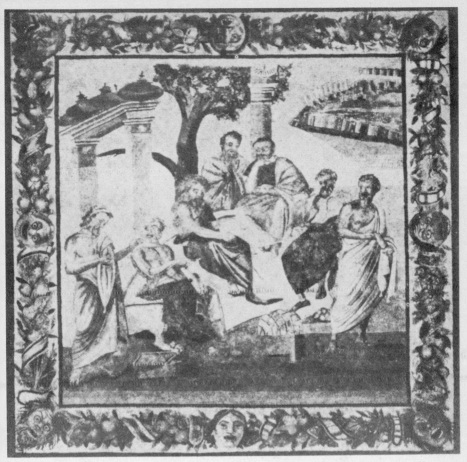

2. Mosaic of the Seven Sages, copy of a late Hellenistic painting, in Naples Museum. Ibid. p 155, no. 1.

II. HINDU MEDICINE

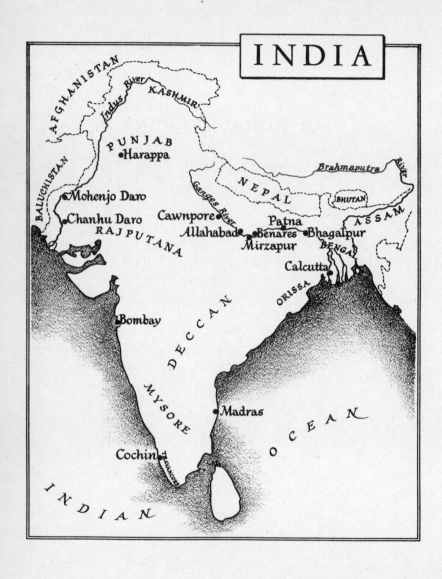

★

1. The Setting

The Indo-European tribes, eastern branch of the Aryans who toward the middle of the second millennium B.C. migrated through the mountain passes of Afghanistan to the valley of the Indus, entered a country that was in every respect different from the Balkan peninsula. More than a mere peninsula, an Asiatic subcontinent rather, extending nearly thirty degrees in latitude from the mountains of central Asia to Ceylon, which is near the equator, and over an equal distance from west to east, from Beluchistan to Burma, it covered a territory of over one and one-half million square miles.[1]

Greece, mainland and islands, is small, and has a great variety of landscapes with its mountains, valleys, creeks, and highly indented shoreline. Here man dominates the landscape. India, on the other hand, is a large country, designed on broad lines, a country in which man feels very small. The Tropic of Cancer which runs one degree north of Calcutta divides the country into two parts of triangular shape. The great plain in the north, the river beds of the Indus and Ganges and their affluents, is a very fertile region which repeatedly attracted invaders; well protected by the Himalaya range, the highest mountains in the world, it nevertheless is accessible from the northwest, and Aryans and Moguls came along the same trails. The southern triangle, the Deccan, consists of a plateau, one thousand to three thousand feet high, bordered on the east and west by hills, the Ghaunts, which fall steeply to the sea on the west, slowly on the east. North and south, however, the land settled by the Aryans and that inhabited by the aboriginal Dravida, were separated not by an imaginary line but by hills, the Vindhya mountains, and by jungles, which are as formidable a barrier as mountains.

India has a sea coast of five thousand miles, but it is very different from that of Greece, being designed in straight lines, with few harbors and very few islands; in many places the shore is rocky and swampy. India's sea is an ocean on east and west, not an inland sea like the Aegean on which one could sail in very small boats. The Indians never became a seafaring nation like the Greeks, although navigation was developed to a certain extent. Many points of the country could be reached much more easily by sea than by land, and we must remember that India colonized Indochina as well as Indonesia. The Indians, however, never possessed the aggressive spirit of the Greeks, who were frequently forced by economic pressure to settle abroad, and who under Alexander endeavored to conquer the world. A large, closed, and self-contained country, India never felt the urge to subjugate her neighbors; only once in the course of India's history did her people go abroad, and this was on a spiritual mission which brought the teachings of Gotama the Buddha to the people of the Far East. Even today, when the pressure of overpopulation on a greatly exhausted soil is tremendous, India has maintained through all trials and tribulations the same spirit of peacefulness, and has demonstrated to the world that great results may be achieved by non-violence.

Since India stretches over more than two thousand miles from north to south it has a great variety of climate. In the north, the mountains are high, the air is thin, the winter is severe, and the summer delightfully cool. In the Punjab, from November to March the weather is dry and the nights are cold. Frosts may occur at Lahore. In the great plain the winter months are very pleasant but from April on the temperature may be unbearable, rising to 110 degrees Fahrenheit. The largest part of the country is tropical, and the Aryans who came from the north were forced to adapt themselves to totally different conditions. They were beef-eaters and became vegetarians. Accustomed to the use of intoxicating beverages they later condemned them.

The rivers of India are unlike those of Greece, which dry out in the summer and become wild torrents during the rainy season. The Indus and Ganges are large rivers which for two thousand miles carry enormous quantities of water very slowly through the Indian plains. The Brahmaputra flows from the heights of Assam and has in Bengal a common estuary with the Ganges. Its valley marks the way from India to China, but with its steep gorges it does not provide easy access; India therefore has never been threatened from that direction. Large rivers are a great blessing for a country. Egypt was a 'gift' of the Nile as Herodotus called it, Mesopotamia the creation of the Euphrates and Tigris. Great rivers bring water that makes the land fertile, and also provide highways for traffic. Great rivers make it possible to irrigate the land, bringing the water where it is needed most; irrigation was practiced in India at an early date. Today great rivers are an inexhaustible source of electric energy, and India's rivers may well become the backbone of her economy. In antiquity, when man had a more personal relation with nature, people were grateful to their rivers for the many benefits they brought; they worshiped them and sacrificed to them. Egyptians prayed to the Nile as to a deity, and to Hindus the Ganges was and still is the holiest of rivers. It gave birth to some of India's most important cities, Cawnpore, Allahabad, Mirzapur, Benares, Patna, Bhagalpur, and Calcutta. Bathing in its water purified sinful men, drinking from its water was to the dying Hindu what extreme unction is to the Roman Catholic, and throwing the ashes of the dead into the river opened the doors of paradise. For thousands of years millions of Indians made pilgrimages to the holy waters of the Ganges.

The large rivers of India, however, are in the northern plain, and the country as a whole would not have had sufficient water to grow the food needed for the population without the monsoon. The monsoon is to India what the inundation of the Nile is to Egypt. It has the same economic effects. For seven months of the year India in most of its sections is a very dry country. The sky is invariably blue, the heat becomes unbearable, the earth is dust; and then the monsoon sets in and brings pouring rains, and for five months the coun-

try is very wet. The monsoon is a wind that hits India from southwest and northeast. The southwest monsoon, which comes from
Africa and was taken advantage of for purposes of navigation as
early as the first century A.D., blows from the middle of February to
the middle of August, reaching its peak in June. The northeast monsoon sets in toward the end of August, becomes strong in October,
and blows heavily for two months. The rains are terrific; water pours
down for days on end in a way never experienced in Europe or North
America. Roads become impassable and for weeks villages are cut
off from the rest of the world. Whatever you touch is damp. Nature
seems to take a deep breath, and the earth which had turned brown
and seemed dead, now all of a sudden becomes green and is teeming
with life, covered with the most luxuriant vegetation. There is
nothing comparable to our spring and autumn. Seasons are violent,
an outburst of nature followed by a collapse.

When the rains stop it is time for sowing, and crops ripen in a few
weeks. India was more industrialized in antiquity and in the Middle
Ages than it is today. It had a flourishing textile industry and
exported fabrics to many countries, but it was always primarily
agricultural. According to some estimates 50 per cent of the territory
is now under cultivation, according to others 34.2 per cent, and the
regional differences are great. While in Sind the sown area is only 16
per cent of the whole territory, it is 58 per cent in the region of
Delhi.[2] The tremendous increase in population during the last few
centuries and the impoverishment of the soil through erosion and
lack of fertilizer have created serious problems and made India a
victim of periodic famines which wipe out tens of thousands of
people. In the beginning of the seventeenth centry A.D. the population
probably numbered about 100 million. It was 130 million around
the middle of the eighteenth century, 150 million around 1850, 294
million in 1901, and today, including Pakistan, must be close to 400
million, an increase in population of 25 per cent in our century alone,
while the area under cultivation with food crops increased by only
10 per cent during the same period.[3] The country is densely populated, with 700,000 villages and large cities in a territory half the

size of the United States. The population per 100 acres of sown land varies from 60 to 300. Sixty per cent of all farmers have less than five acres of land, the minimum needed for the support of a family. In sections of East Bengal the density of the population exceeds 1000 per square mile.[4] Even in good years local agricultural production is not sufficient to feed the entire population adequately, and cereals must be imported. Moreover, the land is overstocked with 200 million cattle and 100 million sheep that require a great deal of grazing land, and the situation is complicated still further by an infinity of religious taboos. Old animals are not killed. Hindus do not eat beef and Mohammedans do not eat pork. Millions of Indians, being strict vegetarians, do not consume any animal parts.

Today's India impresses the traveler as a very poor country, and there is no doubt that the per capita income and the general living standard are very low. India was much more prosperous in the past when it had a smaller population and a better balanced economy. Animals were domesticated at an early date—the camel, the donkey, the buffalo, and even the wild elephant. Wide use of animal power was made thousands of years ago. India still is a potentially wealthy country with large deposits of iron, with coal, oil, copper, manganese, some gold and silver, diamonds, and pearl fisheries. There are still deserts which can be irrigated and thus brought under cultivation, swamps that can be drained, jungles that can be cleared.

There is one point that we should always bear in mind when we talk about the wealth or poverty of a country; namely, that the valuation of material goods varies a great deal. Nobody likes to starve or to see his family starving; nobody cares for physical pain or to see his children suffer and die. Every civilized society endeavors to secure for its members a certain material standard which seems necessary for the pursuit of happiness, but the degree of and the emphasis on what seems important and what does not, vary from culture to culture, and there could be no greater difference than that between the ancient Greeks and the Indians. The Greeks as a whole cherished the good life on this earth. Health and wealth seemed highly desirable goods, and science and technology provided the means to master nature. There were philosophical schools which opposed such an attitude, but they were not very successful; in spite of centuries of Christian austerity and spirituality, we in the West have inherited from the Greeks this worldly outlook and the burning desire to master the forces of nature for material advantages. Nature, however, can also be mastered differently. The Indian yogi who, naked and motionless, sits meditating under a tree or under a primitive roof is mastering nature also, but through the spirit. Why be afraid of death when we have been reborn many times before, and when our goal is to be relieved from the cycle of reincarnations? In our own times Gandhi the Mahatma taught the people through word and example that a simple frugal life was the best path to happiness, that the quest for material goods was vain, and that real freedom could only be attained through freedom from material needs and freedom from passions. We must never lose sight of such basic attitudes, for they explain a great deal and were determining factors in medicine too. The Indian attitude toward animals is also such a basic factor. We mentioned that old cattle are not killed; we must add that Indian philosophy does not consider animals essentially different from man. My cat, my buffalo, the monkey that ravages my storeroom, may house the soul of one of my ancestors; and what will my next reincarnation be? This belief explains the lack of historical sense which is so outspoken in India. We should look in vain for chronicles and annals such as the Chinese wrote. There is no Indian Thucydides, Tacitus, or Sze Ma-chien. Why write history when the past is still alive, when the heroes of a bygone age are still with us? Fact and fiction are blended almost inextricably in Indian historiography, and we shall see later what enormous difficulties Indian chronology presents. This view toward the animal world also explains the great difficulty medical men experience when they try to destroy insects and other animals that are a menace to the people's health.

Health conditions are very bad in India today, and here, as in the case of Egypt, we are inclined to wonder if they were not better in antiquity, if there has not been a steady decline, particularly during the past few centuries. The enormous growth of population on the same land area, with resulting chronic malnutrition and miserable housing in crowded cities, would indicate such a decline. On the other hand, the very fact that the population increased so rapidly, that more children were born and apparently fewer died, would speak for improved conditions. We shall probably never be able to answer the question, since we have no statistics for the past and modern statistics are incomplete and inaccurate. They usually cover only the territory of former British India, are collected by untrained people, and the causes of deaths registered cannot be more than approximate in view of the great shortage of medical personnel. Yet with all their defects they still speak eloquently.

The birth rate in 1938 was 34.1 per 1000 population. In 1943, it dropped to 25.6;[5] this does not mean that the standard of living rose, but rather that 1943 was a year of war and famine. For comparison we may look at the birth rates of England and Wales, and the United States, which in 1937 were 14.9 and 17.0 respectively.[6] The general death rate in India per 1000 population was 22.4 in 1937, 23.4 in 1943. Infant mortality per 1000 births was 162 in 1937; in the period 1932-37 it averaged 173 while it was 61 in England and Wales,[7] 57.1 in the United States. In the city of Bombay infant mortality averaged 218 in the period 1938-42, and the same figure is reported for Madras for the period 1941-42. The general death rate of England and Wales was 12.4 in 1937, that of the United States 11.3. Maternal mortality is also very high; it varies from province to province and probably averages about 20 per 1000 live births. It was 2.1 in the United States in 1945. In India, in those places where maternity and child welfare work is carried on vigorously, conditions have greatly improved, but the country is so large and many areas are still so underdeveloped that only a small section of the population can be reached. As a result of these high death rates the expectation of life at birth was only 27 years in India at a time when it was 67 in

Australia, 63 in England and Wales, 63 in Germany, and 47 in Japan.[8] In other words, in India today conditions are similar to or even worse than what they were in Europe before the Industrial Revolution and before the public health movement. Indian authorities are making great efforts to improve conditions and results have been achieved, but the handicaps are enormous.

India is a tropical country and therefore has all diseases peculiar to the tropics. Malaria probably presents its chief health problem today, as it did in the past, not only because it kills and disables large numbers of people, but because it saps the vitality of the population. It is endemic in all parts of the country except the mountainous regions of Kashmir, Nepal, and Bhutan; in some sections it breaks out in fulminant epidemics. In 1939, in British India alone, no fewer than 1,400,000 cases of death were attributed to 'fevers,' most of which undoubtedly were malaria, and many cases may not have been reported at all.[9] Insects are a plague in all tropical countries, and insect control is difficult where irrigation is necessary, where rice is cultivated, and where religion forbids the killing of animals. Fevers have been the major disease of India throughout its history. Modern methods of combating malaria are effective when and where they can be applied. This was demonstrated on the tea plantations [10] and in the region of Delhi, where the anti-malaria operations of the Malaria Institute of India were highly successful.[11] But the country is so large, and the average peasant still so ignorant in health matters, that malaria will remain the country's chief disease for many years to come.

Another group of diseases less deadly but probably with an even greater prevalence includes the various forms of enteric fever, dysentery, and diarrhea. In 1939, 260,000 deaths from dysentery and diarrhea were reported in British India,[12] and this obviously must be an understatement. In 1941, Calcutta had a reported death rate per 100,000 population of 250 from dysentery and diarrhea, and of 90 from typhoid; the figures for Bombay were 252 and 40, and for Madras in 1940, 436 and 16.[13] The morbidity rates cannot be ascertained, but it is likely that almost the entire population suffers from an intestinal disease at some time during the course of the year. The number of people, moreover, who have a chronic enteric disease must be very large.

For thousands of years India, like China, was an endemic focus of some of the world's most fatal epidemic diseases, diseases which are preventable today but still occur and take a heavy toll of lives in India. It was from the East that the plague spread to the West many times in the course of history, invading one country after another and killing millions of people. The plague is an acute disease of rodents, rats mostly, and is transmitted from them to man. Epidemics flare up suddenly. India is still one of the reservoirs of infected rodents from which epidemics may be generated. Some years the casualties are low, others very high, and no year passes without an outbreak of the disease in some part of the country. Close to 5000 people died from plague in the first six months of 1944.[14] It has been estimated that ten million people were killed by plague from 1903 to 1921. The social and economic distribution of casualties is highly characteristic in this disease also. Thus in one outbreak the deaths per 1,000,000 population were:[15]

Low caste Hindus	53.7
Brahmans	20.7
Mohammedans	13.7
Eurasians	6.1
Jews	5.2
Parsees	4.6
Europeans	0.8

Modern methods of control have reduced the incidence of plague and may ultimately eradicate it altogether, but in the meantime India remains an active focus which constantly threatens the country and also its neighbors.

There is no excuse for the fact that smallpox still kills thousands of people every year and disfigures many more. India was one of the first countries to practice inoculation against smallpox; Jenner's vaccine reached India and was used successfully a few years after its discovery.[16] Yet the vastness of the country, the lack of sufficient personnel, and the low educational standard of the villager have so far prevented vaccination of the entire population. Many births are not registered, and thus many children cannot be reached. It is difficult to carry out revaccination where children do not go to school at all, or go for only a few years. In the Bombay Presidency, vaccination was introduced in 1830. A vaccination department was established in 1858. Primary vaccination is compulsory but is enforced in only 4.9 per cent of the rural areas.[17] In the period from 1880 to 1940 the death rate of smallpox varied from 0.1 to 0.8 per thousand population in British India, but this figure is undoubtedly an understatement. Children are particularly affected, and in the period 1937-41 from 12.1 to 19.7 per cent of all casualties were infants under one year of age. Many cases of blindness are the result of smallpox. The disease frequently flares up in five-year cycles. In the northwest it is sometimes brought by nomads, powindahs, who migrate into the province during the cold season. Progress has been achieved, and the average number of reported annual deaths dropped from 40 per thousand in the period 1902-11 to 25 in the period 1932-41. The problem is still a serious one, as it must have been throughout the course of Indian history, but the example of the Soviet Union shows that smallpox can be eradicated entirely even under difficult conditions once a country has a system of medical care that reaches the population.

The third major epidemic disease of India is cholera.[18] It has endemic foci in the country, in Bengal, and in the Cauveri Delta of the province of Madras. There the disease flares up every year, and from there it takes its course into other sections of the subcontinent. Religious festivals are an important factor in the spread of cholera. Tens of thousands of people from all parts of India gather at one place. Much water is consumed and spilled, and if the water or the food becomes contaminated an epidemic may break out and be carried into remote provinces. Deaths from cholera are reported every year, but there is a wide range of variation in its incidence. Thus, from 1877 to 1941, the average number of annual deaths calculated for five-year periods varied from 141,000 to 444,000. In the province of Madras, 2,115 deaths from cholera occurred in 1939 and 117,039 in 1943. The control of such a disease is difficult in a country like India, for it requires the protection of water supplies, sanitary disposal of nightsoil, and strict food control. Once the disease has broken out, patients should be isolated, infective material must be disinfected, and the population of the area must be immunized by anticholera inoculation; such measures may be easily carried out in economically advanced countries, but not in Asia, where general sanitation is still very poor. Cholera was a new disease to Europe and America when it reached these continents in the nineteenth century, but it was an old disease to Asia.

It is highly probable that tuberculosis existed in ancient India as it did in antiquity in the Mediterranean world. We do not have the skeleton material from India—a country where most cadavers were burnt—that we have from ancient Egypt, but passages in the early texts point to the disease. There can be no doubt, however, that tuberculosis has increased in the course of our century.[19] The rapid growth of the population, malnutrition and undernourishment, the crowding of an increasing number of people in city slums, and industrialization, together with the employment of women and children in unhygienic working places, are all factors that favor the spread of tuberculosis. There are no statistics available, but on the basis of local surveys it has been estimated that the annual number of deaths from pulmonary tuberculosis in former British India must be at least half a million, and the number of people suffering from the disease at least two and one-half million. It is to be expected that the incidence of pulmonary tuberculosis will not decrease but on the contrary increase in the near future, as industrialization develops and the general standard of living remains low.[20]

Syphilis, in all probability a gift from the West brought by Portuguese sailors in the beginning of the sixteenth century, was first recorded as *Phirangi Roga*,[21] literally *morbus Gallicus,* but meaning quite generally European disease. How widespread it was at that time we do not know, but there can be little doubt that the incidence of venereal diseases has grown considerably as a result of the crowding of people in the cities and the promiscuity that unavoidably follows. And as most city people come from the land and return to the native village at some time or other, venereal diseases increase in the rural sections of the country too. There is no compulsory reporting of these diseases, hence no statistics are available. The only figures we have are based on questionnaires sent by the health authorities to general practitioners and specialists. On the basis of these findings it has been estimated that 5.5 million of the village population suffer from syphilis and 7.6 million from gonorrhea.[22] Conditions are particularly bad in Bengal and Madras, but apparently much better in the Punjab. In Calcutta, where the number of prostitutes is supposed to be about 40,000, the incidence of venereal diseases is estimated at about 40 per cent. From 1933 to 1940 the number of recorded cases of still births in Bengal increased by over 33 per cent.[23] In a general hospital of Bombay it was found that 18.7 per cent of the in-patients and 29.8 per cent of the out-patients showed evidence of venereal diseases.[24] And another hospital in Bombay similarly found that 29 per cent of the patients of its Female Outdoor Clinic had some venereal infection.[25] Many cases of blindness—and India has over a million blind people—must be the result of gonorrhea.

While syphilis was a newcomer to India, leprosy must have been endemic in the sub-continent from earliest times.[26] It may be that Africa is the home of the disease, but in that case it must have spread to India and from there to China at an early date. The disease is described and recognized as an entity in itself in the earliest medical literature. It was pictured as being contagious and transmissible from parent to child, and the position of the leper in society was very similar to that in the ancient Near East, familiar to us from Leviticus. The sick man was an outcast. People avoided contact with him and did not marry into families where the disease occurred. Huts were built outside the village for the lepers, who lived as beggars. A stigma was frequently attached to the disease, since it seemed to be punishment for sin committed in a previous incarnation.

Of the estimated five million lepers in the world at least one million are in India. They are scattered everywhere, and are found even in the high mountain regions. But the chief endemic centers are along the east coast and in the south, that is, in West Bengal, South Bihar, Orissa, Madras, Travancore, and Cochin. There the incidence is over 0.75 per cent of the population, and some villages may have as high as 15 to 20 per cent incidence. Since most of the lepers are beggars they migrate a great deal, invading the cities. The problem presented by leprosy in India is of such magnitude and requires such far-reaching social and economic measures that the chances of bringing the disease under control are very slight so long as there is no effective medical treatment.

Like all tropical countries India has a high incidence of worm diseases.[27] Worms are frequently mentioned in the early medical literature and must have been parasites that plagued man at all times. It has been estimated that 60 to 80 per cent of the population of certain provinces on the east coast are infected with hookworm, and the incidence is particularly high among miners and workers on tea plantations. The disease is very well known, but its eradication requires social measures which are difficult to carry out in a country such as India.

Filariasis caused in India by two worms, *Filaria bancrofti* and *Filaria malayi,* the embryos of which are introduced into the human body by mosquitoes, is widely prevalent in Bihar and Orissa, and also affects other provinces of the east and south. The disease is characterized by permanent swellings of the legs and genital organs, and hence was known in antiquity as elephantiasis. It also causes attacks of fever and inflammation of the lymphatic system, and while it is not deadly, yet it is a highly disabling disease. So also is the guinea-worm disease, prevalent in the Northwest Frontier Province and certain sections of central India. Infection occurs through the drinking of water that contains embryos of the worm. It takes almost a year for the embryo to develop into an adult worm, which settles under the skin, usually in the legs. There it causes a blister which bursts, setting the worm free to discharge its numerous embryos whenever it comes into contact with water.

And finally we must mention starvation as a major cause of death and of numerous diseases. Conditions may have been better in the past when the country had a much smaller population and a better balanced economy, but, like China and Europe in previous centuries, India has always felt the threat of famine. At a time when transportation was slow, crop failures in some sections of the country invariably led to famines which killed large numbers of people outright and affected many more indirectly. In most countries famines lead to social disturbances. Exasperated by hunger, people take food where they can find it. Criminality, brigandage, and prostitution are well-known symptoms of famine, and hunger makes people take to the road in search of lands where food is, or is said to be, plentiful.[28] The Indian's reaction is different. His resignation is such that he may lie down and die of starvation in front of a food store without rebelling. To most Indians famines are still natural catastrophes; they do not see the human failure which is always involved; poor administration, an antiquated economic system, the breakdown of the means of transportation, lack of international co-operation—all these factors are as much responsible for the people's sufferings as is the shortage of crops. The famine of 1770 in Bengal killed one-third of the population. One million people succumbed to the famine of 1899-1900;[29] the recent Bengal famine of 1943 wiped out over a million people, and disabled many for a long time, because famines always produce a fertile breeding ground for diseases. Lack of food not only causes edemas, anemias, ulcers, and specific deficiency diseases, but by lessening the people's resistance makes them an easy prey to all kinds of infections. Famines, furthermore, disorganize normal life. Even if they do not succumb, people are impoverished, living conditions deteriorate, the louse thrives, rodents move into empty granaries (thus getting closer to man), water systems go out of order, and conditions are created for the rise and spread of epidemics which will take a further toll of lives.

India thus is a country which by its mere geography presents many more and much more serious health problems than Greece and the shores of the eastern Mediterranean basin. And we shall see that social and economic conditions resulting from historical developments in this large territory created still more problems. We shall talk about India's diseases again when we analyze its classical medical literature, but when considering its geography we had to discuss some of the major diseases here, particularly those characteristic of a tropical country as contrasted with those of the temperate zone.

NOTES

1. On India in general see the still useful *Grundriss der indo-arischen Philologie und Altertumskunde,* begründet von Georg Bühler, fortgesetzt von F. Kielhorn, herausgegeben von H. Lüders und J. Wackernagel, Strassburg, 1895 ff., and the recent book by Louis Renou and Jean Filliozat, *L'Inde classique,* Paris, 1947 ff. On geography see A. Cunningham, *Ancient Geography of India,* London, 1871; C. A. Morrison, *A New Geography of the Indian Empire,* London, 1909; S. G. Burrard and A. M. Heron, *The Geography and Geology of the Himalaya Mountains,* Delhi, 1932.
2. *Proc. of the Food and Nutrition Conference held at Delhi in January 1944,* p. 33.
3. Ibid. p. 4; see also Radhakamal Mukerjee, *Population and Food Supply,* Delhi and Lahore, 1944, p. 3ff. About population in general see S. Chandrasekhar, *India's Population, Fact and Policy,* Indian Institute for Population Studies, Annamalai University, Chidambaram, India, 2nd ed., 1950.
4. The figures are taken from the two pamphlets mentioned in notes 2 and 3.
5. C. A. Bozman, 'Health Conditions in India in 1943,' *Ind. Health Gaz.,* 1944, p. 4.
6. John B. Grant, 'The Health of India,' *Oxford Pamphlets on Indian Affairs No. 12,* Bombay, 1943, p. 3.
7. These and the following figures are taken from J. N. Morris, 'Health of Four Hundred Millions,' *Lancet,* June 16, 1945, p. 743.
8. Grant, op. cit. p. 3f.
9. M. C. Balfour, 'Some Impressions of Public Health in India,' *Ind. Med. Gaz.,* 1943, 78:3.

10. *Annual Report of the Public Health Commissioner with the Government of India for 1940,* Delhi, 1944, p. 13f.

11. G. Covell, 'Antimalaria Operations in Delhi,' *J. Malaria Inst. India,* vol. 2, pp. 1–61, 315–40, vol. 4, pp. 1–13.

12. Balfour, op. cit. p. 3.

13. Grant, op. cit. p. 21.

14. Bozman, op. cit. p. 1.

15. Quoted from C. Vaughan, *Epidemiology and Public Health,* St. Louis, vol. II, p. 781.

16. Jean de Carro, *Histoire de la vaccination en Turquie, en Grèce et aux Indes orientales,* Vienna, 1804; *Report on the Progress of Vaccine Inoculation in Bengal, from the Period of Its Introduction in November, 1802, to the End of the Year 1803,* Calcutta, 1804; *Report on the State and Progress of Vaccination during the Years 1804–6,* Calcutta, 1805–7.

17. These and the following figures are taken from *Report of the Health Survey and Development Committee,* Delhi, 1946, vol. I, p. 109ff.

18. Ibid. p. 111ff.

19. *Annual Report . . . for 1940,* Delhi, 1944, p. 22ff.

20. Ibid.

21. D. V. S. Reddy, *'Phirangi Roga' or Syphilis in India,* Bombay, 1943.

22. *Rep. Health Sur. Dev. Com.,* vol. I, p. 123.

23. *Control of Venereal Diseases in Bengal,* Report 1944 issued by the Director, Social Hygiene, Government of Bengal.

24. Socrates Noronha, *Venereal Diseases and Their Prevention,* Byculla, Bombay (Tata School of Social Work), n. d.

25. Ibid.

26. Government of India, Central Advisory Board of Health, *Report on Leprosy and Its Control in India,* New Delhi, 1942; R. G. Cochrane, 'Leprosy Control, with Particular Reference to the Madras Presidency,' *Ind. Med. Gaz.,* 1944, 74:438.

27. About worm diseases see *Rep. Health Sur. Dev. Com.,* vol. I, pp. 125–8.

28. H. E. Sigerist, *Civilization and Disease,* Ithaca, N. Y., 1943, p. 7ff.

29. R. C. Dutt, *Famines in India,* 1900.

★

2. Early Indus Civilizations

When the Greeks invaded the Eastern Mediterranean basin they
came into contact with the highly developed civilization of Crete.
They destroyed it but not without taking over and assimilating
many of its elements. A similar process took place in India. When
the Aryans entered the Indus Valley they found the region settled,
and their earliest literature, the Vedas, reports the battles they had
to fight with the Dâsas, the dark-skinned inhabitants of the region
whom they gradually drove to the south. As a matter of fact, the
Indus Valley had been the seat of a flourishing civilization for many
centuries before the advent of the Aryans, a civilization that had
already completed its course and left a deep imprint on what was
to become the culture of India.

The discovery in the 1920's by Indian archaeologists of large cities
in the Indus Valley was a thrilling event.[1] It revealed a civilization
totally unknown before and closely related to those of Sumer and
Crete. The chief sites excavated so far are Mohenjo Daro, which
was built on the Indus but is no longer on the shores of the river;
Harappa on an affluent of the Indus, 450 miles northeast of
Mohenjo Daro; Chanhu Daro; and a few minor places. Many
others have not yet been excavated. The territory covered by the
Indus civilization, as it is commonly called, was very large, twice
as large as that of Egypt, and four times as large as that of Sumer
and Akkad. These modern excavations explained findings that had
been made in Elam and Mesopotamia, where amulet seals of Indian

origin had been unearthed. There could be no doubt of their origin, not only because their style pointed to India, but also because the animals represented—elephant, rhinoceros, and a certain species of crocodile—were Indian. These seals assumed great importance in dating the Indus civilization. Indeed, some were found at Djemdet Nasr with objects that could be dated at about 3000 B.C., others were discovered at Tell Asmar in layers of about 2500 B.C. Hence the culture of Mohenjo Daro and Harappa must have flourished in the third millennium B.C., and thus was contemporary with the Old Kingdom of Egypt, the period of Sumer and Akkad in Mesopotamia. Like the Egyptians and Sumerians, the Indus people had a pictographic script which, however, has not yet been deciphered. So far no bilingual inscription has been found, so that we are completely in the dark about the language. All we possess are short inscriptions on seals. Longer texts may have been written on wood, leather, or palm leaves, materials later used for such a purpose in this region and, of course, highly perishable.

Excavations have unearthed four different cultures, characterized chiefly by their pottery. During the golden age of Mohenjo Daro and Harappa ceramics were monochrome, black on polished red ground. Before that time—that is, before 3000 B.C.—the sites were occupied by a more primitive people whose pottery was decorated with geometrical ornaments in three colors. Another culture, dating probably from the end of the third millennium, had again a different style, polychrome pottery with ornaments in the form of ribbons on yellowish, pinkish ground.[2] The top layer of the excavated site reveals that the last flourishing culture of the valley was destroyed by a barbaric people whose gray pottery, not made on the potter's wheel, had very primitive ornaments, mere scratch lines.

The fact that the same type of pottery was found in other parts of western Asia points to migrations, and gives us a better idea of the history of this region than anthropological findings can. Corpses were cremated and the ashes perhaps thrown into the rivers, as was done in India later. The number of skeletons found is small, certainly not large enough to give conclusive evidence on racial characteristics. What seems to have happened is that northern Syria, northern Mesopotamia, and Persia were settled in the fourth millennium B.C. by a people who had developed a civilization, one feature of which was its polychrome pottery, and that this people also settled part of the Indus Valley, where it produced the civilization named Amri after the site where it was first discovered. Another migration from the same center must have taken place toward the end of the fourth millennium, extending its reach as far as Crete in the West, to southern Mesopotamia, and still further into the valley of the Indus. The period around 3000 B.C. was the time when progress was greatest, when tools of metal began to replace those made of stone, when people invented signs to record events and a pictographic script was thus discovered, and when the stars were observed and a calendar established to regulate agricultural work and the cult of the gods. India had a great share in this development, and common origin may well be the explanation for the similarity of many cultural traits of India, Sumer, and Crete.

Since we have no literary records that we can read, our knowledge of the Indus civilization, like that of Crete, is derived entirely from archaeological findings. They are so rich, however, that they give us a picture of life in ancient India, and also illustrate some aspects of great medical interest. The people were primarily farmers and merchants. They grew wheat, barley, melons, dates, cotton, and lotus, and raised cattle, sheep, pigs, and poultry. The rivers and the sea supplied fish. Stone implements have been found which were used for the grinding of spices and condiments. Food may have been prepared with curries then as it is today. The women spun cotton and wool to make textiles. Clothing was simple in such a tropical country—a short skirt with ornamented belt, and, for women, much jewelry, necklaces and bracelets, made of gold, silver, electrum, copper, bronze, and ivory. Then as today jewels were worn in the sides of the nose, and women wore their hair in plaits with a ribbon. As might be expected, mirrors have been found, and chemicals that served cosmetic purposes, kohl for the eyes, the same kind of rouge that was found in Sumer, lead carbonate to whiten the face, and cinnabar, probably also applied as a cosmetic. The number of small, double-edged razors found is so large that they must have been used by both men and women.

These few remarks indicate that the country had skilled craftsmen. They made the pottery of which so many beautiful fragments have been preserved. They carved of steatite the numerous amulet seals which served the double purpose of identifying the owner and of protecting him against evil spirits. Every ancient civilization developed its special type of seal. In Mesopotamia the cylinder seal was most popular, in Egypt it was the scarabaeus seal, while the Indus people preferred plates. Many of them are extemely beautiful, revealing an exquisite taste, a keen sense of proportion, and delicate craftsmanship. Next to the name of the owner the seal as a rule showed the picture of an animal, the bull mostly, but also other animals, buffalo, elephant, rhinoceros, tiger, crocodile, or imaginary animals. Obviously these were not mere ornaments but had a magic purpose. They were holy animals, deities whose protection the owner of the seal sought. Deities appear also on seals with human bodies and animal heads, or entirely in human form but with horns. On some seals we find a combination of woman and tiger which reminds us of a centaur.[3] This woman-tiger is also seen fighting and being defeated by the bull-god. The bull here as in Crete was the symbol of generative power. In Greece the bull-god became identified with Zeus, in India with Shiva. A very interesting seal represents a three-faced deity with horns, sitting in Indian fashion on a platform, surrounded by various animals.[4] Shiva is still frequently represented with several faces, and he undoubtedly is one of the oldest deities of the Indian pantheon. On other seals we see holy trees, the *peepul* or holy fig-tree which still plays an important part in Indian rituals. On one seal a horned goddess appears in such a tree and is worshiped by another deity. Some seals show highly dramatic scenes which cannot be anything but mythological.

If we had nothing but the seals we would have ample evidence of the fact that the early inhabitants of the Indus Valley, like their western cousins in Elam, Sumer, and Crete, had a rich pantheon, a colorful mythology, and a highly developed religious life. But we have other evidence than the seals, notably a large number of statuettes of a woman alone or with a child, dressed in a short loincloth and belt, with an elaborate hairdress. Serpent and dove are her attributes, and she holds a cup in one or both hands. On some of these cups we still find traces of smoke caused by the burning of oil or incense.[5] This is the Great Mother, the goddess worshiped all over the Near and Middle East, the goddess who is still closest to the heart of millions of Indians of lower caste. In the Indus Valley she was apparently worshiped in every home; her statue was kept in a niche; people prayed and sacrificed to her. She embodied all the friendly forces of nature, protected the home and its inmates, notably the women and children, made the womb fertile, and assisted in childbirth. It is interesting to note that the cult of the mother, the one who is always ready to help her children unselfishly, is almost universal in some form or other, and the greater the stress and strain and anxiety in a society, the greater the wish for the help of the mother.

Statuettes of male deities have also been excavated, although in far smaller quantity than those of the Great Mother. Some have animal horns; others are animals entirely. Most of these statues are badly mutilated, probably by some conquering tribe. Phallic symbols—cone-like stones, symbols of male fertility—were worshiped in ancient India as they are today in connection with the cult of Shiva, and the swastika and Greek cross were engraved on amulets here, as also in Elam. Votive offerings representing a pregnant woman or a woman feeding her infant were deposited in sanctuaries, a custom common to most ancient cults. We know little enough about the religion of these early Indian civilizations, but whatever evidence we have tends to show that many elements survived the destruction of this culture, were taken over and assimilated by the Aryans, and are still alive today.

Of course, we should like to know what kind of medicine the Indus people practiced, but since we have no texts, no documents of any kind pertaining to the subject, we can merely guess that their medicine must have been similar to that of other peoples who were civilized in the third millennium B.C.—that is, a combination of religious, magical, and empirical rites and procedures. Amulets were worn to protect the owner against evil, hence also against disease; prayers must have been said here as in Mesopotamia and Egypt to placate the gods; incantations were probably performed to drive out evil spirits; and, like all peoples, the inhabitants of the Indus Valley must have known drugs and house remedies with which to treat the sick. Substances have been found that are used in Indian medicine today—cuttlebone, staghorn, a black substance, *silajit*—and it is quite possible that they were used as drugs in remote antiquity too.

While we cannot do more than speculate in this matter on the basis of analogy with contemporary and related civilizations, we stand on firm ground when we look at another aspect of the Indus civilization, one which has a profound influence on the people's health, namely, the construction and sanitation of their cities.

The excavation of Mohenjo Daro brought to light a city in many ways different from those of Egypt and Mesopotamia. There the cities consisted of temples, palaces, mansions of the rich, and mud huts of the poor. Here the early excavations uncovered no palaces, no temples, no slums, but a large number of what we would call middle-class, fairly comfortable, two-story houses built of baked bricks. At first, archaeologists were inclined to believe that the Indus city was a kind of ideal democratic community which had lived in peace for centuries. Later excavations, however, revealed traces of city walls, sanctuaries, palaces, and barracks, and it seems more likely that the Indus communities were theocratically ruled city-states, similar to those of Sumer. It would have been difficult to build such cities without a strong state power.

Mohenjo Daro antedates Kahun in Egypt, and is probably the oldest planned city of which we know, and one of the best-planned ancient towns. Its public health facilities were superior to those of any other community of the ancient Orient.[6] The streets ran in north-south and east-west directions. Some were very long, one avenue measuring as much as 800 yards. Their width varied from narrow lanes of four to five feet to wide avenues of over ten yards.

The houses, different from those of Egypt and Mesopotamia, were neither court houses nor block houses. They impress us as being highly functional, and remind us of today's settlements of an industrial suburb. Bricks baked in the oven were the chief building material. Sun-baked bricks were used only sparingly, and only in combination with other bricks, in spots that were not exposed to the weather. Small houses measured about 26 by 30 feet, larger houses twice as much. Roofs were probably flat, and rain water was drained into the street through gutters of pottery and probably also of wood. No traces of windows have been found, and light and air entered the house through the doors. Cooking was frequently done out of doors, as it still is done in the East, but indoor kitchens have also been found. Supplies were kept in large pottery jars, and rubbish was drained by chutes through the wall into tanks that must have been emptied periodically.

Almost all houses had bathrooms. Bathrooms were not uncommon in Egypt, Mesopotamia, and Crete, but there we find them only in palaces or in the houses of the rich. The fact that they were so numerous in the Indus cities perhaps means that bathing had not only a hygienic but also a ritual purpose, as it still has in India today. The bathrooms were built near the wall that faced the street, and the water was drained through pipes into covered sewers that ran under the street. Many Indian cities today have open sewers. Bathrooms were square or rectangular, had a sloping floor with an opening in one corner through which the water escaped. In several houses latrines have been found, water closets with a drainage system similar to that of the bathrooms. Most houses had their own wells, the walls carefully built of bricks. Houses which did not have their own wells probably got water from a neighbor.

The most monumental building found in Mohenjo Daro so far is a public bath house, 108 by 180 feet in size. Its center was a basin measuring 23 by 39 feet with a sloping floor that reached a maximum depth of eight feet. Water came from a large well, and the basin was surrounded by a gallery with pillars. Eight small private bathrooms were located at the northern end of the building, and were probably connected with an equal number of cells on an upper floor. This again points to the possibility of a ritual rather than hygienic purpose of the baths, and the building may have been inhabited by priests or members of a religious order. The large basin either served those who had no bath at home, or was perhaps used during festivals. It would be easy to find parallels in later Hindu rituals.

The sewerage system of Mohenjo Daro is truly impressive. The openings in the houses through which water and nightsoil were drained were carefully constructed in such a way that pedestrians would not be molested, and this is not the case in many Indian cities today. A system of covered and vaulted sewers and canals, small and large, drained refuse and sewage into the river. Our illustrations give a fair idea of these constructions, and make us realize that not until Roman days do we find cities with equally good public health facilities.

This flourishing culture was brutally destroyed by barbaric primitive tribes who invaded the Indus Valley around 2000 B.C., coming perhaps from Beluchistan, seat of savage tribes until very recently, or from the northwest through the mountain passes of Afghanistan, or possibly from the north through Kashmir. They killed, looted, and broke the statues and statuettes of the gods. Their gray handmade pottery with its most primitive ornaments betrays the low standard of their civilization, and we may well imagine that the elaborate public health system of the cities deteriorated very rapidly. For a period of about five hundred years—that is, until the Aryan migration—we know very little about the fortunes of India. We have no written and very few archaeological records. But a great civilization never perishes entirely, no matter how savage the conqueror may be. Egypt was invaded by the Hyksos, Babylonia by the Kassites, but both civilizations survived the shock; and there can be no doubt that in a similar way gods and rites, customs and art forms of the early Indus civilizations survived the barbarian invasion and ultimately became elements in India's Aryan culture.

NOTES

1. The literature on these early Indus civilizations is very considerable. The findings were first reported in *Annual Reports of the Archaeological Survey of India*, 1923–24 to 1928–29. The basic publication is Sir J. Marshall, *Mohenjo Daro and the Indus Civilization*, London, 1931, 3 vols. An excellent survey which includes later findings is E. Mackay, *Early Indus Civilization*, London, 2nd ed., 1948. A good study from the point of view of the history of art with bibliography and illustrations is II. Mode, *Indische Frühkulturen und ihre Beziehungen zum Westen*, Basle, 1944.

2. Mode, op. cit. p. 9.

3. Ibid. p. 68.

4. Ibid. pl. VI.

5. Ibid. p. 36.

6. See Sir J. Marshall and E. Mackay quoted above, and also W. von Brunn, 'Von einer bisher unbekannten früh-indischen Kultur,' *Sudhoffs Arch. Gesch. Med.*, 1935, 28:347–58.

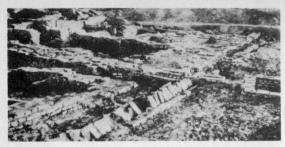

1. Pent-roofed drain in middle of street, Mohenjo-Daro. From Sir John Marshall, *Mohenjo-Daro and the Indus Civilization*, Arthur Probsthain, London, 1931, vol. 3, pl. LXVII a.

2. Floor of eating-house, Mohenjo-Daro. From E. Mackay, *Early Indus Civilization*, Luzac, London, 1948, pl. XV, no. 1.

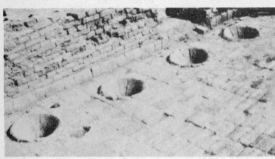

3. Pottery drain-pipes, Chanhu-Daro. Ibid. pl. XIII, no. 2.

4. Sump-pit, Mohenjo-Daro. Ibid. pl. XIII, no. 5.

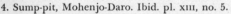

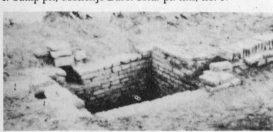

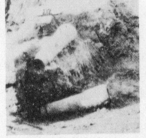

5. Rain-water culvert, Mohenjo-Daro. Ibid. pl. XIII, no. 4.

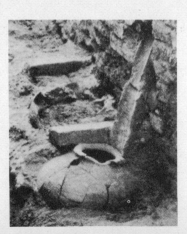

6. Water chute from house, Mohenjo-Daro. Ibid. pl. XIII, no. 3.

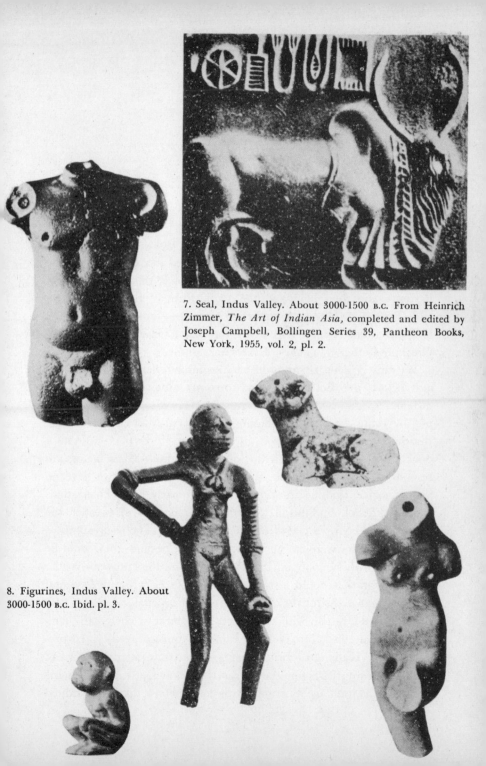

7. Seal, Indus Valley. About 3000-1500 B.C. From Heinrich Zimmer, *The Art of Indian Asia,* completed and edited by Joseph Campbell, Bollingen Series 39, Pantheon Books, New York, 1955, vol. 2, pl. 2.

8. Figurines, Indus Valley. About 3000-1500 B.C. Ibid. pl. 3.

3. Vedic Medicine

The Aryans, the most eastern branch of the Indo-European family, migrated into the Indus Valley and conquered it toward the middle of the second millennium B.C.[1] They were closely related to the early Persians, and their language, the Vedic form of Sanskrit, was an Indo-European language that had much in common with old Iranian, and of course had many roots that we encounter also in Greek and other languages of the same family.

We must emphasize, from the very beginning, that Indian chronology before the Buddhist period presents almost insurmountable difficulties, and the dating of events by various scholars may differ not by centuries but by thousands of years. And even after the Buddhist period we sometimes find it extremely difficult to date a book, or to determine the lifetime of an individual. Many factors are responsible for this state of affairs. One is that so far we have no archaeological findings from the time of the early Indus civilizations to the time of Buddhism, and the campaign of Alexander the Great—that is, for a period of fifteen centuries. The excavations of early Indus sites were extraordinarily helpful, because they could be correlated with Mesopotamian chronology, and thus proved that the Aryan migration could not have taken place before the second millennium B.C. As for the early literature, the Vedas, we find it very difficult to date them with any degree of accuracy. There can be no doubt that the literature of India is old. Hymns, prayers, ritual prescriptions, records of historical events, were transmitted by word of mouth for centuries before they were written down, just as the Homeric hymns were sung by itinerant bards long before they were edited and collected to form the books known to us today. The oral tradition was more highly cultivated in India than in any other country, and was considered the authentic version of a text to a much higher degree than any written book. Even the Buddhist canon was transmitted orally long before it was written down. Today we can still find Brahmans who know the 1028 hymns of the Rigveda by heart. The dating of an oral tradition is obviously not easy, and in India an additional factor increases our difficulties. The Egyptian, Babylonian, and Greek civilizations have completed their courses. Their languages have become dead languages today. No Homeric hymns are heard in today's Greece, no Babylonian astrologer is active in Iraq, and Egyptian surgeons are trained in Paris. In India, however, the ancient culture is still alive. The sacred books of the early Aryans are still the canons of Hinduism. Vedic hymns are still recited, old rites still performed, and the classics of medicine are reprinted and commented upon not only as historical documents but for the instruction of physicians. When a literature is preserved in writing after centuries of oral tradition, and when it remains alive for several thousand years, it obviously undergoes changes. Passages are left out, others are added, commentaries become part of the text, and after a few thousand years it is almost impossible to assign a definite date to a book or parts of it.

Nevertheless, it seems highly probable that the Aryans migrating from the high plateau of Iran through the mountain passes of Afghanistan entered the Indus Valley arround 1500 B.C. They found the region occupied by tribes of dark-skinned, flat-nosed people whom they called Dâsas, slaves, while they spoke of themselves as Aryas, as lords. These early dark inhabitants of India, of whose early history hardly anything is known, the Mundas and Dravidas, spoke agglutinative languages, and may have entered India from the east. They were not barbarians but had cities which the Aryans conquered, pushing the inhabitants gradually to the south. From the Indus Valley the Aryans moved east and conquered the valley of the Ganges, until they finally held a territory that reached from coast to coast and from the Himalaya to the Vindhya Mountains. They never conquered the whole subcontinent: in the course of its entire history India was never united under one rule. The Vedas reflect these early struggles between Aryans and Dâsas, and also battles between one Aryan tribe and another. The conquerors were not a united nation but tribes, each led by a chieftain, or a king—political conditions very similar to those of early Greece.

Language and religion were the bonds that united them, and from the very beginning the Aryans in India appeared as a highly religious people. Religion has dominated Indian life throughout the course of its history, and even in our days of crude materialism India maintains its spirituality; its greatest political leader, Gandhi the Mahatma, was a saint. It is no wonder that the priest who stood next to the king gradually became the most important man in society. He was the intellectual, knew rites that became ever more complicated, was in contact with the spiritual powers that seemed to determine the fate of man on earth, the outcome of battles, prosperity or misery of the kingdom, and life in the hereafter. The priestly caste, the Brahmans, therefore became the highest of all social classes, while king and nobility constituted the next upper class, that of the warriors, or Kshatriya. The mass of the people were farmers and merchants; their caste was that of the Vaisyas. At the bottom of the social scale were the Sudra, the conquered Dravidas, kept at first as slaves, later as free men engaged in humble occupations. The caste system so highly characteristic of Indian society must have been developed around 1000 B.C.—that is, when the Aryans had conquered the entire north of India and Brahmanism had become strong.[2]

Our chief sources of archaic Indian culture and also medicine after the Aryan invasion are the four Vedas.[3] The word Veda means knowledge, sacred lore, and the Vedas were thought to be revealed by the godhead, by Brahma, and received by inspired sages who passed them on by word of mouth. The texts consisted of hymns, prayers, incantations, chants, ritual formulas. They were organized into collections, Samhitas, and later commentaries were written for various purposes, the Brahmanas, Aranyakas, and Upanishads, about which we shall have to say more in a later chapter.

The chronology of these writings, as I said before, presents very great difficulties. There is general agreement that the Rigveda, a collection of 1028 hymns recited in connection with sacrifices brought to the gods, is the oldest of the four Vedas, but it is obvious that not all the hymns date from the same period.[4] Some, probably the majority, must have been brought by the Aryans when they entered the Indus Valley, and the gods are the same that we also find in old Iran and Mitanni. Other hymns may have been composed at the time of the conquest, and others again may have been added to the collection later. At any rate, there can be no doubt that the Rigveda preceded the other collections. Thus the Yajurveda[5] contains many hymns taken from the Rigveda.

The Yajurveda consists of five samhitas, five collections of prayers and ritual texts in verse and in prose; four of these collections known as the Black Yajurveda also contain explanatory glosses in prose incorporated in the text, while in the fifth, the White Yajurveda, litanies and commentaries are separated. The texts deal with the various sacrifices, with the role of him who brings the sacrifice, with the royal consecration, the construction of the fire altar, and similar subjects. The Samaveda [6] is also derived from the Rigveda. Most of its 1810 stanzas can be traced to the Rigveda as their source. It is a collection of chants to be sung on special occasions, in the village or in the woods. Unfortunately the original music has not been preserved, and we only know the melodies recorded at a later time.

Rigveda, Yajurveda, and Samaveda are very closely related. They were the backbone of India's religious life for over three thousand years, and today are still the most important canonic books of Hinduism. Slightly different, not in language and style but in intention, is the Atharvaveda,[7] a collection of 731 hymns, prayers, incantations, and charms in twenty books. It is somewhat later than the Rigveda and may have been composed around 1200 B.C. Because of its outspokenly magic character it was not immediately accepted as a canonic book, and it is still not recognized as such by some schools of southern India. As a source of archaic medical history, however, it is the most important book, for it reflects better than any other collection popular views and practices. Most of its verses were not recited for the glorification of the great gods or on the occasion of formal sacrifices but to protect the people against enemies, witchcraft, lightning, worms, and all kinds of disease, or to provide for them welfare and long life, freedom from fear, recovery of virility, the love of a girl, a husband, fecundity, successful pregnancy, a male child, relief from insanity and other diseases, or even to take care of such trivial matters as 'to fasten and increase the hair.' In other words, this is a book which reminds us very strongly of certain Egyptian and Mesopotamian texts.

As the earliest literary documents of India the Vedas give us an idea of what conditions were like in the second and in the beginning of the first millennium B.C. The life of the Aryan settlers was very similar to that of the Indo-European tribes who occupied Greece at about the same time. People lived in villages in wooden houses. Agriculture and cattle-breeding were their main occupations. Industries were home industries, and the family produced the textiles for clothing, tools, and weapons, and whatever else was needed. Commerce must have flourished as it had done before in the days of Mohenjo Daro and Harappa. Trade routes once established are seldom abandoned. Peoples may change but the demand for goods remains and, if conditions permit, is satisfied in much the same way. Trade obviously was by barter, and the cow, the most treasured possession of a cattle-breeding society, was the measure of all values. However, precious metals, notably gold, and jewelry, were also used as a medium of exchange then as they are today. Millions of Indians still invest their savings in bracelets, rings, and other jewelry, upon which they draw in case of need.

The main foods of the early Aryans were milk, ghee—that is, clarified butter—various kinds of grain, and the meat of oxen, sheep, and goats and on certain occasions also horse meat—meat probably was consumed only on festive occasions after it had been sacrificed to the gods. To most people all over the world, then as today, meat is a luxury. An alcoholic beverage, *sura,* prepared from grain, and another intoxicating liquor, *soma,* brewed from an unidentified herb, played a very important part in the cult, very much as *peyotl* did in Mexico. The early Aryans were not vegetarians nor did they abstain from alcoholic beverages.

The family was the social unit. There was no child marriage, and widows were not burned with their deceased husbands. Women held an honored position in the family and were not confined to the interior of the house. The tribe elected a king, but it seems that kingship soon became hereditary, although the king's decisions had in many cases to be approved by the tribal assembly. Wars were fought with swords and with bow and arrow, and like the Homeric heroes the chiefs went to war in chariots and met their opponents in fierce single combats. Chariot races were held just as in Greece; games and athletic contests seem to have been common to all Indo-European peoples. Hunting, dancing, and singing were other forms of recreation; lutes, flutes, and drums were the chief musical instruments. Whoring was considered a recreation also, and prostitutes were respected. Like other Orientals outside the Semitic orbit the Indians developed love-making into a great art, which had its textbooks, such as the famous *Kamasutra* of Vatsyayana.[8] Heterosexual love was glorified, and it seems that pederasty never played the part it did in Greece and later in Mohammedan countries.

We mentioned before that the early Aryans were a highly religious people, and indeed religion was to play a dominant role in Indian life throughout its history.[9] People in tropical countries are more inclined to lead a contemplative life than people in the north, and in no country has the art of meditation been brought to such perfection as in India.

The Aryans brought with them their gods, chief among them Dyaus, the sky god, equivalent to the Greek Zeus. His place was gradually taken by Varuna who personified the cosmic and moral order, and he was in turn superseded by Indra, originally the god of battles who became the national god of ancient India. Many of the Vedic hymns are addressed to Agni, who appears as sun in the sky, as lightning, and as fire on earth. In every house, on every hearth, a

sacred fire was kept burning, and numerous sacrifices were brought
to Agni. Frequently mentioned in connection with him were the
Maruts, storm gods, 'born from the laughter of lightning,' sons of
Rudra, himself a storm god, malevolent as storms are but also
benevolent at times, for do not storms bring the much-needed rains?
A whole book of the Rigveda was devoted to Soma, and the sacrifice
to him took a central place in Vedic ritual. Drinking of soma brought
ecstasy, protection from disease, and cure of many ailments. The
Ashvins, twin brothers riding their chariots in the sky and announcing dawn and twilight, were also healers—the physicians of the gods
who were invoked by sick mortals. They restored eyesight to the
blind and performed many miraculous cures. They correspond in
origin and function to the Greek Dioscuri, who in turn were succeeded by the Christian saints Cosmas and Damian. It is interesting to
note that healers frequently appear as twins, and we are inclined
to think of surgery and medicine as being twin crafts, but this is
probably a late interpretation; I do not know of any valid explanation
for the twin gods in their relation to medicine.

At all times India has had a rich and colorful pantheon; people still
pray and sacrifice to Vishnu, Shiva, or some other individual god to
whom they feel particularly close. However, at a very early time it
was vaguely felt that this immense multitude of gods represented but
various aspects of one, *the* divine being.

What medicine did the Vedic Aryans practice? [10] What did they
think of health and disease, of the human body and its place in the
whole of nature? We have no medical book from that early period and
could not possibly expect one. All the literature we possess is religious,
but just as it tells us about life in general in those early days so it
gives us a great deal of information about medical views and practices. We must keep in mind, however, that medicine was a craft,
and that treatments must have been performed which were not
described in writing but were passed on from father to son, from
master to pupil, and appeared in medical books only centuries later.

Vedic medicine, as we may call it for brevity's sake, was archaic
medicine, and as such it was very similar to that of other early civiliza-

tions: that is, it was a combination of religious, magical, and empirical views and practices. The gods were thought to make a mortal sick as a punishment, either directly or through the intermediary of demons; treatment consisted in placating the irate deity and in driving out and fighting the demons. Or a man could become ill as a result of witchcraft, and a magic cause of disease had to be eliminated by magical means. Finally the Indians, like all other peoples, had a considerable store of knowledge of drugs and other rational treatments gained empirically.

We discussed the basic ideas of primitive and archaic medicine in great detail in the first volume of this book. There is no point in repeating what we said in dealing with Egyptian and Mesopotamian medicine. What we shall do instead is illustrate the basic aspects of Vedic medicine by quoting a few texts. Like Greece but unlike the ancient civilizations of the Near East, India soon outgrew the archaic stage and developed a scientific system of medicine whose roots obviously reach far back. Our chief source will be the Atharvaveda, and we shall also have to consult the *Kaushika Sutra,* a commentary which is particularly important, since it indicates the manual rites that had to be performed when hymns were recited.[11]

Sin, the breaking of a norm, the wanton cursing of a fellow man, and similar transgressions result in illness, for the gods and particularly Varuna, guardian of law and order, punish the offender. But also other gods—Rudra, Soma, any one of the nineteen gods invoked in these texts—may send illness.[12] Here, as in the Near East, we also encounter the view that a patient may suffer for the guilt of his parents, 'in consequence of a sin committed by thy mother or thy father.'[13] The remedy is prayer and sacrifice:

From the sins which knowingly or unknowingly we have committed, do ye, all gods, of one accord, release us!
If awake or if asleep, to sin inclined, I have committed a sin, may what has been, and what shall be, as if from a wooden post, release me!
As one released from a wooden post, as one in a sweat by bathing (is cleansed) of filth, as ghee is clarified by the sieve, may all (the gods) clear me from sin![14]

While this prayer does not mention disease specifically but is a general prayer for release from sin and, as is tacitly assumed, its consequences, the following text is without question to be recited by a sick man:

O Soma-and-Rudra, eject asunder the disease that has entered our household; drive far to a distance perdition; any committed sin put away from us.

O Soma-and-Rudra, do ye put all these remedies in our bodies, untie, loosen from us what committed sin may be bound in our bodies.[15]

Varuna could send all kinds of disease, but one was attributed to him in particular, namely dropsy:

Thy golden chamber, King Varuna, is built in the waters! Thence the king that maintains the laws shall loosen all shackles!

From every habitation (of thine), O King Varuna, from here do thou free us! If 'O waters, inviolable ones,' if 'O Varuna' we have said, from this (sin) O Varuna, free us ...

Loosen from us, O Varuna, all fetters, the uppermost, the nethermost, and those imposed by Varuna! Evil dreams and misfortune drive away from us: then may we go to the world of the pious![16]

A hut was built at a point of land where two rivers come together. The dropsical patient was placed in it. An offering was made while the prayer was recited, and the patient was washed with three bunches of grass which had been dipped in water during the recitation.[17]

Rudra's special way of inflicting illness was to shoot arrows at the victims, thus causing acute pains. The arrow was removed by prayer and incantation:

The arrow that Rudra did cast upon thee, into (thy) limbs, and into thy heart, this here do we now draw out away from thee.

From the hundred vessels which are distributed along thy limbs, from all of these do we exorcise forth the poisons.

Adoration be to thee, O Rudra, as thou casteth (thy arrow); adoration to the (arrow) when it has been placed upon (the bow); adoration to it as it is being hurled; adoration to it when it has fallen down![18]

The gods sent illness directly or through the intermediary of demons. Like Babylonia and Egypt, India knew of demons whose very function it was to cause illness. They had to be placated or driven out. Such an evil spirit was Takman,[19] a demon of fire, who caused the various kinds of fever. The following charm, with its mythological introduction, reminds us in many ways of Babylonian incantations:

When Agni having entered the waters, burned, where the (gods) who uphold the order (of the universe) rendered homage (to Agni), there, they say, is thy origin on high: do thou feel for us, and spare us, O Takman!

Whether thou art flame, whether thou art heat, or whether from licking chips (of wood) thou hast arisen, Hrudu by name art thou, O god of the fiery,[20] do thou feel for us, and spare us, O Takman!

To the cold Takman, and to the deliriously hot, the glowing,[21] do I render homage. To him that returns on the morrow, to him that returns for two (successive) days, to the Takman that returns on the third day, homage shall be! [22]

In this charm, which has more the character of a prayer, Takman appears almost as a god to whom tribute is paid, but in the following he is a demon, driven out of the patient, and transferred to an animal:

Homage (be) to the deliriously hot, the shaking, exciting, impetuous (Takman)! Homage to the cold (Takman), to him that in the past fulfilled desires!

May (the Takman) that returns on the morrow, he that returns on two (successive) days, the impious one, pass into this frog! [23]

Finally we have several texts in which an unidentified mountain plant *kushtha*[24] is prescribed for the patient suffering from fever. A prayer gives it the magic power to destroy the disease; a few stanzas may be quoted in illustration:

1. Thou art born upon the mountains, as the most potent of plants, come hither, O Kushtha, destroyer of the Takman, to drive out from here the Takman!

7. Thou art born of the gods, thou art Soma's good friend. Be thou

propitious to my in-breathing and my out-breathing, and to the eyes of mine!

9. 'Superior' O Kushtha, is thy name; 'superior' is the name of thy father. Do thou drive out all disease, and render the Takman devoid of strength!

10.   Pain in the head, affliction in the eye, and ailment of the body, all that shall the Kushtha heal—a divinely powerful (remedy) forsooth![25]

According to the *Kaushika Sutra* the powdered drug was made into a salve with butter and then applied to the sick man from head to foot.[26]

We know of other similar demons, such as Yakshma, who caused fever.[27] Jaundice was attributed to several demons, and its magic treatment consisted in banishing the yellow color to yellow creatures and objects, and in bringing redness to the patient from red objects and creatures, notably from a red bull. An elaborate ritual was developed to that end. The patient was to drink water mixed with hair from a red bull. An amulet consisting of a piece of bull's skin steeped in cow's milk and anointed with the dregs of ghee was tied around his neck. He must drink milk and eat prescribed foods; another amulet, consisting of hairs from the breast of a red bull glued together and covered with gold,[28] was tied on him while the following hymn was recited:

Up to the sun shall go thy heart-ache and thy jaundice: in the colour of the red bull do we envelop thee!

We envelop thee in red tints, unto long life. May this person go unscathed, and be free of yellow colour!

The cows whose divinity is Rohini, they who, moreover, are (themselves) red (rohinih)—(in their) every form and every strength we do envelop thee.

Into the parrots, into the ropanakas (thrush) do we put thy jaundice, and, furthermore, into the haridravas (yellow wagtail) do we put thy jaundice![29]

Cough was besought to 'fly forth along the soul's course of flight,' to 'fly forth along the expanse of the earth,' to 'fly forth along the flood of the sea.' [30] The flow of blood was stopped with a very poetic incantation beginning, 'The maidens that go yonder, the veins, clothed in red garment, like sisters without a brother, bereft of strength, they shall stand still!' [31] At the same time, as the manual part of the ritual, a poultice of dust, sand, and mud was applied. [32]

Yet disease was caused not only by the gods but also by fellow men through witchcraft, 'in that men have bewitched thee, one of thine own people (or) a strange person.' [33] And magic had to be fought by magical means: a white lump of earth was given to a dog, a certain amulet was attached to the patient, an oblation was poured, and faggots of a certain wood were laid on the fire [34] while the following hymn was recited:

The thousand-eyed curse having yoked his chariot has come hither, seeking out him that curses me, as a wolf the house of him that owns sheep.

Avoid us, O curse, as a burning fire (avoids) a lake! Strike here him that curses us, as the lightning of heaven the tree!

He that shall curse us when we do not curse, and he that shall curse us when we do curse, him do I hurl to death as a bone to a dog upon the ground! [35]

Diseases and desires of women play a large part in this literature. Women are more burdened by sex than men and need added protection. They have sought it in religion and magic at all times, and particularly in antiquity. Hence it is no wonder that a woman's whims and ailments figure in the earliest literature, religious, magic, and medical. One of the earliest medical monographs of Egypt is gynecological. [36] Women are mentioned repeatedly in the *Odyssey* as magicians who have an expert knowledge of drugs, poisons, and philters. In the Atharvaveda we have a number of hymns and charms to ensure conception, [37] but also to make one sterile, [38] conceive a son, [39] prevent miscarriage, [40] or secure easy parturition. [41]

The methods of preventing illness are determined by the views held on the causation of disease, and therefore religious and magic means will be resorted to in archaic medicine. At night when man is asleep he is an easy prey to evil spirits. He will seek protection before going to sleep by praying to the night: 'O night, the earthly space hath been filled with the father's orderings; great, thou spreadest thyself to the seats of the sky; bright darkness comes on ... Uninjured may we, O wide darksome night, attain thy further limit ... Let no demon, (no) mischief-plotter master us; let no evil-plotter master us ...' [42]

For the long life of a boy the parents would pray: 'For thee alone, O (death from) old age, this (boy) shall grow up: the other hundred kinds of death shall not harm him! Like a provident mother in her lap Mitra shall befriend him, shall save him from misfortune! ... Lead this dear child to life and vigour, O Agni, Varuna and King Mitra! As a mother afford him protection, O Aditi, and all ye gods, that he may attain to old age!' [43]

Evil omens which came in the form of pigeons,[44] owls,[45] black birds,[46] or evil dreams [47] were warded off by the recitation of hymns, and here as everywhere else amulets were made and worn for protection. The pearl, 'born of the wind, the atmosphere, the lightning, and the light,' [48] the shell, 'born in the sea, at the head of bright substances,' [49] and gold, 'which is born from fire, the immortal ... bestowed upon the mortals,' [50] were powerful substances, able to conquer disease and poverty and to grant long life. Witchcraft was destroyed by an amulet made from wood of the gangida, an un-identified tree,[51] and amulets combined with incantations were powerful remedies,[52] very similar in character to those so graphically described in the Egyptian papyrus Berlin 3027.[53]

The diseases mentioned in the Vedic books are numerous.[54] They are not described in any detail: religious books are not the place for elaborate descriptions of disease symptoms. Fever occurs frequently, and the term, in addition to meaning malaria, must have been used to designate many other infectious diseases such as typhoid and cholera. The diarrheas, so frequent in India today, were probably due to various forms of dysentery. Jaundice is a symptom that never escapes attention, being frequent in all tropical countries, where many people suffer from diseases of the liver. Heart disease and dropsy are mentioned, but we have no possibility of determining the nature and character of such diseases. Cough is an easily apparent symptom of bronchitis and pneumonia, while consumption is the end stage of a disease that may be tuberculosis, cancer, or anything. Eye diseases and skin diseases such as pustules, sores, and leprosy could not fail to attract attention. The light spots of the initial stages of leprosy are much more striking on dark than on white skin, and a dark plant was given to restore the color. Addressing the plant the priest said, 'The leprosy and the gray spots drive away from here— may thy native color settle upon thee—the white spots cause to fly away! ... The leprosy which has originated in the bones, and that which has originated in the body and upon the skin, the white mark begotten of corruption, I have destroyed with my charm.' [55] Tumors, abscesses, retention of urine, excessive discharges from the body, snake poisoning, and worms, as well as paralysis and mania, are objects of incantations. An interesting hymn of the Atharvaveda pictures the loudly jabbering manic patient who is 'bound and well secured.' Agni is invoked to quiet down his mind which 'has been maddened by the sin of the gods, or been robbed of sense by the Rakshas.' 'May the Apsaras restore thee, may Indra, may Bhaga restore thee; may all the gods restore thee, that thou mayest be freed from madness.' [56]

These few examples suffice to give us a picture of the magico-religious system of Vedic medicine. The texts quoted remind us vividly of Mesopotamian and Egyptian medicine. The prayers, incantations, and charms are very similar to those analyzed in detail in the preceding volume of this book, and the underlying views are very much the same. We may raise the question why there is no corresponding literature in ancient Greece.

Greek archaic medicine had religious and magic elements, to be sure, and we found traces of them in the Homeric epics. Greece also developed a complete system of religious medicine with magic elements in the cult of Asclepius and other healing deities. Everyday magic, the belief in the power of amulets, the belief in omens and in the importance of their correct interpretation, and many other magic ideas and procedures were always extant in Greece, but for centuries remained under the surface or were in the background; we have no early Greek book comparable to the Atharvaveda. One might argue that the Egyptians, Sumerians, Babylonians, Assyrians, and Indians were Orientals, that mysticism finds a more fertile soil in the hot climates of the East than in the temperate zone where people are more sober, and that all great world religions originated in the Orient. Such an explanation, however, would be too simple. In such matters the factor of time is of considerable importance. There is no old Greek literature, that is, no literature written before 1000 B.C. The Homeric epics reflect reminiscences of the Mycenaean period but were composed at a much later date. Literature of the type of the Atharvaveda, however, flourished in the third and second millenniums B.C. It was the expression of the aspirations and endeavors of men of a culture earlier than the Greek.

It would be a mistake to asssume that Indian medicine in the Vedic period was only magical and religious. Like all archaic medicine it also had empirical and rational elements, and probably many more than we can ascertain, since we have no medical books from that period. But the classical medical literature was the outgrowth of an old tradition, and there can be no doubt that much of its factual content could be traced back to the Vedic period. Medicine was not practiced by priests exclusively, but here, as everywhere else, also by laymen who knew symptoms of disease, had knowledge of drugs, and were able to perform certain operations. Even in the Vedic Samhitas, purely religious books, we find a reflection of anatomical, physiological, and pathological views which are neither magical nor religious, and we hear of treatments which impress us as being rational. We shall discuss them later, however, when we examine the classical medical literature of India and its Vedic roots.

NOTES

1. About the Vedic period of Indian civilization see the general histories and reference books quoted before. A book recently written by Indian scholars may be consulted profitably: *The Vedic Age,* ed. by R. C. Majumdar and A. D. Pusalker, London, 1951.

2. About the caste system see E. Sénart, *Les Castes dans l'Inde,* Paris, 1896; S. V. Ketkar, *The History of Caste in India,* Ithaca, N. Y., 1909; N. K. Dutt, *Origin and Development of Caste in India,* vol. I, London, 1931.

3. For the history of Indian literature M. Winternitz, *Geschichte der indischen Literatur,* Leipzig, 1909–20, 3 vols., is still authoritative. Louis Renou, *Anthologie sanskrite,* Paris, 1947, gives a cross section through Indian literature in French translation.

4. Sanskrit editions of the Rigveda by T. Aufrecht in A. F. Weber's *Indische Studien,* vols. 6–7, 1861–3, new ed. Bonn, 1877, and by Max Müller, 2nd ed., 1890–2, 4 vols.; German translations by H. Grassmann, Leipzig, 1876–7, 2 vols., and by A. Ludwig, Prague, 1876–88, 6 vols.; English translation by R. T. H. Griffith, Benares, 1896–7, and a partial translation by Max Müller and H. Oldenburg in the *Sacred Books of the East,* vols. 32 and 46, Oxford, 1891 and 1897.

5. Maitrayani Samhita, ed. by L. von Schröder, Leipzig, 1881–6, 4 vols., reprinted 1923; Taittirya Samhita, ed. by A. Weber, Berlin, 1871–2; Kapishtala Katha Samhita, ed. by Raghu Vira, Lahore, 1932; Kathaka Samhita, ed. by L. von Schröder, Leipzig, 1900–10, 3 vols.; Vajasaneyi Samhita, ed. by A. Weber, London, 1852. English translation of the White Yajurveda by R. T. H. Griffith, Benares, 1899.

6. Ed. with English translation by T. Benfey, Leipzig, 1899.

7. Sanskrit edition by R. Roth and W. D. Whitney, Berlin, 1856. English translation by W. D. Whitney, Cambridge, Mass., 1905, 2 vols. Partial translation by M. Bloomfield in *Sacred Books of the East,* vol. 42, Oxford, 1897. The quotations are from this edition unless indicated otherwise.

8. Sanskrit edition by Pandit Durgaprasada, Bombay, 1891. English translation published from manuscripts at Benares, 1883; German translation by R. Schmid, Leipzig, 5th ed., 1915.

9. On Vedic religion see: A. Bergaigne, *La Religion védique d'après les hymnes du Rig-Veda,* Paris, 1878–83, 3 vols.; A. Hillebrandt, *Vedische Mythologie,* Breslau, 1891–1902, 3 vols.; H. Oldenberg, *Die Religion des Veda,* Berlin, 1894; E. W. Hopkins, *The Religions of India,* Boston, 1895; M. Bloomfield, *The Religion of the Veda,* New York, 1908.

10. Recent publications that discuss Vedic medicine are: R. F. G. Müller, 'Die Medizin in Rg-Veda,' *Asia Major,* 1930, 6:315–76; R. F. G. Müller, *Grundlagen altindischer Medizin,* (Nova Acta Leopoldina, N. F., vol. 11, no. 74), Halle, 1942; H. R. Zimmer, *Hindu Medicine,* Baltimore, 1948; J. Filliozat, *La Doctrine classique de la médecine indienne,* Paris, 1949.

11. Sanskrit edition by M. Bloomfield, 'The Kauśika-Sūtra of the Atharva-veda,' *J. Am. Orient. Soc.,* vol. XIV. Partial German translation by W. Caland, *Altindisches Zauberritual,* Amsterdam, 1900.

12. They are listed and discussed in W. A. Jayne, *The Healing Gods of Ancient Civilizations,* New Haven, 1925, p. 145ff.

13. E. g. Ath., V, 30, 4 although the passage may also mean that father or mother bewitched the son.

14. Ath., VI, 115.
15. Ibid. VII, 42, transl. by Whitney.
16. Ibid. VII, 83.
17. *Kaushika Sutra*, 32, 14–16.
18. Ath., VI, 90.
19. About him see R. F. G. Müller, 'Der Takman des Atharvaveda,' *Artibus Asiae*, 1937, 6:230–42.
20. Most translators render *harita* by 'yellow,' but it also means 'fiery.'
21. The passage refers to the chill and heat experienced in fevers.
22. Ath., I, 25.
23. Ibid. VII, 116.
24. The plant, its origin, and effects are described in three hymns of the Atharvaveda, V, 4; VI, 95; XIX, 39. It has sometimes been identified with the Greek *kostos,* a drug that came from the East, the root of which was used as a spice, but the identification is uncertain.
25. Ibid. V, 4.
26. *Kaushika Sutra*, 28, 13.
27. See Rigveda, X, 163.
28. *Kaushika Sutra*, 26, 14–21.
29. Ath., I, 22.
30. Ibid. VI, 105.
31. Ibid. I, 17, 1.
32. *Kaushika Sutra*, 26, 10–13.
33. Ath., V, 30, 2, transl. by Whitney.
34. *Kaushika Sutra*, 48, 23–26.
35. Ath., VI, 37.
36. One of the Kahun papyri. See this book, vol. I, p. 302ff.
37. Ath., VI, 81.
38. Ibid. VII, 35.
39. Ibid. III, 23; VI, 11.
40. Ibid. VI, 17.
41. Ibid. I, 11.
42. Ibid. XIX, 47, transl. by Whitney.
43. Ibid. II, 28.
44. Ibid. VI, 27.
45. Ibid. VI, 29.
46. Ibid. VII, 64.
47. Ibid. VI, 46.
48. Ibid. IV, 10, 1.
49. Ibid. IV, 10, 2.
50. Ibid. XIX, 26, 1.
51. Ibid. II, 4.
52. Ibid. II, 9; IV, 36.
53. See this book, vol. I, p. 272.
54. They are listed in H. R. Zimmer, *Hindu Medicine,* Baltimore, 1948, p. 31f.,

and W. A. Jayne, *The Healing Gods of Ancient Civilizations,* New Haven, 1925, p. 150ff.

55. Ath., I, 23.
56. Ibid. VI, 111.

1. Vishnu, second god of the Hindu triad, marble, carved in relief. About eighth century A.D., in Wellcome Historical Medical Museum, no. 209/1946.

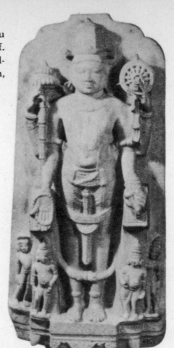

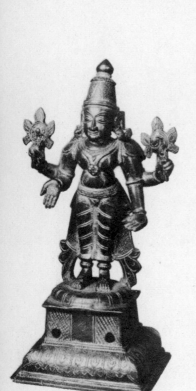

2. Vishnu, second god of the Hindu triad, copper, in Wellcome Historical Medical Museum, no. A 5432.

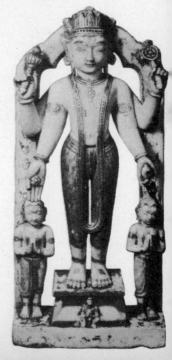

3. Vishnu, second god of the Hindu triad, marble, carved in relief, in Wellcome Historical Medical Museum, no. A 23956.

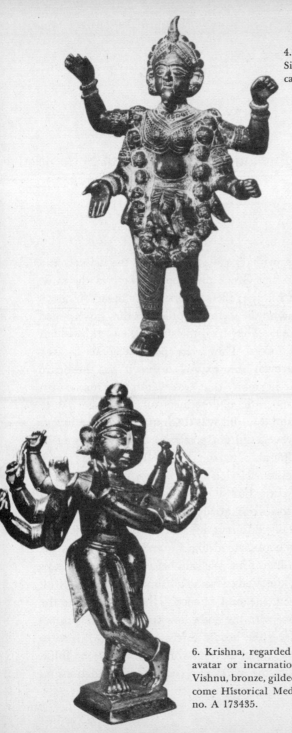

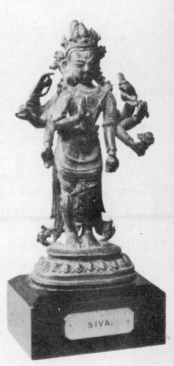

4. Devi, wife of the Hindu god, Siva, bronze, in Wellcome Historical Medical Museum, no. A 212190.

5. Siva, the third god of the Hindu triad, brass, in the Wellcome Historical Medical Museum, no. 16633.

6. Krishna, regarded as the eighth avatar or incarnation of the god Vishnu, bronze, gilded, in the Wellcome Historical Medical Museum, no. A 173435.

4. Indian Philosophies and Early Medical Schools

Greek philosophy began with speculations about the nature and origin of the world. The first Greek philosophers were at the same time the first scientists of Europe; their theories were based on observation of everyday life and on the technical processes they saw applied in the workshops of the cities. They tried to explain the world without resort to transcendental forces. They were not irreligious by any means, and the view has even been expressed that it was the desire to find in the cosmos the harmony that was wanting in man's own soul that drove the pre-Socratic philosophers to investigate nature beyond practical needs, and that this was the Ionian form of religious experience.[1] Greece, however, did not possess at the beginning of its literature anything comparable to the Veda. The earliest Greek literature consisted of epics. Hesiod's *Theogony* was a piece of religious writing, to be sure, but it was a mortal man's work, a collection of myths and stories told about the life of the gods.

The situation was totally different in India. There the Veda, a collection of old religious books, stood like a grand monument at the very beginning of Indian literature. We said before that Veda means knowledge, and, indeed, the Veda was at all times the source of all knowledge, including medicine and science. The Veda taught the people how to live at peace with the gods, how to secure their protection, how to be safe among the hostile forces of the world, how to maintain or restore their health, how to win a girl's love or fulfill other wishes. But hymns of the Veda also contained speculations on

168

the origin of the world, on the essence of the divine, and on man's nature and purpose in life. They became the starting point of all Indian philosophy as it was developed, notably in the Upanishads,[2] from the seventh century B.C. on, and in the Bhagavadgita,[3] a philosophical poem inserted into India's great epic, the Mahabharata.

In the course of the centuries various philosophic systems developed, among them six major systems considered orthodox because they all were based upon the authority of the Veda and accepted the social order of Brahmanism.[4] Much as they differed in detail they had some basic concepts in common. The primary element that constituted the universe was not water, fire, or air, as Greek philosophers believed, but Brahman, the universal spirit of which Atman, man's individual spirit, was a part, since Brahman was the source of origin of all forces of nature. The world was not matter but spirit.

Another old concept of the early Upanishads which became universal in India and spread far beyond its borders was that of reincarnation, which is closely linked up with the idea of Karma. It means that man's present and future life, his happiness or misery, are determined by his own actions. We are not burdened with an original sin for which we cannot be held responsible, nor do we depend on the grace of a personal god. The sum total of all our actions, good and evil, constitutes our Karma and determines whether we shall be reborn in a higher or lower station, where a new chance is given to us to improve our Karma. The goal of philosophy is to teach man how he should live in order to liberate his soul from the cycle of reincarnations. Moral perfection is the only way to salvation. Thus a transcendent philosophy has very practical consequences. If I am sick and suffer it is nobody's fault but my own, the result of mistakes committed by me in this or previous lives; it is my Karma. I am not punished for sin, but sin results logically in suffering. Hence if I wish to enjoy good health, be free from pain, and ultimately enter into what the Buddhists were to call Nirvana, I must lead a strictly moral and pure life and must help my fellow men, and not only them but all fellow creatures, the humblest animal as well as man. Indians have been guided in their behavior by these basic principles through-

out the centuries, irrespective of schools and sects. And in our days
they have been taught to live in an exemplary way by such men as
Ramakrishna [5] and Mahatma Gandhi.[6] It goes without saying that
these ideas influenced medicine very strongly, and to our day medicine
in India has maintained an outspokenly philosophical character.
Western medicine will succeed in India only if it is not applied
mechanically but is spiritualized so as to conform to the Indian mind.

It cannot be our task to discuss here in any detail the various
philosophic systems that were developed in India. We shall mention
only a few and those very briefly, in particular those which had a
deeper influence upon problems of health and disease.

The earliest philosophy worked into a complete system was the
Samkhya philosophy,[7] which was decidedly pre-Buddhistic—that is,
elaborated before the sixth century B.C. It is strictly dualistic. On one
side there are the eternal souls in their multiplicity, and on the other
the material world, essentially different, gradually evolved from the
still undifferentiated primordial element into which it will ultimately
dissolve. This philosophy is frequently called atheistic, although it
readily accepts the gods, demigods, and demons of the traditional
religions. It accepts them but declares that they, like all other
beings, are subject to death and reincarnation, and may enter into
the condition of complete redemption only through their own deeds.
The aim of this philosophy is to lead its adepts to the recognition of
the antagonism between soul and matter, and to teach them how to
divorce the soul completely from all that is material, and notably
from the organs of the body.[8]

The Samkhya philosophy had strong repercussions on medicine,
primarily through one of its late offshoots, the philosophy of Yoga.[9]
The date of its classic work, the *Yoga Sutra* of Patanjali [10] is
still controversial. The first three books may have been written in the
second century B.C., but the fourth cannot be so early as it reflects
late Buddhistic thought.[11] Yet there can be no doubt that the basic
ideas and techniques of Yoga are old. We find them in some of the
early Upanishads, we find them presented beautifully in the
Bhagavadgita, and some elements may even be traced back to the

Atharvaveda. We mentioned previously that a seal from Mohenjo
Daro represented a god in the characteristic position of a yogi.
This would be a further confirmation of the view that Samkhya and
Yoga have strong non-Aryan elements taken over at an early date
from the pre-Aryan civilizations of India.[12]

Yoga is sometimes called the theistic form of Samkhya, since it
accepts a personal god who is not subject to the cycle of reincarnations. But the two systems are not in any way antagonistic; on the
contrary, they supplement each other. Like Samkhya, Yoga is
dualistic and its goal is the same: namely, the liberation of the mind,
the true self, from material bonds. The mind is in continuous motion
like the surface of a lake, agitated from without by sense impressions
and from within by memories, emotions, urges, attachments to the
world. And as long as the mind is in motion we cannot come to the
true realization of our self. Hence Yoga endeavors to still the mind. It
teaches how to control the waves of the mind, for ignorance is the
chief obstacle in the path of Yoga. Our self is by nature pure and
divine, but ignorance covers it as with a veil, and ignorance leads to
egoism, attachment, aversion, and clinging to life, all of which become 'pain-bearing obstructions.' [13]

Yoga's most positive accomplishment and the one most influential in the control of health and disease was its development of a
method which could be taught and learned, a method of inward
concentration by which an individual's mind undoubtedly gained
far-reaching control over the body. The method consisted in psychosomatic practices which were to lead to a gradual detachment from
the world, and ultimately to the supreme ideal, renunciation, when
Yoga would be attained, and the true nature of the self would
stand revealed.[14] These practices began with posture *(asana)*, defined as that which is firm and pleasant. The chief requirement was
that the spine be kept straight. It is well known how later a whole
system of physical culture was developed with exercises intended to
benefit all parts of the body,[15] a system which can compete with the
best Swedish systems of gymnastics, although their physiological explanations may differ.[16]

The next step was regulation of breath through breathing exercises *(pranayama)*. The very correct idea was that there is a relation between breathing and thought. When we are afraid, nervous, or angry, the rhythm of our breathing is different from what it is when we are serene and at peace with the world. Hence the logical deduction was that if we are able to control our breathing we may thereby gain control over our thought. Yoga developed an elaborate system of breathing, postures, and exercises. Again, correct breathing takes an important place in all modern systems of physical culture.

The third practice named *pratyahara* is a mental exercise by which we learn to steady our mind, to apply it to our endeavors while withdrawing it from disturbing sense perceptions. Just as the tortoise draws in its limbs and is all by itself, protected from the outside world, so we must learn to withdraw from without unto ourselves.

Once the student yogi has learned to control his postures and breathing, and has steadied his mind so that it will not be distracted at every opportunity, he may proceed to the higher exercises, the first of which is concentration *(dharana)*. He will need the guidance of a *guru,* a teacher, since these exercises are very difficult and cannot be performed mechanically but must be varied according to the student's development. With a mind now firmly under control the student concentrates upon some ideal—a vision, a dream, an image, such as the light within the heart—and once he has mastered the technique of concentration he is ready for the next step, meditation *(dhyana),* which is a condition of perfect concentration upon one idea. At this stage the outside world vanishes, the senses no longer perceive it, and the next stage, *samadhi,* is entered into when the mind merges with the object of contemplation. The mind is now set free, time and space have been overcome, the door to the transcendental world has been opened, the yogi has visions; a feeling of elation, of ecstasy, fills his heart, and some are even said to acquire occult powers. The final stage reached by only a few is that of transcendental consciousness, the complete awareness of the divine self, complete liberation, and merging with the godhead. 'Supreme happiness comes to the yogi whose mind is peaceful, whose passions are at rest, who is stainless and has become one with God.' [17]

All religions know ecstatic conditions, the mystic communion with the deity. In our previous volume we discussed the Siberian shaman who falling into a trance acquired healing powers. The prophets of all civilizations were mystics, the prophets of the Old Testament as well as the Pythia of Delphi. Mystic communion with God was the central part of the Greek mystery religions; Christian and Mohammedan saints experienced the state of supreme ecstasy. But nowhere was the technique of meditation developed to such a high degree of perfection as in India, and spreading from India with Buddhism, it was developed in Tibet, China, and as far as Indian influence reached.

Nobody will deny that the mind has an enormous power over the body. Every cell of our organism is controlled by the nervous system which conveys impulses of the mind. Every physician knows that the mere will power of a patient, his determination to get well, is a strong and in many cases decisive healing factor. How much more potent must be the effect of a mind concentrated in meditation. We may think of auto-suggestion, auto-hypnosis, but whatever the mechanism may be there can be no doubt that a philosophy such as that of Yoga had great medical potentialities. A German Sinologist, Eduard Erkes, who learned Taoist methods of meditation, reported that even a beginner could cure light colds, headaches, neuritic pains, and similar ailments by meditation, as he had experienced personally.[18]

A few words should also be said about Vedanta, although its influence on medicine was no stronger than that of other systems. Vedanta has spread to the West recently and has been called the scientific approach to religion.[19] Vedanta societies have been founded in various cities of America and Europe. Meetings are held and a bi-monthly journal, *Vedanta and the West,* is published in California. There was a time when Buddhism made a strong appeal to Europeans, so much so that Buddhist monasteries were founded in Berlin, Lausanne, and a few other cities. Now Vedanta is spreading.[20] What is the cause of its appeal? Is it the lure of a pure voice from the East that attracts a war-weary society becoming tired of useless, mechanical gadgets, and finding no satisfaction in its traditional religion? The best we can do to answer these questions is to listen to a modern European interpreter of Vedanta, Christopher Isherwood.[21] According to him the essence of Vedanta can be summed up in three basic propositions, namely, that man's nature is divine, that the aim of life is to realize this divine nature, and that all religions are essentially in agreement. It is the simplicity, rationalism and tolerance of Vedanta that give it its wide appeal, as is also the case with Buddhism. Vedanta became the orthodoxy of Brahmanism, and was developed from the teachings of the Upanishads, the Brahma Sutras, and the Bhagavadgita. Other philosophies and many religious sects emerged in India in the course of the centuries, but Vedanta remained the basis of all of them, or, at least, of most of them.

Unlike Samkhya, Vedanta is a monistic philosophy. There is but one reality and nothing else. This reality is Brahman. It is beyond sense perception, is omnipresent. Within the creature it is Atman, and Atman and Brahman are identical, the divine, eternal, all-permeating essence from which objects emerge just as we pass from dreamless sleep to dream and finally awaken. But all objects, the very universe as we perceive it with our senses, are unreal, a mere appearance, an illusion, what the Indians call Maya, for there is but one reality and that is Brahman. Man's aim is to realize Atman, his true and essential nature, and thus to merge with Brahman, to realize his identity with it. This obviously is not easy, since we are born with our Karma, the accumulated sum of our deeds in previous lives. We must improve our Karma in our present life until at some time in some future life it becomes completed and we may then experience Samadhi, the bliss of having realized our divine nature. Thus Vedanta has the doctrine of Karma and reincarnation in common with most Indian philosophic systems.

These idealistic philosophies did not remain unopposed. As early as pre-Buddhist days a purely materialistic school of thought arose; it went under the name of Lokayata, which means literally 'belonging to the world of sense' and was attributed to Charvaka as its founder. No greater contrast could be imagined than between this philosophy and the idealistic systems mentioned before. To quote Garbe, one of the greatest scholars on Indian philosophy, 'Lokayata allows only perception as a means of knowledge, and ... recognizes as the sole reality the four elements, i.e., matter, and teaches that, when a body is formed by the combination of the elements, the spirit also comes into existence .... With the destruction of the body the spirit returns again into nothingness.' [22] There is no room for Karma in this system: the spirit is destroyed with the body. There is no reincarnation, and no authority of any kind is ascribed to the Vedas. The ritual of the Brahmans is declared a fraud intended only to enrich the priestly caste. The school undoubtedly had a following, but it was considered heretic and was opposed. Its writings are lost. We know about its doctrines only from the arguments of its opponents. Had it prospered it might have led to a scientific development similar to that which was initiated in the schools of the Milesian philosophers in Greece, but its approach to the problems of life and death was so diametrically opposed to the traditional Indian way of thinking that it hardly had a chance to succeed. Other schools which denied the law of Karma did not fare much better. Thus the school of Makkhali Gosala, a contemporary of the Buddha, stood for a rigid determinism, denying free will and moral responsibility of the individual. It is not our actions that determine our fate but circumstances and the environment.[23]

Many reform movements sprang up in the sixth century B.C. How can man free himself from the inexorable cycle of reincarnations? Brahmanism and the various philosophical schools had answered the questions, but other answers, other solutions were sought. No country in the world produced more religious sects and philosophic schools than India. Its very nature provides a fertile breeding ground for them. The cold of the northern world can be overcome through action only, while the intense summer heat of the Indian plains leads to inward contemplation, as do also the months of monsoon when communications are frequently interrupted and the individual seeks refuge under a roof.

One reform movement was the sect founded by Vardhamana, who became known as the Great Hero, Mahavira, or as the Victor, Jina. His school, known as Jainism, urged its members to seek Nirvana through most severe ascetic discipline, rigid fasts, and even death from starvation. Jainism still has over a million followers in India but at all times it remained a local sect. On the other hand, the reform initiated by Siddhatta Gotama Shakyamuni, who was to be known to the world as the Awakened-One, the Buddha, became one of the great world religions and a universal philosophy that had close affinities to medicine and influenced its course considerably. What gave it its strong appeal, not only to the people of India but to those of the entire Far East? Let us first consider the life of the founder, as it appears when it is divested of the infinity of legendary embellishments.[24]

The cradle of Buddhism was northeastern India, the region south of Nepal at the foot of the Himalaya Mountains. Toward the middle of the sixth century B.C.—that is, at the time when the Buddha was born—the region was made up of states ruled by hereditary or elected clan chiefs or rajas. In one of the small states, in the capital Kapilavatthu, about one hundred miles north of Benares, the future Buddha was born, the son of the local king, Suddhodana, and his wife Maya. The child grew up in luxury, carefully protected, as became a prince and future ruler. Following the custom of the country he was married young to princess Yasodhara and had a son Rahula, who later became his disciple.

Tradition tells us how he discovered the misery of the world. One day wishing to go to his garden-house, he had his driver make ready the chariot. On the way he saw 'a decrepit old man wasted by age, broken-toothed, grey-haired, bowed and bent-bodied, holding a staff and trembling ... "Fie on earthly existence," he cried, "in which to him who is born decay will be known!" Then with agitated heart he turned back and re-entered his mansion.'[25] Again, one day driving to the garden-house, he saw a sick man covered with ulcers, a poor

leper, and again he drove back deeply shaken by what he had seen.
After a while he had a third experience: he saw a dead man
whose body was entering the stage of decomposition. He suddenly
realized that he who lived in health and luxury was also subject to
old age, disease, and death. 'As I thus thought all intoxication (with
youth ... with health ...) with life utterly left me.' But then again
on another day 'going towards his garden-house he saw one who
had retired [from worldly life], duly robed and covered.' That day he
went to the garden-house and took pleasure in the thought of giving
up rank and wealth, of retiring from worldly life too, like the mendicant brother he had just encountered on his path. Man is born,
suffers illness, old age, and death, only to be reborn and to experience again the whole cycle of miseries. Was there no remedy?
What was the evil, its cause, its chance of being overcome? This
he must find out. Disease, old age, and death—in other words,
phenomena that belong to the physician's realm—were the starting
point of the Buddha's thinking, and he was to become the spiritual
doctor of mankind.

And so on a night when the moon was full, after a last look at
his sleeping wife and young son, he secretly left the palace, had his
hair and beard cut, assumed the yellow robes of the mendicant
brothers, 'and went forth from the household to the homeless life.'
He first did what an Indian does in such a case; he sought a guru,
a teacher, a wise man who would instruct him in the rituals and
disciplines, and who might be able to quiet his doubts. Begging for
his food he wandered to the Kingdom of Magadha, near the capital
of which two famous Brahmans lived. He became their disciple,
but was disappointed in both. They taught him prayers, rites, sacrifices, and methods of meditation, but he found that this was not
the path that leads to tranquility, highest knowledge, full enlightenment, Nirvana. Again he departed; 'pursuing the good, seeking the
supreme path of tranquility, I journeyed by stages among the Ma-
gadhas and came to where Uruvela, the army-township, was. There
I saw a delightful spot and a fair grove, and a clear flowing river,
delightful and easy of approach, and finally a village near by in

which to beg food.' [26] There he remained for six years, thinking, meditating, fasting to the point of starvation, submitting himself to the most rigorous ascetic disciplines. His example attracted disciples who looked upon him as a great yogi. But after six years of exercises and trances he found that this was not the right path to salvation either. Then one evening he sat cross-legged under a fig tree, which from then on was called Bodhi or Bo Tree, tree of enlightenment. The god Kama-Mara (Desire and Death) approached him and tempted him, but he remained in meditation, reaching immeasurable heights of thought, and ere the night was out, he experienced the Great Awakening and became the Buddha. And he sat there for seven days under the Bo Tree, living in the bliss of liberation. Now he knew he had the answer to his problems and had a mission, to teach his fellow men the Noble Truths and guide them on the path that leads to the Great Peace, to Nirvana. From then until his death around 477 B.C. he wandered through the lands of northeastern India, preaching to an ever-growing crowd of followers, organizing his Order. He addressed himself to high and low, irrespective of caste. Kings, like Bimbisara, King of Magadha, joined the movement, and after the master's death his teachings were carried far and wide by his disciples. He himself never wrote a book; he preached and taught, but his sermons were preserved by his closest students, who passed them on by word of mouth until they were written down and became the Buddhist Canon.

Heinrich Zimmer has pointed out that the Buddha proceeded exactly as the physician of his time did when he was called to the sickbed of a patient.[27] The physician was instructed to examine first whether the patient was actually sick, whether his complaints were justified. He then proceeded to make a diagnosis ascertaining the nature and origin of the disease. In the next stage he gave the prognosis. Is the disease curable or not, are we at least able to alleviate it? If there was no cure or hope, the physician would withdraw and make way for the priest. Otherwise, the physician's fourth task was to determine the treatment and to instruct the patient how to carry it through. The Buddha's four Noble Truths corresponded exactly to these four major tasks of the physician, and in announcing them in his famous first sermon delivered to his first five disciples in a deer park near Benares he became the spiritual doctor of mankind. Illness, he found, was very real indeed. 'Earthly existence indeed is sorrowful, decay is sorrowful, disease is sorrowful, death is sorrowful, union with the unpleasing is sorrowful, separation from the pleasing is sorrowful, the wish which one does not fulfil is sorrowful—in brief, desirous transient individuality is sorrowful.' [28] In other words, life is instrinsically sorrowful.

And what is the nature and origin of all this suffering? The Buddha answered the question with his Second Noble Truth. The origin of sorrow 'is this recurring craving associated with enjoyment and desire, seeking enjoyment everywhere, namely, the craving for sense-pleasures, the craving for individual existence, the craving for super-existence.' Thus, ignorant craving is the cause of suffering, not guilt or a hypothetical original sin. Because we are ignorant, we constantly crave for lust, for satisfaction of our many appetites, for life as individuals now and after death. What is the prognosis? Is it at all possible to suppress this endless suffering? Yes, it is and the Third Noble Truth declares: the cessation of 'sorrow is the cessation of this very craving, so that no remnant or trace of it remains—its abandonment, its renouncement, liberation from it, detachment from it.' So it is possible to overcome this craving, cause of all sorrow, but what is the remedy? The remedy is 'that Noble Eightfold Path, namely, right outlook, right will, right speech, right action, right self-discipline, right activity, right self-knowledge, right self-transcendence.'

Buddhism thus placed chief emphasis on high morality. Not the rituals of the Brahmans, nor prayers, nor sacrifices to the gods will lead to final liberation from sorrow, but only a life that is pure and moral in thought, word, and deed. In his First Sermon the Buddha declared explicitly that the Noble Eightfold Path was the middle road to peace which avoids both extremes. 'Which two? On the one hand that which is linked and connected with lust through sensuous pleasures, and is low, ignorant, vulgar, ignoble, and profitless; and on the other hand that which is connected with self-mortification, and is painful, ignoble and profitless. Avoiding both these extremes ... the middle road ... bringing insight, bringing knowledge, leads to tranquility, to highest knowledge, to full enlightenment, to Peace (Nirvana).' [29] It is the road from ignorance to Buddhahood.

There was no room for a personal god, a creator or divine providence, in such a system. The Buddha did not speculate about the soul, about Brahman and Atman. The law of Karma was inexorable. What we are and experience is the logical result, the iron consequence of our thoughts, words, and deeds in this or previous lives. If we lead a highly moral life along the Eightfold Path we improve our Karma, we may expect a better reincarnation and may ultimately hope to enter Nirvana, the condition of perfect peace, beyond thought and consciousness, released from the law of Karma and from the cycle of reincarnations.

The Buddhist community consisted of laymen and monks. Everybody could join it by taking the 'Triple Refuge,' pronouncing the words, 'I take refuge in the Buddha, I take refuge in his Doctrine, I take refuge in his Brotherhood,' [30] and by observing the fivefold morality: abstinence from the destruction of life in all its forms, abstinence from taking what is not given, abstinence from unholy living (meaning particularly the observance of conjugal fidelity), abstinence from false speaking, and abstinence from intoxicating wine and spirits causing negligence. It was even more meritorious for the laymen also to observe, at least for certain periods of time, three additional rules: namely, abstinence from eating at wrong times; abstinence from dancing, singing, music, and watching entertainments; abstinence from wearing garlands and using scent and unguents for adornment and ostentation. In addition to these eight pledges the monks had to observe two more, abstinence from high or large beds—that is, soft beds—and abstinence from receiving gold and silver—in other words, a vow of poverty. The monks were supported by the laymen of the Buddhist community, who earned merit by attending to their professional duties, by carefully observing the Fivefold Morality, and by giving alms liberally. The monks, on the other hand, were the spiritual advisers of the lay members. They lived in complete chastity and poverty, strictly observing all the other pledges and preaching to the community. Membership in the Brotherhood was open to all irrespective of caste, which was a revolutionary move, bound to arouse the hostility of the Brahmans. Membership in the Order, on the other hand, was not irrevocable. If a monk felt that he was unable to live up to his pledges he was free to relinquish the Order and to live henceforth as a lay member, taking a wife and engaging in a profession or trade. By leading a meritorious life both monks and lay members were improving their Karma and getting closer to the path that leads to Nirvana.

We usually think of Buddhism as a religion, and in the course of time it did become the religion of almost the entire Far East. But in the beginning it had much more the character of a philosophy. As a matter of fact, it had many elements in common with Samkhya, Yoga, and Vedanta, although it differed from these in some decisive points. Buddhism never took the place of Brahmanism, and never developed a ritual of its own. When people married, had children, or cremated their dead, they observed Hinduist rites. This was a strength and at the same time a weakness of Buddhism. It was very adaptable and, as a matter of fact, was superimposed upon existing local religions all over the Far East. But this very adaptability made it also highly vulnerable, and in many countries Buddhism became so inextricably interspersed with local rites and superstitions that little was left of the pure philosophic doctrine of the Buddha. And just as we in the West had a Counter-Reformation from which the Roman Catholic Church emerged purified and stronger than before, so there was a strong Hinduistic counter-movement. Shivaism and Vishnuism acquired an active clergy,[31] and Buddhism was finally driven from the Indian continent, to survive in Ceylon, Tibet, and in the Far East. But before its disappearance it was a rich source of inspiration for many centuries, and exerted a profound influence on the fine arts, literature, music, statesmanship, the art of living and dying, and also on medicine. With its tolerance, its principle of non-violence, its universal compassion extended to all living creatures, its high morality and humanity, Buddhism had and still has a great message for the world.

The ways of Indian philosophy were different from those of Greece, and since medicine always reflects the philosophy of its time we may also expect differences in the systems of medicine of the two areas. Yet medicine is a highly practical matter. Its purpose is not theoretical knowledge of nature, although the physician's experience has at all times contributed to the understanding of nature. The physician's task is earthbound, spiritual though his philosophic outlook may be. Diseases are very much the same everywhere, producing the same symptoms in different countries, and individuals react to them in similar ways. Like problems call for like or, at least, similar solutions, and this is why we shall find great similarities in the procedures and achievements of Greek and Indian doctors.

The Hippocratic writings can be dated with fair accuracy, or at any rate assigned to a certain century. The great Indian medical collections of Charaka, Susruta, and Vagbhata which correspond to the Hippocratic writings, like so many other Indian books, present great chronological problems to be discussed in detail in another chapter. There can be no doubt that they were written relatively late, not before the beginning of our era, but it is equally certain that their content must be much older, the result of a long, for the most part oral, tradition.

Indians look to the Veda as the source of all their science and learning. Just as the philosophy of Vedanta was considered derived from the Veda, so also was the medicine of the Golden Age. We saw that the Rigveda and particularly the Atharvaveda were concerned with matters of health and disease. There a Vedic medicine that must have flourished for several centuries, and Indian medicine thereafter was named Ayurveda, 'Knowledge of Long Life,' or 'Wisdom of Long Life,' a very good term since it puts the emphasis not on healing but on the prolongation of life, and that includes the promotion of health and the prevention of illness.

What was medicine like in the thousand-year period from the time when the Veda was written to the time when the great medical compilations were given literary form? We have no medical books from that period, nothing comparable to the Upanishads or to the great epics Mahabharata and Ramayana. All we have are traditions which must be legendary to a certain extent, but in all probability also relate historical facts. In all ancient civilizations the origin of medicine was traced back to the gods or at least to culture heroes. Thoth revealed the healing art to the Egyptians, Apollo to the Greeks, and in a similar way the Indians attributed the invention of medicine to Brahma, creator of the world and all that is in it, fount of all knowledge. He instructed other gods in the 'Wisdom of Long Life' and they passed it on to heroes of old from whom mortal men finally learned it. Let us hear the story of the origins of Ayurveda as it is related in the opening paragraphs of the Charaka Samhita: [32]

Bharadvaja, the mighty ascetic, in search of (the science of) longevity approached Indra, having deemed him, the lord of the immortals, worthy of suit. Daksha Prajapati (the progenitor) first obtained the Science of Life in its entirety as promulgated by Brahma (the Great One, the Creator) and from him in turn the Ashwin Twins obtained it. From the Ashwin Twins the god Shakra (Indra) acquired it. Therefore Bharadvaja bidden by the sages approached Shakra. When diseases arose like so many impediments to the austerity, fasting, study, continence and the vows of the embodied souls, then the great sages, the doers of good, keeping compassion for creatures foremost, met together on the sacred slopes of the Himalayas.

A list of names follows, names of great sages of old, 'all of them veritable mines of the Brahmic lore, and of restraint and discipline, and resplendent with the glow of austerities, like to fires fed with oblations—seated at ease there, (they) initiated the following inquiry:

"Health is the supreme foundation of virtue, wealth, and enjoyment and salvation. Now diseases are the destroyers of health, of the good of life, and even of life itself. Thus has arisen the great impediment to the progress of humanity. What shall be the means of remedying it?" Having observed thus they sat in meditation.

Then they saw with the eye of understanding, their refuge in Indra. "He, the lord of the immortals, shall tell us rightly the means of overcoming disease."

Bharadvaja was delegated to approach the god, and Indra, 'knowing his wide understanding, propounded in a few words the Science of Life. He taught the science of causes, symptoms and medication, the supreme refuge of both the healthy and the ailing, the tripartite science, eternal and holy, which the Great Father (Brahma) knew.' Bharadvaja 'soon learned correctly, by single-minded devotion, the whole Science of Life, tri-based and extending without end . . . and (in his turn) taught it to the sages, without either adding or withholding any part. . . . These great sages perceived this science with the eye of discernment; the nature of the general and the particular; the substances, their qualities, action and inherent relation.' Then one of them, Punarvasu, more commonly known under the name of Atreya or Krishna Atreya, 'the most benevolent, moved by compassion for all creatures, bestowed the science of life on his six disciples. Agnivesha, Bhela, Jatukarna, Parasara, Harita, and Ksharapani received the teaching of the sage.' Agnivesha became the foremost compiler of Ayurveda. But Bhela and the others made their own compilations and read them to Atreya and the assembly of the sages. And these compilations approved by the great masters obtained currency in the world for the well-being of the multitudes of living beings.

This undoubtedly is a legendary account of the beginnings of Ayurveda intended to demonstrate its divine origin and its great age, but it is intrinsically true. The great medical compilations that contain the main body of India's classical medical lore must have been created in some such way. At all times India had physicians who were

not necessarily priests.[33] An enormous amount of medical experience
must have been gained empirically in the course of the centuries
and passed on orally from master to pupil. Religion and philosophy
provided the methods of correlating the empirical facts in thought,
and of developing medical theories. Then the day came when somebody wrote down what he had learned and the great compilations
of the Ayurveda took shape.

It is beyond doubt that India had early medical schools before
and at the time of the Buddha, and by 'schools' we do not mean
institutions and buildings but teachers and their disciples. A great
physician and medical teacher named Atreya is mentioned in the
Mahabharata, and quite possibly he played a part similar to that
of Hippocrates in Greece.[34] In the Charaka Samhita every chapter
begins with the words, 'Thus spake the worshipful Atreya.' Why
should this be mere fiction; why not a historical reminiscence?
Atreya, it was said, instructed six students who wrote down his
teachings, and in fact the works of two of them are known to us.
The great encyclopedic treatise of Agnivesha finally became the
Charaka Samhita, and the book of another of the six disciples, the
Bheda Samhita, was found not so long ago in a south-Indian manuscript.[35] The tridosa theory of disease about which we shall have
more to say later was conceived before the fourth century B.C. That
there was rational medicine, not only magico-religious medicine,
at the time of Buddhism, is evidenced by the fact that Indian
medicine spread to neighboring countries together with Buddhism.
Jivaka, a son of the Buddhist king Bimbisara, was reported to have
been a famous physician who performed spectacular cures. Stories
were told about him in all Buddhist countries.[36] The great epics
Ramayana and Mahabharata contain as many references to health,
disease, and treatments as do the Homeric poems. We have not
analyzed them for medical content [37] as we have the Greek epics,
because the dating of the constituent parts of the two Indian poems
presents many difficulties.[38] While some are undoubtedly very old,
others are late and may reflect medical conditions for which we
have better sources.

There were other traditions of the divine origin of Ayurveda. According to Sushruta it was Dhanvantari, the god of medicine, who revealed the 'Wisdom of Long Life' to a group of sages who approached him when he was on earth incarnated as Divodasa, king of the city of Benares, living in a hermitage. They addressed him with the following words:

'O Sire, it grieves us much to find men, though otherwise well befriended by their kin and relations, falling a prey to diseases, mental, physical, coming to them from outside or from their inner being, and piteously wailing in agony like utterly friendless creatures on earth; and we supplicate thee, O Lord, to illumine our minds with the truths of the Eternal Ayurveda so that we may faithfully discharge the duties allotted to us in life, and alleviate the sufferings of humanity at large. Bliss in this life and hereafter is in the gift of this eternal Ayurveda, and for this, O Lord, we have made bold to approach thee as thy humble disciples.' To them thus replied the holy Dhanvantari, 'Welcome to all of you to this blissful hermitage. All of you are worthy of the honor of true pupilship or tutelage.' [39]

Dhanvantari is an interesting deity. He does not appear in the Vedic pantheon and was probably taken over from aboriginal antiquity.[40] Mythology depicts him as being born from the depths of the ocean when the gods and titans joined forces to churn the Milky Ocean in order to extract from it *amrita,* the universal life fluid, the nectar of immortality. One deity after another arose from the depths of the ocean, Shri Lakshmi, goddess of life, beauty, and riches, the elephant of Indra who brings the rain, and many others, until, as the last and fourteenth 'jewel,' Dhanvantari appeared carrying the nectar of immortality in a white bowl. Zimmer pointed out that Dhanvantari is closely related both to Vishnu, maintainer of the world, and to Shiva, conqueror of King Death and lord of destructive forces, combining thus 'the two main elements of Hindu medicine: the wisdom which increases life-strength and maintains life-length to its full extent (Ayurveda), and the wisdom of cures and remedies (Bhaishajya) for diseases and demons.' [41]

Dhanvantari was the god of classical Indian medicine, the

tutelary divinity of physicians, and as such he is still held in high esteem wherever classical medicine is studied in India today. In the beautiful new building of the Ayurveda Medical College in Jamnagar his statue stands at the entrance. In the left hand he holds the bowl of nectar, in the right hand a medical text, an herb, a leech, and a knife, thus symbolizing the whole range of medicine. There he stands, the savior of man, bestowing health and immortality.

NOTES

1. E. Howald, *Die Kultur der Antike,* Zurich, 1948, p. 31.
2. Consult *The Upanishads,* Katha, Iśa, Kena, and Mundaka, by Swami Nikhilananda, New York, 1949, vol. I.
3. Most convenient is the edition by S. Radhakrishnan, The Bhagavadgītā, with an introductory essay, Sanskrit text, English translation, and notes, London, 1948.
4. On Indian philosophy in general see P. Deussen, *Philosophie des Veda,* Leipzig, 1894; *Die Philosophie der Upanishads,* Leipzig, 1899, (Engl. trans. Edinburgh, 1929); H. Oldenberg, *Vorwissenschaftliche Wissenschaft. Die Weltanschauung der Brahmana-Texte,* Göttingen, 1919; S. Radhakrishnan, *History of Indian Philosophy,* London, 1923-7, 2 vols.; 'Hinduism,' *The Legacy of India,* Oxford, 1937; A. B. Keith, *Religion and Philosophy of the Veda and Upanishads,* Cambridge, Mass., 1925; S. N. Das Gupta, 'Philosophy,' *The Legacy of India,* Oxford, 1937; H. Zimmer, *Philosophies of India* (Bollingen Series 26), New York, 1951.
5. See Romain Rolland's beautiful study, *La Vie de Ramakrishna,* Paris, 1930; and also his study on Ramakrishna's chief disciple, *La Vie de Vivekananda et l'évangile universel,* Paris, 1929.
6. Gandhi can be best studied in his own works such as *Young India, 1919–1922,* Madras, 1922, 2 vols.; his *Autobiography: The Study of My Experiments with Truth,* Washington, 1948; most biographies I have seen so far are utterly inadequate.
7. R. Garbe, *Die Sāṁkhya Philosophie,* 2nd ed., Leipzig, 1917; *Sāṁkhya und Yoga,* Strassburg, 1896; A. B. Keith, *The Sāṁkhya System,* New York, 1918.
8. See Zimmer, *Philosophies,* p. 326ff.
9. S. N. Das Gupta, *Yoga as Philosophy and Religion,* London, 1924; *Yoga Philosophy in Relation to Other Systems of Indian Thought,* Calcutta, 1930; K. T. Behanan, *Yoga: A Scientific Evaluation,* London, 1937; A. Daniélou, *Yoga: The Method of Re-integration,* London, 1949.
10. *The Yoga-System of Patañjali,* Engl. transl. by J. H. Wood, Harvard Oriental Series 17, Cambridge, Mass., 1914.

11. See Zimmer, *Philosophies,* p. 282f.
12. Ibid. p. 280ff.
13. Swami Prabhavananda, 'The Goal of Yoga,' in Christopher Isherwood, *Vedanta for the Western World,* London, 1948, p. 48ff.
14. Prabhavananda, 'The Yoga of Meditation,' in Isherwood, op. cit. p. 81.
15. Ibid. p. 85f.
16. For a good modern presentation see Yogi Vithaldas, *The Yoga System of Health,* London, 1936.
17. Bhagavadgita, VI, 27.
18. E. Erkes, 'Die taoistische Meditation and ihre Bedeutung für das chinesische Geistesleben,' *Psyche,* 1949, 2:371–9. One of the great classics of Chinese meditation is *Das Geheimnis der goldenen Blüte,* transl. by R. Wilhelm with a commentary by C. G. Jung, Zurich, 1929 (reprinted 1944); Engl. trans. from the German, *The Secret of the Golden Flower,* London, 1931.
19. Gerald Heard, 'Vedanta as the Scientific Approach to Religion,' in *Vedanta for the Western World,* pp. 51–6.
20. In 1948 there were thirteen Vedanta centers in the United States, one in England, and one in Argentina.
21. See his introduction to *Vedanta for the Western World.*
22. Hastings, *Encyclopaedia of Religion and Ethics,* vol. VIII, p. 138.
23. S. N. Das Gupta in *The Legacy of India,* p. 114.
24. The literature on Buddhism is enormous and no attempt can be made here to list even the basic publications. The reader is referred to M. Winternitz, *Geschichte der indischen Literatur,* vol. II, Leipzig, 1920, where he will find the literature published up to 1920, and to H. von Glasenapp, *Die Literatur Indiens,* Wildpark-Potsdam, 1926. I mention a few recent books which I consulted with benefit: most convenient collections of texts in translation are H. C. Warren, *Buddhism in Translations,* Harvard Oriental Series, vol. III, Cambridge, Mass., 1922, and J. G. Jennings, *The Vedantic Buddhism of the Buddha,* London, 1948 (quoted in the following as Jennings); E. J. Thomas, *The Life of Buddha as Legend and History,* New York, 1927; R. Grousset, *Sur les Traces du Bouddha,* Paris, 1929; C. H. Hamilton, *Buddhism in India, Ceylon, China and Japan,* Chicago, 1931; H. von Glasenapp, *Der Buddhismus in Indien und im Fernen Osten,* Berlin-Zurich, 1936; A. Foucher, *La Vie du Bouddha,* Paris, 1949; De la Vallée Poussin, 'Buddhism,' in *The Legacy of India.*
25. For this and the following passages see Jennings, p. 9f.
26. Ibid. p. 22.
27. H. R. Zimmer, *Hindu Medicine,* Baltimore, 1948, p. 32ff.
28. The Four Noble Truths in the translation of Jennings, p. 44ff.
29. Jennings, p. 43.
30. Cf. ibid. p. 65 and 101f.
31. *Legacy of India,* p. 184.
32. I use the edition and translation published in six volumes by the Shree

Gulabkunverba Ayurvedic Society at Jamnagar, India, 1949.

33. See, for example, Rigveda, IX, 112.

34. See the discussion of the Atreya problem in the introductory volume to the Charaka Samhita, p. 45ff.

35. The Bheda Samhita, Sanskrit text published by the University of Calcutta, 1921.

36. Liacre de Saint-Firmin, *Médecine et légendes bouddhiques de l'Inde,* Paris, 1916.

37. But see D. V. S. Reddy, 'Glimpses of Medicine in the Age of Ramayana,' *Indian Med. Record,* 1943, vol. 63, no. 1; and 'Clinical Descriptions and Case Sheets from Ramayana,' *The Indian Physician,* 1943, vol. 11, no. 15.

38. About their dating see M. Winternitz, op. cit. pp. 403, 439; H. von Glasenapp, *Die Literatur Indiens,* pp. 89, 104.

39. The Sushruta Samhita, Engl. trans. ed. by Kaviraj Kunja Lal Bhishagratna, Calcutta, 1907, vol. I, p. 1ff (slightly changed).

40. See H. Zimmer, *Hindu Medicine,* p. 36ff., where the legend is discussed in detail. See also W. A. Jayne, *The Healing Gods of Ancient Civilizations,* p. 166ff.

41. H. Zimmer, op. cit. p. 37f.

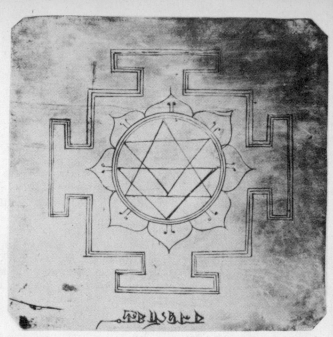

1. and 2. Yoga prayer patterns. From Heinrich Zimmer, *Kunstform und Yoga im indischen Kultbild*, Berlin, Frankfurter Verlags-Anstalt A-G, 1926, pl. 33, 34.

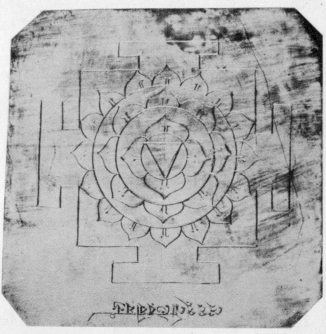

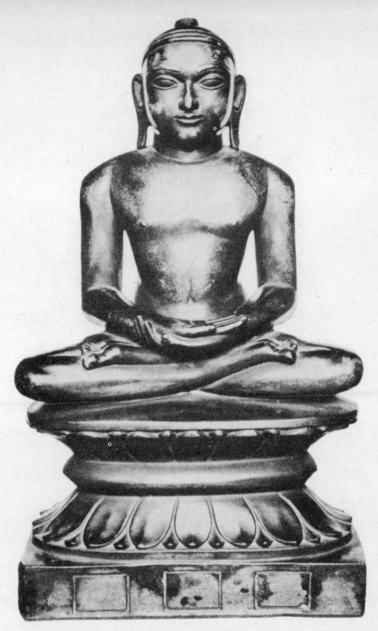

3. Jina in Yoga posture. Ibid. pl. 1.

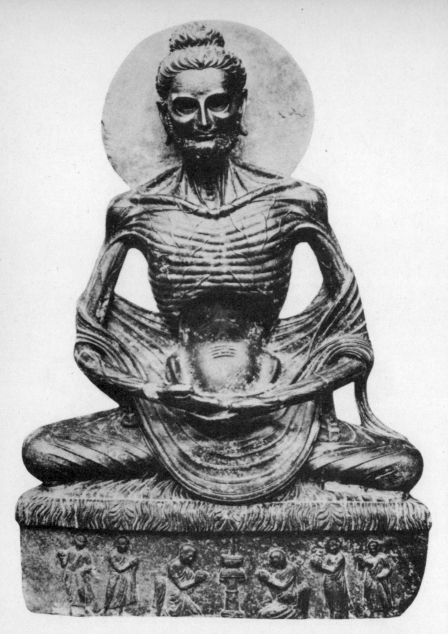

4. The fasting Buddha, Gandhara, second or third century A.D. From Zimmer, *The Art of Indian Asia*, pl. 65.

5. Buddha on the lion-throne, Gandhara. From Zimmer, *Kunstform und Yoga*, pl. 6.

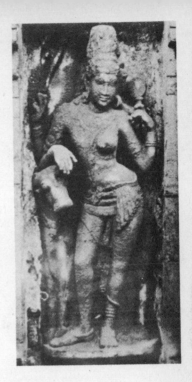

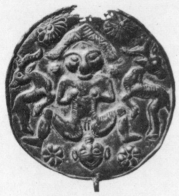

6. Silver needle showing birth-scene, from Luristan, first millennium B.C. Photo supplied by Dr. F. Merke, Basel.

7. Mother and child, Pathari, seventh century A.D. or later. From Zimmer, *The Art of Indian Asia*, pl. 105 a.

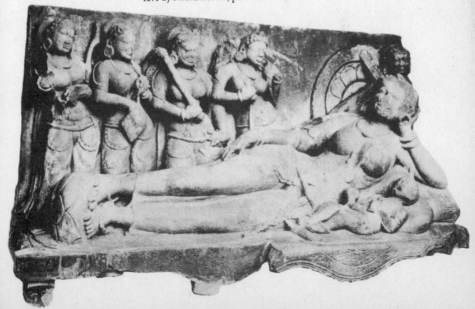

III. MEDICINE IN ANCIENT PERSIA

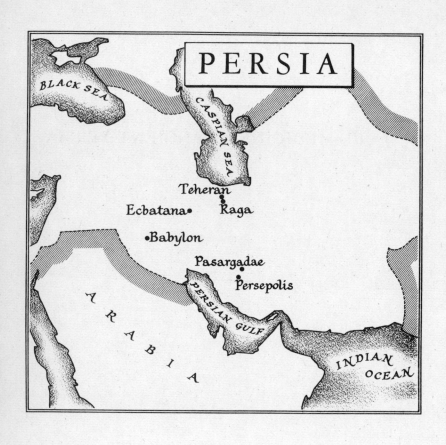

★

Ancient Persia

Although we have reached the point at which we might begin to discuss the Golden Ages of Greek and Indian medicine, the blossoming forth of systems of medicine such as the world had not seen before, yet we must insert here a brief interlude. Between India and Greece lie the highlands of Iran, where a strong and aggressive empire had developed in the sixth century B.C.—a menace to both Greece and India.[1] We spoke of the Persians as the conquerors of Babylon and Egypt in the first volume of this history, and we pointed out that there was constant intercourse between the Greek colonies of Asia Minor and the Persian state, sometimes friendly yet more often hostile. Persia was a formidable military power which with every decade extended its frontiers further. When Cyrus died in 529 he left an empire that reached from the Aegean Sea to the Indus, from the Black Sea, the Caspian Sea, and the mountains of Central Asia to the Persian Gulf and the Indian Ocean. And Cyrus' successor Cambyses II added Egypt to the empire. Under Darius, and perhaps even earlier, Persia had two satrapies in the Indus Valley. But India was a large country that could develop its culture even while some border regions were occupied by a foreign power. To small Greece the aggressive policy of Persia was a question of life and death, and not until the Persian peril had been averted could Greek culture develop freely and produce its most beautiful creations.

It is well known how the Persian menace was strong enough to unite the Greek city-states temporarily for common defense, how in a war that lasted almost half a century the Greeks succeeded in

197

maintaining their independence and defeated the superior might of
the Persian army and navy in the decisive battles of Marathon,
Thermopylae, Salamis, Plataea, Mycale, and others, battles which
even after two thousand years are still an inspiration to mankind,
since they were the heroic battles of a brave, small people in a great
war of independence. One hundred years later Alexander the Great
destroyed the Persian empire, and himself marched against India,
spreading Greek culture in the wake of his armies.

The giant empire of Persia collapsed after only two centuries,
because it had no culture of its own. The Persians were Indo-
Europeans like the Greeks and the Indians, but most of their cultural
creations reflect foreign influence. Every young nation borrows from
its neighbors in the beginning, but it assimilates foreign modes and
one day finds its own means of expression. Persia never did, with
one exception to be discussed presently. The gigantic structures,
tombs, temples, and palaces erected by the Great Kings at Pasarga-
dae, Persepolis, and Susa and decorated with monumental reliefs are
most impressive even in ruins, but they remind us of Babylonia and
Assyria. They are not copies, to be sure, yet the inspiration is foreign.
And the Great Kings wrote their triumphant inscriptions recording
their great victories in cuneiform script, while they also used the
Aramaic alphabet and even the language for their diplomatic
correspondence. The calendar they took over from Egypt. They were
not barbarians by any means, but learned from their neighbors
wherever they could, and ruled and administered their large empire
wisely. The Greeks obviously had a grudge against them, and the
accounts they gave of Persian life were neither entirely accurate nor
fair. But the fact remains that Persia never developed a civilization
of its own strong enough to influence the course of human culture or
leave a permanent mark on it, except in one respect, religion.

Before the sixth century B.C. and long thereafter, Medians and
Persians had a nature religion with a colorful pantheon, similar to
that of other Indo-European immigrants. Their priests were the
Magi. They brought animal sacrifices to the gods, among whom
Mithra held a prominent place. They did not bury the dead but

exposed them to be torn by birds and dogs. But in the sixth century
B.C. a reformer arose, Zoroaster or Zarathustra, who preached a
purified religion and attacked the traditional gods.[2] He was a
Median nobleman born in Raga, south of the Caspian Sea, son of a
daughter of the last Median king, Astyagas, and of Spitama, chief of
a Median clan. Through his mother he was also related to the
ruling Persian house. But he was a revolutionary who strove for liberation of the peasants. Proscribed by his home town and indicted by
Cambyses, he wandered through the lands teaching and preaching
until Hystaspes, father of Darius, gave him protection and asylum.
When Herodotus traveled in Persia toward the middle of the fifth
century B.C., he never heard the name of Zoroaster; the religion he
met with was that of the Magi. In other words, the teachings of
Zoroaster were not accepted widely, and his followers were few until
Darius embraced the new faith, which then gradually spread from
the court to other strata of the population.

The tenets of the new religion are to be found in the Avesta, a
collection of the holy books of the Persians.[3] Like the Old Testament,
it contains writings by different authors and from very different
periods. The oldest part, the Gathas, hymns, are Zoroaster's own
work, written in a Median dialect—a language as artificial as Homer's Greek—the traditional language of ancient Persian poetry.
Other books contain prayers, invocations, moral precepts, tales of the
origin of the world, and similar matters that are found in so many
ancient religious books. One, the Videvdad, is a code similar in intent
to the biblical Leviticus. Although it is a late book it is most
important to us, for it reflects many hygienic views, and also gives
valuable information about the physicians, their training and
practice.

The whole Avesta is Zoroastrian and post-Zoroastrian, and it has
come down to us in late editions, but it obviously contains much
ancient material, old myths, reminiscences of old views, customs, and
practices. Together with the archaeological findings and Greek
reports it is the most important source of our knowledge of Persian
culture and also medicine. The Avesta, moreover, contains many

elements that are not purely Zoroastrian, for the old nature religion did not die. Driven into opposition, the Magi worked their way into the new religion, and even became its priests. The Zoroastrian Great Kings were buried, not exposed, but gradually the old custom of exposing corpses was generally re-introduced, and today the Parsees of India have their 'Towers of Silence' in Karachi, Bombay, Calcutta. The old gods also came back gradually, first of all Mithra, who was to play such an important part in the Roman empire, and was to become a serious competitor of Christ. Homa took a position similar to that of Dionysus.

The word 'homa' is linguistically the same as the Vedic word 'soma,' but while 'soma' is the juice of an undefined plant, 'homa' is simply wine.[4] Students of Indo-European linguistics have taken great pains to search for identical words and concepts in the old Iranian languages and Vedic Sanskrit. Where such words and ideas can be found, they are considered to point to common Indo-European origin or to influence from one country on another. I think that this has been greatly overdone[5] and that great caution is necessary here. All archaic civilizations have a great deal in common, and archaic medicine is very much the same everywhere. Water, fire, air, or wind play an important part in the thinking of many peoples, and such views need not necessarily be borrowed from neighbors. Similarly, I think there is no need to assume that the humoral theory of disease originated in India and reached Greece by way of Persia,[6] for the important part played by blood and other humors was recognized everywhere.

Zoroaster's religion in its pure form was monotheistic. It does not have the many gods of the Magi, only the one god Ahura Mazda, the Wise Lord, the Creator who upholds the cosmos and directs its course. His world is the world of light, purity, and goodness. But he is opposed by the spirit of evil, Angra Mainyu, whose world is one of darkness, where the daevas are attached to him, not demons but the old nature gods of the Magi who now are condemned to a life of darkness. Thus there are two primordial principles, good and evil, light and darkness, and man must make a choice between the two.

If he chooses Ahura Mazda, the life of light, the true creed—'In our profession of faith is embodied: Right, shall be strengthened; Evil, shall be destroyed! I desire the union with Good Will, I renounce every communion with the evildoer' [7]—then his will be a happy life in this world and the hereafter; but if he chooses the world of darkness and continues to worship the daevas, his lot will forever be Hell. Christianity has much in common with the religion of Zoroaster: God and the Devil, Heaven and Hell, Good and Evil, man's obligation to make a choice between the two.

The Videvdad in its present form was probably written in the beginning of the Arsacid period—that is, between 250 B.C. and A.D. 224—but since it undoubtedly embodied much older material, we may be justified in studying it in this chapter.[8] The Videvdad is a law book, a code, which states what is allowed and what is forbidden, and indicates the penalties for transgressions. It reminds us of Assyrian codes, particularly in its attitude toward sex life. Girls were to marry past their fifteenth year.[9] Women were highly respected. Marriage with relatives was recommended and seems to have been customary, as it was in Egypt and still is in Arab countries.[10] Abortion was considered a great crime, tantamount to manslaughter, and if a girl was made pregnant and had recourse to an abortionist woman, she, the woman, and the man were all considered equally responsible,[11] and if a child was born, the father had to support it until it had grown up.[12] Sodomy was rated one of the greatest crimes. The passive and unconsenting victim was to be whipped to death;[13] for the active and consenting pederast there was no way of atoning— he was a daeva and worshiper of daeva forever.[14] Assault with battery was punished with whipping, which was increased whenever the criminal relapsed.[15] Bodily injury was punished by retaliation, not only injury inflicted on men but also that inflicted on dogs, for dogs were holy animals, firmly protected by law.[16]

Much space was devoted to purity regulations. Fire, earth, water, and vegetation were not to be defiled, prescriptions similar to those we found in Hesiod's *Works and Days*. Man became unclean as a result of physiological processes such as menstruation, childbirth, ejaculation of sperm, and death. Whoever touched a corpse, whether of man or dog, became unclean and had to purify himself through elaborate rites,[17] views very similar to those of Leviticus. Strange was the position granted to the dog, which in most of the other civilizations was very low in the scale of living beings. But since the dog, like the vulture, was allowed to devour the dead, he was privileged among other animals.

We mentioned in another connection that the Persian Great Kings had Egyptian body physicians, and that Darius thought so highly of them that he had the medical school of Sais restored. Yet we also saw that Greek doctors became very serious competitors of their Egyptian colleagues.[18] Why were foreign physicians so popular with the Persian court and nobility? Had they not physicians of their own? They had indeed, but what the Persian physicians practiced was mostly magico-religious medicine. They never reached the level of Egyptian medicine as it had developed in the late centuries of the New Kingdom, or of medicine as the Greeks practiced it as early as the sixth century B.C. They were priests, specialized priests like the Babylonian physicians, and as priests they belonged to the client class of Persian society, a society of four classes—nobility, clients, peasants, and slaves.[19] They were trained in temple schools, the most famous of which seems to have been at Raga. Three types of physician were distinguished: 'If several healers offer themselves together, O Spitama Zarathustra, namely, one who heals with the knife, one who heals with herbs, and one who heals with the holy word, it is this one who will best drive away sickness from the body of the faithful.' [20]

In other words, Persia had surgeons, herb doctors, and incantation priests. Filliozat and others have pointed out that these three methods of treatment are the same ones that Pindar mentions in the ode where he speaks of Chiron instructing Asclepius,[21] and from that analogy they concluded that this threefold division of medicine must be Indo-Iranian.[22] They overlooked the fact that the division of medical treatments into pharmacology, surgery, and magic is universal in archaic medicine, and may be found in Egypt and

Mesopotamia as well as in China. The great Greek contribution was the development of dietetics, which raised the standard of medicine far beyond the archaic stage.

Physicians, as a rule, were not licensed to practice in antiquity. Everybody could claim to be expert in matters of health and disease, and treat sick people for a fee. In ancient Persia, however, there seems to have been some kind of licensing of surgeons. Ignorance is more immediately fatal in surgery than in medicine, or rather, mistakes are more easily apparent to the laymen. The Babylonians protected society against malpractice of the surgeon by making him liable for his actions.[23] The Persian document dealing with the admission of physicians to the practice of surgery is the earliest preserved regulation of this kind. It reads:

O Maker of the material world, thou Holy One! If a worshipper of Mazda want to practice the art of healing, on whom shall he first prove his skill? On worshippers of Mazda or on worshippers of the Daevas?

Ahura Mazda answered. On worshippers of the Daevas shall he first prove himself, rather than on worshippers of Mazda. If he treat with the knife a worshipper of the Daevas and he die; if he treat with the knife a second worshipper of the Daevas and he die; if he treat with the knife for the third time a worshipper of the Daevas and he die, he is unfit to practice the art of healing forever and ever.

Let him therefore never attend any worshipper of Mazda; let him never treat with the knife any worshipper of Mazda, nor wound him with the knife. If he shall ever attend any worshipper of Mazda, if he shall ever treat with the knife any worshipper of Mazda, and wound him with the knife, he shall pay for it the same penalty as is paid for wilful murder.

If he treat with the knife a worshipper of the Daevas and he recover; if he treat with the knife a second worshipper of the Daevas and he recover; if for the third time he treat with the knife a worshipper of the Daevas and he recover; then he is fit to practice the art of healing forever and ever.

He may henceforth at his will attend worshippers of Mazda; he may

at his will treat with the knife worshippers of Mazda, and heal them
with the knife.[24]

Physicians practiced mostly [25] as itinerants, just as the Greek
doctors did at that time. The population was scattered over a wide
area and large cities were few, so that this was the best way for the
doctor to serve the people and, at the same time, to make a living.
Like the Code of Hammurabi, the Videvdad had a fee tariff, and
here as in Mesopotamia the fee was determined by the social status
of the patient. Since this is another document of very great importance, I quote it here:

A healer shall heal a priest for a holy blessing; he shall heal the
master of a house for the value of an ox of low value; he shall heal
the lord of a borough for the value of an ox of average value; he shall
heal the lord of a town for the value of an ox of high value; he shall
heal the lord of a province for the value of a chariot and four.

He shall heal the wife of the master of a house for the value of a
she-ass; he shall heal the wife of the lord of a borough for the value
of a cow; he shall heal the wife of the lord of a town for the value of a
mare; he shall heal the wife of the lord of a province for the value of a
she-camel.

He shall heal the son of the lord of a borough for the value of an
ox of high value; he shall heal an ox of high value for the value of an
ox of average value; he shall heal an ox of average value for that of an
ox of low value; he shall heal an ox of low value for the value of a
sheep; he shall heal a sheep for the value of a meal of meat.[26]

This text shows that the physician treated not only his fellow men
but also animals and was remunerated for his veterinarian services.

What kind of medicine did these priest-physicians practice? We
have no medical writings from ancient Persia, and the books of the
Avesta—religious books—are our only source. All evidence, however, points to the fact that ancient Persian medicine was archaic
medicine, a blend of religious, magical, and empirically grounded
rational views and practices very similar to those we have encountered in other civilizations and have discussed in great detail.
Hence, we shall be very brief here.

Diseases are named in various passages of the Videvdad and of other Avestan books. They are diseases of the skin, scabies perhaps, filth diseases which itch,[27] and also leprosy; here as in Mesopotamia the lepers were considered unclean and were excluded from society.[28] Fevers are mentioned very frequently,[29] and this generic term obviously designated a great variety of disease entities that we distinguish today. The heat or chill of fever were the outstanding symptoms. Nervous and mental diseases here as in other civilizations were the favorite object of magico-religious treatments.[30] Epilepsy was in all probability one of them, but it would be futile to attempt a diagnosis of other nervous diseases. Cripples are mentioned, hunchbacks,[31] dwarfs, the deaf and the blind, and individuals who have the evil eye.[32] We have entire lists of diseases, but unfortunately they contain only names not symptoms, so that we have no way of even attempting identifications.[33] The number of evils which beset mankind was very large. Ahura Mazda had created the world with all that was good and beautiful and bright in it, but the evil one, Angra Mainyu, created '9 and 90 and 900 and 9000 and 9 times 10,000 diseases.' [34] They had to be fought with the holy word, with sacred formulas, incantations which are described as divine, strong, victorious, and healing. They are not different in character and style from those of Egypt, Mesopotamia, or Vedic India; therefore, one example will suffice: [35]

To thee, O Sickness, I say avaunt! to thee, O Death, I say avaunt! to thee, O Pain, I say avaunt! to thee, O Fever, I say avaunt! to thee, O Disease, I say avaunt!

By their might may we smite down the Drug (the evil angel)! By their might may we smite the Drug! May they give to us strength and power, O Ahura!

I drive away sickness, I drive away death, I drive away pain and fever, I drive away the disease, rottenness, and infection which Angra Mainyu has created by his witchcraft against the bodies of mortals.

Incantations were the chief means of treating patients in a system of magico-religious medicine, and the priest who knew the right

charms and spells was the most important physician. He was called
in all serious cases of illness. But like all other ancient peoples, the
Persians also made wide use of drugs. Medicinal plants were the gift
of Ahura Mazda,[36] and there can be no doubt that potions were
drunk, pills were swallowed, salves applied to aching limbs, in most
cases of minor ailments. Homa—that is, wine—was drunk for therapeutic as well as religious reasons, and here as everywhere else in
archaic medicine pharmacological treatment was frequently nothing
but the manual procedure of an otherwise religious rite. Being a
collection of religious books, the Avesta naturally does not give any
information on which drugs were used for which diseases, just as it
does not describe surgical operations. Yet we know that Persia had
surgeons since severe tests were prescribed for them before they
could practice their craft. The armies of Persia needed surgeons, and
there is no doubt that they knew how to treat battle wounds, perhaps just as well as their Greek and Babylonian colleagues, because
operations are easily learned from neighboring countries.

All in all, it can be said that ancient Persia did not in any way
contribute to the advancement of medicine. It did produce great
rulers, great soldiers, and above all a prophet and poet who taught a
pure and highly ethical religion. Medicine, however, remained
primitive. Persia's time to make its contribution to world medicine
came much later, in the tenth and eleventh centuries of our era.
Again it was a foreign impulse, Islam, that activated latent forces.
At that time Persia gave to the world great physicians as well as
immortal poets.

NOTES

1. About Persian history in general see *Cambridge Ancient History,* vol. IV,
   The Persian Empire and the West, Cambridge, 1926.
2. The basic study on Zoroaster is E. Herzfeld, *Zoroaster and His World,*
   Princeton, 1947, 2 vols.; see also J. Hertel, *Die Zeit Zoroasters,* Leipzig,
   1924.
3. Edition of the text by K. Geldner, Stuttgart, 1889–95; English translation
   by James Darmesteter and L. H. Mills in *Sacred Books of the East,* ed. by
   F. Max Müller, vols. IV, XXIII, XXXI, Oxford, 1880–87 (our quotations

are from this translation) ; French trans. by James Darmesteter, *Le Zend-Avesta,* traduction nouvelle avec commentaire historique et philologique, Paris, 1892–3, 3 vols.; German trans. based on Bartholomae's Dictionary by F. Wolff, *Avesta, Die Heiligen Bücher der Parsen,* Strassburg, 1910 (reprinted Berlin and Leipzig, 1924).

4. Herzfeld, op. cit. p. 543ff.
5. E. g. by Filliozat, *La Doctrine classique de la médecine indienne,* Paris, 1949, p. 35.
6. As is claimed by C. Elgood, *A Medical History of Persia,* Cambridge, 1951, p. 19f.
7. Herzfeld, op. cit. p. 412.
8. On ancient Persian medicine see H. Fichtner, *Die Medizin im Avesta,* Leipzig, 1924, and Elgood's first chapter.
9. Videvdad, 14, 15.
10. Yasna, 12, 9; Videvdad, 8, 13.
11. Videvdad, 15, 14.
12. Ibid. 15, 15.
13. Ibid. 8, 26.
14. Ibid. 8, 31.
15. Ibid. 4, 17f.
16. Ibid. 13, 10ff.
17. Ibid. 9, 1ff.
18. See this book, vol. I, pp. 324 and 357.
19. Herzfeld, op. cit. p. 110ff.
20. Videvdad, 7, 44. See also Yasht, 3, 6, where in addition to these three types of healers two others are mentioned, 'one may heal with Holiness, one may heal with the Law.'
21. *Pythiae,* III, 91.
22. Filliozat, op. cit. p. 33; see also his note 4.
23. See this book, vol. I, p. 428f.
24. Videvdad, 7, 36–40.
25. Visprat, 9, 2.
26. Videvdad, 7, 41–3.
27. Yasht, 8, 56; 13, 131; 14, 48; Videvdad, 7, 58.
28. Yasht, 5, 92; Videvdad, 2, 29.
29. E. g. Yasht, 3, 8; 13, 131; Videvdad, 20, 7.
30. Yasht, 5, 92–3; 13, 131; Videvdad, 2, 29, 37; 7, 57.
31. E. g. Videvdad, 2, 29.
32. Ibid. 20, 3.
33. Ibid. 20, 3, 6, 7, 9.
34. Ibid. 22, 2.
35. Ibid. 20, 7–9.
36. 'And I Ahura Mazda brought down the healing plants that, by many hundreds, by many thousands, by many myriads, grow up all around the one Gaokerena,' Videvdad, 20, 4.

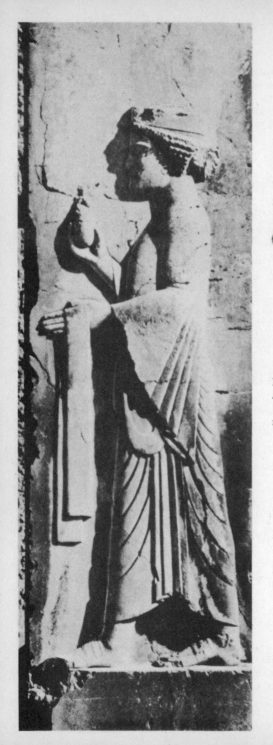

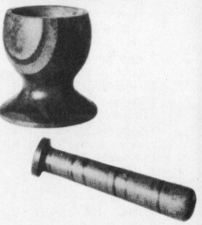

1. Mortar and pestle, Treasury, Persepolis. From Erich F. Schmidt, *The Treasury of Persepolis*, University of Chicago Press, 1939 (Oriental Institute Communications, no. 21), fig. 41.

2. Beardless attendant with cosmetic bottle and towel, Palace of Darius. Ibid. pl. 149.

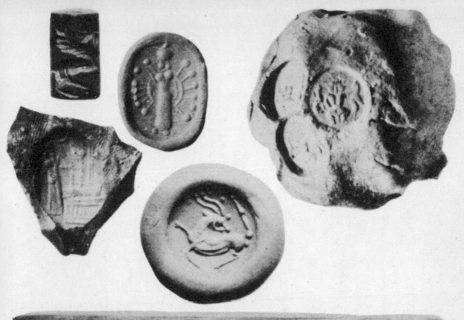

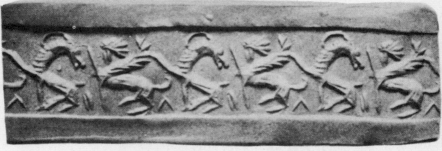

3. Seals, showing animals, Ibid. fig. 25.

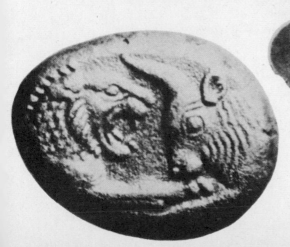

4. and 5. Coins, Treasury, Persepolis. Ibid. fig. 56.

IV. THE GOLDEN AGE OF
GREEK MEDICINE

1. Life in the Greek City-States

The fifth century B.C. was the Golden Age of Greek culture, the time to which Greeks and Romans always looked back as their classical age, the time that formulated ideas and ideals and set the style for centuries to come. In this cultural development Athens was foremost, a small town with a small hinterland, Attica, and a total population which probably never exceeded 300,000, including over one-third slaves and about 40,000 metics or resident aliens.[1] Pericles made the city one of the most beautiful the world had seen. Architecture, sculpture, painting flourished as never before. Even in its present ruined state the Acropolis of Athens presents an overwhelming sight, with its stairway over which the processions marched; the Propylaea, a monumental gateway; the graceful temple erected to Nike, goddess of victory; the Erechtheum, house of a mythical king of Athens, with its 'Porch of the Maidens'; and the noble structure of the Parthenon, of Pentelic marble which today looks and feels like old ivory, built and decorated by the best artists of the time to house the protectress of Athens, the virgin goddess Athena.

At the same time that Athens became a city of marble monuments decorated with priceless statues and paintings, the great tragic poets had their plays produced as part of the spring festival of Dionysus, tragedies which are still performed in the Western world. And somewhat later Aristophanes won a high reputation with comedies which are still read today with great enjoyment. In Thucydides Athens produced one of the great historians of all times, and with Socrates

213

Greek philosophy took a new turn from the investigation of nature to the study of man, problems of morality and the conduct of life. His method of obtaining results by questioning people, which is so beautifully pictured in Plato's *Dialogues,* remained a method of investigation in the West, and is still used in the seminar courses of our universities.

Athens was the cultural center of Greece in the fifth century B.C. and attracted visitors from all over the Greek world, but it was by no means the only center, and it was not and never became a center of medical studies. Athens had drawn much inspiration from Ionia, the flourishing cities of Asia Minor, and from the Aegean Islands. The Athenians were Ionians and basically spoke and wrote the dialect of the pre-Socratic philosophers and Hippocratic physicians. Close ties of blood and civilization united these two peoples, yet scientific and medical research continued to be cultivated primarily in the periphery, from Asia Minor to North Africa, Sicily, and southern Italy. There the great medical schools developed, and from these centers came the famous physicians of the period, who were known and practiced not only in their homeland but all over the Greek world. Hence, to find the Golden Age of Greek medicine we must turn our eyes not to Athens but to the Greek periphery, and more particularly to the small island of Cos and to the Asiatic peninsula of Cnidus.

Before we discuss and analyze fifth-century medicine we should find out what kind of society the physicians were serving. We gave a brief sketch of the physical environment in which the Greeks lived, of its influence on health and disease; we must now inquire into the social environment and its effect on man's condition. It is obviously impossible for us to give here a detailed picture of Greek life as it unfolded in the various sections of the country. What we must know, however, is in what respect Greek life differed from life in Egypt and Babylonia, the two great civilizations we studied in the previous volume of this work.

Egypt and the states of Mesopotamia were, or at least soon became, absolute monarchies. The king was all-powerful, god or highest priest of the gods. The administration was centralized, and districts and provinces were ruled by governors appointed by the king to enforce the laws of the land and the king's wishes. The land belonged to a feudal aristocracy, or at times to freeholders or soldiers. Laborers in industry and agriculture were to a large extent serfs and slaves. Free and unfree played hardly any part in the political life of the country. The king with his advisers and officials held the power and the others were mere subjects.

Greek life in the period under consideration was totally different. It centered on the *polis,* a man's city and at the same time his state, or in other words, his city-state.[2] The polis was everything to the citizen. His thoughts and actions, his entire life were devoted to the community. Greeks in all parts of the country were very politically-minded, and a citizen's time was directly or indirectly almost entirely spent in the service of his polis. Yet there was a great difference between the Dorian and Ionian way of life as exemplified by Sparta and Athens. In both, people lived for the state, but in a totally different manner.

Sparta in the fifth century B.C. was a conservative, aristocratic, authoritarian, military state. There had been a period, in the eighth and seventh centuries, when the arts had flourished in Sparta too.[3] The city produced and attracted great poets: Tyrtaeus, whose songs praised the fighting qualities of the brave man, and Alcman, whose hymns were sung by choirs of maidens on festive occasions. Sports and games were cultivated here perhaps more than anywhere else, and no city could boast of more Olympic victors in those days Thucydides tells us that the Spartans were the first to exercise in complete nudity and anoint their skin with oil,[4] a custom which soon became universal. But as time went on, Sparta's development stopped; it became archaic, even reactionary, A small, half-literate upper class, the Spartiates, controlled the state. They did not work for a living but were supported by the labor of others, by tributes of subjugated peoples. They lived on government funds as soldiers who formed the core of a formidable army, or engaged in official duties, or hunted and exercised to keep fit. They were an aristocratic master-class far above the *perioikoi,* the free-born peasants who had certain civil rights and were permitted to serve in the army; and the helots, serfs and slaves who were the property of the state. Since the very large number of the latter was a constant threat to the ruling class, they were watched and kept in check by a secret police.

Double kingship was a traditional institution in Sparta, but the kings had no actual power. They were advised by a Council of Elders, composed of twenty-eight men over sixty years of age, elected by acclamation by the Assembly of Spartiates. The actual power was vested in five magistrates, the ephors, who exercised executive, judiciary, and disciplinary power in an almost dictatorial way. The Assembly was very different from that of Athens. Officers were elected by acclamation, and the Assembly could only approve or disapprove of proposals brought before it. One is indeed reminded of the sham parliaments of modern authoritarian states.[5]

For us the word Spartan has assumed the connotation of 'hardy, undaunted, frugal, laconic, severe,'[6] and such indeed was the Spar-tan's life. Education in Sparta had only one purpose, to toughen boys and girls so as to make them hardy soldiers and strong mothers of soldiers.[7] Principles of eugenic breeding were applied in the pro-creation of children. According to Plutarch, boys and girls exercised in the presence of each other in the nude, not only to harden their bodies but also to enable the young man to select the right mate. When the time came he raped the girl and carried her into his house. Her hair was cut, and from then on she was primarily a breeding machine who might sleep with other men, if eugenic reasons made it seem desirable.[8] We do not know how far we can trust Plutarch's statements, but once a society has accepted the principle 'everything for the state, nothing against the state,' such customs may easily develop, as recent history has taught us. When a child was born it was inspected by government experts, who decided whether it should be brought up or not. If it was weak or crippled, it was thrown into a deep pit on Mount Taygetus and thus destroyed. There was no reason to bring it up, since it would be useless to the state and a mere burden to society. Children belonged to the state but were brought up by their families until the age of seven. Even at home they had a hardening education. Plutarch tells that a new-born child was bathed not in water but in wine, since it was thought that sickly children would get faint by such bathing while healthy children would become even stronger under such treatment.[9] Infants were not swaddled as in other parts of Greece; children were trained to eat any kind of food and like it, to stay in the dark without being afraid, and to stop crying.

At the age of seven the collective education of boys began. The state then took them over. They continued to remain with their families up to the age of twelve, but became members of youth organizations where, apart from some rudiments of elementary education and some singing, they were given mostly physical training. The aim was to detach them gradually from the family, so that they would never aspire to a private life but live like bees,[10] perfectly adjusted to the requirements of a totalitarian state. At the age of twelve education became more severe. From then until the age of thirty youths and men lived in barracks, even when they were married. Their hair was cropped short. They walked barefoot, wore no undergarment, only a simple cloak. Their meals were extremely frugal, and since the basic necessities were provided by the state they owned practically no property. Physical exercises and drills filled the day. They were trained to be obedient, good, and tough fighters. Whatever served the state, including lying and stealing, was morally good and justified. Young people were encouraged to steal food, but they must not be caught. If they were caught they had to expect severe whippings, which were to be endured without uttering a cry. As in all totalitarian states citizens were not allowed to travel abroad without urgent reasons, and foreign visitors were not welcome. The depersonalization of the individual went so far that his name was not recorded on his tomb, except in the case of men who had died on the battlefield, and in the case of priestesses.[11]

The goal of male education was to train the perfect soldier, the perfect hoplite or heavy infantryman. And this goal was certainly attained. The Lacedaemonian armies were formidable and at Thermopylae, in 480 B.C., when King Leonidas and his Spartans were killed to the last man defending the pass against the Persian army, they left a record of heroism which will be remembered forever. Their feat was glorified in a simple monument bearing the names of the fallen heroes with the epigram:

> Tell them in Lacedaemon, passer-by,
> That here obedient to their word we lie.

Like all true soldiers the Spartans had a high code of chivalry. Thus they never killed enemies in flight. They would pursue an enemy until there was no doubt that he was completely defeated, but then let him go, for they considered it unworthy of a Greek soldier to kill an opponent once he had admitted defeat. Plutarch adds that such an attitude was not only noble but profitable, for defeated enemies would take to flight rather than be killed while resisting.[12]

The education of girls was regimented also. They were taught songs and dances, but were trained physically first of all, so as to be prepared for the bearing of children, their chief purpose in life. In Greece they had the reputation of being strong, courageous women who were not without influence over their husbands. They were proud women, and the story was told that when a foreigner said to Gorgo, the wife of Leonidas, hero of Thermopylae, 'You Lacedaemonians are the only women who have power over men,' she answered, 'Yes, and we are the only ones who give birth to men.' [13] They were also known for the short skirts they wore which made them look like Amazons or Artemis the huntress. At least in the early days they enjoyed more freedom than women in other Greek states.

For over two thousand years, from the time of Plato to our own, the Spartan mode of living has been condemned, ridiculed, or praised to excess. Democratic societies that valued individual freedom and artistic creation could not approve of a regimented society that held spiritual matters in deep contempt. Sparta, on the other hand, had a strong appeal to militaristic nations. The simplicity of its life, its denial of all luxuries, and its military virtues set an example that was followed eagerly by nations intent upon regimenting their population for military ends.[14] Jaeger recently stated that Sparta's real contribution to the history of culture, a contribution the importance of which can scarcely be overestimated, was the postulate that education should be the concern of the state.[15] Nobody will deny the validity of this postulate which today is generally accepted, and it is equally true that Sparta fulfilled it in a most thorough way. But I think that in doing so Sparta set an evil example, because it matters a great deal to what end the state assumes responsibility for education. The fact that the first European country to have a complete system of state education used it to regiment its people in a totalitarian, militaristic, anti-artistic, and anti-spiritual way is most unfortunate, and apt to discredit rather than encourage state education.

I should also mention here an aspect of Greek life not limited to the Dorians but universal, one that may seem strange to us who were brought up in the orbit of the Judaeo-Christian civilization. It is hardly ever mentioned in our schools, no matter how many years we devote to humanistic studies, and yet it is an essential part of Greek culture. Without the knowledge of it we could not possibly understand the ancient world or its Eastern successors. We must write about it here also, because it had definite psychological and, to a certain extent, medical implications. I refer to the fact that to a Greek of the upper classes the ideal relation between two human beings was the love between an adult male and an adolescent boy. Pederasty was an accepted and universal institution in the Greek world during the period under consideration and long thereafter.[16] This does not in any way imply that all Greek men were homosexuals or inverts. In fact, the majority of them were married, had normal sexual relations with their wives, with slave girls, and with courtesans at times. A boy of the upper classes could satisfy his sexual need as soon as it was felt and without any social reprobation. It is important to know this, because it means that so many of the frustrations encountered in young people today were non-existent in antiquity. Girls were married off young, and the only bachelor girls we hear of were courtesans, many of whom were highly intellectual women whose company was eagerly sought, or who became the mistresses of great men; the Milesian Aspasia for many years was the mistress of Pericles. Yet the ideal relationship was between man and man, adult and adolescent. It was a form of education, to be sure, and a very important one. The youth followed the example of his older lover, who was responsible for him, and felt a strong moral obligation to live up to what was expected of him. Plutarch said that Spartan boys' lovers shared in their honors as well as in their disgrace. And when a boy once cried out during a fight, his lover was punished.[17] Thus far did responsibility extend. Pederasty was general in Athens, too, and we actually know the names of the friends of many of the great Athenians. There was no secrecy about it. A man never appeared in public with his wife, but he did with his boy.

The origin of this custom is probably to be sought in the comradeship between warriors as it existed for many centuries in the feudal period of Greece. Homer does not mention sex relations between men, which does not mean that they did not exist at his time. But the custom certainly spread in the warlike centuries that preceded the period we are studying, and was generally accepted in the fifth century B.C. Experience in the two world wars, when millions of men were thrown together in armies, prison camps, and concentration camps, have shown how sex relations between men developed first as a result of the extraordinary circumstances. But we also saw how many deep and lasting love relations were engendered by this war camaraderie. It was also interesting to watch how pederasty greatly increased in fascist countries, particularly in Germany.[18]

Fascism wanted to create a men's world, relegating women to the home and to the bearing of potential soldiers. Spartan ideals were revived, and homosexual relations became an accepted matter. It is very likely that there is more pederasty in Europe today than before the wars. Yet once war is over, prison camps closed, fascist societies broken up, and the individual reintegrated into a society in which Judaeo-Christian taboos are still strong, the homosexual relations of camp life die together with the memory of other war experiences. This was not the case in ancient Greece where these taboos did not exist outside of certain religious sects and where homosexual love became highly ethical and a pure source of inspiration. The so-called Hippocratic Oath, about which we shall have to say more very soon, presupposes the custom of homosexual intercourse, in that it requires the physician to pledge himself to abstain from sexual relations with both female and male persons, be they free or slaves.

Sex relations between adult and adolescent males necessarily call for their counterpart, for relations between women and girls. Plutarch explicitly states that in Sparta homosexual love was so completely accepted that respectable women had relations with girls.[19] Here, as in the case of males, the educational element was probably very strong. Lesbian practices must have been common in Athens, where women were confined to the house and men spent the entire day in the streets, the market place, porticoes, barbershops, or wrestling places. Women therefore sought their own pleasures; and Greek leather workers were very clever. In one of his delightful mimes Herondas reveals the secrets of two friends, one of whom had procured a certain contraption which gave more pleasure than the strongest male. The cynicism of their conversation could not be surpassed. [20] Lesbianism had a great tradition in Greece, where it had been glorified by such a great poetess as Sappho, whose passionate lyrics expressed in immortal verses the joys and burning pains of a woman's love for a beloved girl. Sappho was a teacher of girls. On the island of Lesbos, toward the end of the seventh century B.C., she had a school for adolescent girls who were instructed in music and dancing, in love, and in the art of living in beauty. And in those days Sappho was certainly not exceptional. Other women had similar schools in the Aeolian world, at a time when women were much freer than in later centuries.

When we study ancient cultures our task is not to judge but to understand them. To that end we must avoid measuring them with the moral yardstick of our own time, realizing that our own morals have no absolute value but are the result of certain historical developments in which we happen to be involved at the moment. This is particularly necessary when we study the sex life of other civilizations. Customs vary; the style of living changes. To the superficial observer it may look as if the Greeks had been highly promiscuous, having intercourse with whoever happened to be around —wife, slave girl, courtesan, boy, man—but this was not at all the case. Affections were at least as deep as they are today. No Don Juan creates an art, literature, and philosophy as the Greeks have. Human relations were broader and deeper, and there was less hypocrisy in matters of sex than in our present world.

Athens was a polis like all other Greek city-states. But in addition to being a polis and the capital of Attica, it was the capital of an empire. And while Sparta kept to herself and remained closed to the world, the Athenian way of life, by sheer force of circumstances, was gradually imposed upon other Greek city-states or rather, imitated by them. This is why we must study it in more detail. Under the threat of Persia the city-states on the islands and coasts of the Aegean Sea formed a confederacy with Athens in 477 B.C. The larger states supplied ships for defense, while the smaller contributed money. And because the treasury was in the temple of Apollo at Delos, the organization became known as the Confederacy of Delos. Later Athens alone supplied the naval power, all confederates contributed money, and the treasury was transferred to Athens. This was very important, for these contributions became a regular tribute which greatly added to the revenue of the state. Otherwise this revenue consisted of taxes paid by metics and gainfully employed slaves, sales taxes, taxes on prostitutes, and people engaged in other occupations, import and export duties, revenue from the state-owned and state-operated Laurium silver mines, court fees, and fines.[21] These high revenues made possible the development of a leisure class, which lived at the expense of the state, despised manual labor and trade on a small scale, and became the carrier of Athens' artistic and intellectual life.

The Athenian citizen lived for the state just as the Spartan did, but in a different, democratic way. He also served in the army and was trained to be a hoplite,[22] and he fought well enough in the Persian Wars, but to be a soldier was not his aim in life. Athens was a democracy in which rich and poor citizens had equal rights. Solon had divided the citizens into four classes according to income from real property, and the higher offices were always held by citizens of wealth. However, the constitution of Cleisthenes in 508 B.C. abolished this class distinction. The state power was vested in the Ecclesia, the Assembly of all citizens. This sounds rather formidable, but we must remember that the number of adult male citizens was very small. Of these a certain number lived outside of Attica, since citizens without means could obtain cleruchies—that is, land in the colonies which they could exploit without losing their citizenship. The metics, the resident aliens, had no political rights and were not allowed to possess real property. They paid regular taxes and a special aliens' tax, enjoyed the protection of the law, and played a very important part in a state whose citizens were mostly engaged in politics. They were the businessmen and industrialists, the ship-owners and bankers, who considerably increased the wealth of Athens. Painters, philosophers, and physicians came from their ranks. They had to be sponsored by a citizen, and served in separate divisions of the army.

The slaves were another social class which played a very important part in the economic life of the country.[23] They did most of the manual work; without their labor it would have been im-

possible for a leisure class that could devote all its time to politics
and intellectual pursuits to develop. Slaves were either born as such
—that is, as children of slaves—or were captives, mostly barbarians,
since Greek captives were usually ransomed. The state owned slaves,
who were needed for public works and who received clothing and
wages. But most slaves were privately owned, purchased on the
market, and used for domestic service or in the other occupations.
The average household had three to twelve slaves; rich people might
have as many as fifty.[24] We must bear in mind, however, that many
commodities which we buy ready-made in department stores today
were made at home in an ancient household. Slaves were employed
in industry. A craftsman, shoemaker, potter, or smith had a few
slaves to help him, or a master craftsman might himself be a slave.
A skilled slave who mastered a craft was more highly valued than
an unskilled one. Industry was on a very small scale, an artisan
industry as it still is in the Orient and in some sections of southern
and eastern Europe. There was no mass production, and the emphasis was on quality and individuality. We hear of a shield-making
factory which employed 120 slaves, but this must have been an
exception.[25]

By far the hardest lot was that of the slaves who worked the silver
mines of Laurium.[26] The mines were rich in galena, a silver-lead
ore. They were state-owned but were exploited by private con-
tractors who leased concessions from the state. The miners were
slaves, either criminals who had been sentenced to this kind of labor
or slaves purchased on the market. Sometimes the contractor rented
slave gangs from individuals who made it a business to own large
numbers of slaves whom they hired out at an obol a day [27] and with
the obligation to replace them in case of casualties.[28] The miners
entered the mine through shafts which went as far down as 386 feet,
and worked ten-hour shifts in ill-ventilated galleries only two to three
feet high. These were kept low and narrow to avoid the necessity
of using props. Kneeling or lying on his stomach, the hewer worked
in a gallery sparsely lit by oil lamps. Carriers brought the ore to the
shafts, whence it was hauled to the surface in amphorae or in

baskets. Discipline was very harsh. Fetters and chains have been found by excavators. The chief reason a contractor had to spare his workers, and even to provide entertainment for them during their free period, was the obligation to replace them in case of death. Still, there can be no doubt that the lot of these mine slaves was a very hard one and that they were ready to revolt whenever they had a chance. Of the 20,000 slaves that went over to the Spartans during the Peloponnesian War,[29] many must have been from the mines. In the second century B.C. they killed their overseers, and captured the acropolis of Sunium, where they entrenched themselves. But such revolts were ruthlessly suppressed. Athens' silver was one of the major assets of its economy, and the mines had to be exploited day and night, without interruption. Slave gangs were also used for quarrying, road construction, and similar undertakings.

We mentioned before that only citizens were entitled to the possession of real property. Hence agricultural land was owned exclusively by citizens,[30] who either worked it personally with the help of farm laborers —slaves as a rule—or leased it to tenants. Most estates were small. Attica was a small territory, and the soil was poor. Agricultural methods were still primitive. The custom to let the land lie fallow in alternate years was still practiced. The threefold rotation of crops was introduced slowly and hesitatingly but was gradually adopted.[31] The cereal chiefly grown in Attica was barley; wheat had to be imported in large quantity, mostly from the Ukraine, and this is why it was so important for Athens to keep the trade route to the Black Sea open at all times.[32] The pastures were not good enough for cattle breeding on any large scale. Horses, mules, and asses were kept here and everywhere else in Greece as means of transportation, and were also needed for the army. Pigs were fattened here as they are on every farm, and sheep and goats had no difficulty in finding sufficient food. One branch of agriculture played an infinitely greater part in antiquity than it does today, namely, apiculture. Honey to us is a luxury; to the Greeks and Romans who had no sugar, honey was the chief sweetening substance and was extensively used in the kitchen and also for the sweetening of medicaments. A very popular, refreshing drink that took the place of our lemonade, Coca Cola, and other 'pops,' was oxymel,[33] a drink prepared from water, vinegar, and honey.

Slaves in agriculture did not fare badly. For them, as well as probably for the slaves in the city, working days were from sunrise to sunset, but undoubtedly there was a long break for the inevitable siesta when the heat was at its peak.Death of a slave was an economic loss, and a sick or discontented slave did not work as well as one who was in good health and satisfied. Moreover, the Athenians were humane toward slaves. A slave might be liberated by his master, or, as happened more often, he bought his freedom. In such a case he became a freedman and had a status similar to that of the metic.

From all that has been said it becomes easily apparent that the actual number of male citizens in whom the state power of Athens was vested was extremely small, between 10,000 and 20,000. Since many of them were absent, the number of citizens who attended the Assembly, where the most weighty decisions were taken, hardly ever exceeded 10,000 and was usually much smaller. For certain decisions a quorum of 6,000 was required. A council of 500 designated by lot prepared the agenda for the Assembly and advised the executive organs, the Magistrate, a body of nine archons, and a secretary who were also elected by lot. The Areopagus was a kind of supreme court which watched over the constitution and handled certain criminal cases. After their term of office had expired, archons became members of the supreme court. Ordinary courts held trial by jury. Six thousand jurors were appointed each year, and panels of five hundred jurors were customary.

In order to protect the young democracy from the return of tyrants, the Assembly was empowered to ostracize a citizen by secret ballot. The victim of such a sentence was banished for ten years, but without disgrace and loss of citizenship or property. It is well known how many deserving citizens—men such as Aristides, Themistocles, Cimon, and many others—became the target of suspicion and were ostracized without justification, for these mass jury courts miscarried justice more than once. The sentencing to death of Socrates on a charge of introducing strange gods and corrupting the youth is merely the best known of many such cases. Democracy, even a limited democracy such as that of Athens, undoubtedly has enormous advantages in that it makes every individual citizen responsible for the welfare of all and guarantees a certain amount of political freedom, but it is not a panacea. Abuses, infringement of civil liberties, and miscarriage of justice under pressure from the mob occurred in Athens as well as in our own days under a democratic regime. The guilt and dishonor of such abuses fall on so many shoulders that they seem light to bear, but they weigh heavily in the verdict of history.

This small group of Athenian citizens became the foremost representatives of Greek culture. They were a leisure class who lived for and on the state. They could afford to do so because other groups of the population tilled the soil, reaped the crops, worked in shops, carried on trade with foreign lands, and brought wealth to the country. Some citizens, probably a good many of them, had means of their own and inherited real estate, and many did not hesitate to invest money in some shipping expedition or other commercial venture, so long as others did the actual work. And all citizens drew funds from the state. Every office, every function was remunerated, and everyone exercised some duty, if only attendance at the Assembly for which every citizen received one obol, later three, a day. Jurors were paid one obol in the beginning, but when the cost of living increased, the pay was raised to two and then three, and we saw that thousands of citizens served as jurors in the courts. Councillors were paid five obols, later a drachma, a day. It has been calculated that in the latter part of the fifth century an Athenian town-dweller could live on two obols a day, husband and wife on three.[34] In other words, a citizen could live on state funds even if he had no means of his own. Material life was simple in those days, much more so than in the Eastern colonies, where the luxuries of decadent Asiatic cultures were adopted all too eagerly. Few Athenians were very wealthy; there could be no latifundia in a country as small as Attica, and riches were not accumulated in a society that despised business actives. (The *nouveaux riches* were metics.) If an Athenian citizen was wealthy, liturgies were imposed upon him—that is, the obligation to finance certain festivals, a public service in which metics shared and which was in effect a high income tax.

Athens set the style for Greek life and was imitated by other city-states. When Alexander the Great conquered large sections of the ancient world, when Greek became the language of civilized societies, it was Athens' ways not Sparta's that were copied, and the whole Western world looked to Athens as the center of culture long after Greece had lost its liberty. We must, therefore, say a few words about private life in fifth-century Athens, emphasizing particularly those aspects which had some bearing on health and disease. Here as everywhere the social environment played as important a part in the genesis of disease as the physical environment.[35]

We mentioned before that women were relegated to the house, while men lived out of doors and came home only for meals and for the night. If the husband brought friends for dinner, the women of the house, wife and daughters, retired. Feasting was a man's affair, and if the presence of women was wanted one sent for flute players and dancers to add color to the banquet. Woman was a necessary evil; she was needed to keep the house in order and to bear children. She had hardly any education, could probably neither read nor write, and was skilled in household duties only. It has frequently been said that the position of the Ionian woman, so different from that of the Dorian, was the result of Asiatic influence. This is possible, although women enjoyed a much freer position in many parts of the ancient Orient.

When a girl had reached the age of fifteen, her parents began to look around for a husband, provided they could raise a sufficient dowry. Marriages were arranged by the parents, and the girl usually met her husband for the first time at the wedding. As a rule, people were older when they married than in Egypt or India, girls from fifteen to even twenty years of age, men from twenty to thirty. It was believed that both man and woman secrete semen, and when the two mix in sexual intercourse and the semen is kept in the womb, then pregnancy will result. Like her Egyptian sister, the Greek woman was curious to know whether the child would be a boy or a girl. There were certain signs to observe.[36] If the skin of her face remained bright and the nipples of her breasts were turned upward, it would be a boy; but if she had freckles on her face and the nipples were turned down, it would be a girl. Or she would take woman's milk and flour, knead it into a dough, bake it on a slow fire. If it burned she would have a boy, but if it split open she would have a girl.[37] And since boys developed in the right part of the uterus, and girls in the left, she watched her breasts and also her eyes. If the right breast was larger, the right eye more widely open, these signs pointed to a boy.[38] There were many such popular notions which were sometimes right and sometimes not.

Children were wanted, particularly a son and heir to whom a man could leave his property. If the wife did not conceive, there was supposed to be some good reason for this. The opening of the uterus might be deviated or closed altogether, or it might be slippery by nature or as a result of ulceration. Again, the uterus might be ulcerated or too large, or contain residual menstrual blood; or the menstrual flow was not normal, too weak or too strong or missing altogether; or the uterus had prolapsed or was anteflected;[39] many of these explanations are still valid today. What is most noteworthy, however, is that infertility was not ascribed to witchcraft or to the wrath of the gods, that it was not considered a punishment for sins, but was considered the result of natural causes and had to be treated by rational means, ointments, fumigations, manipulations, and other measures. There is no doubt that many a woman in such a case sacrificed to Artemis, Hera, or Eileithyia, just as sterile women today pray for children, make vows, and wear medals and amulets. But the great step forward was taken when in addition to religious and magic rites —or instead of them—women consulted the midwife or the physician who had anatomical and physiological explanations for the condition, and endeavored to treat it rationally.

Sometimes women did not want a child. They used contraceptive devices, or, if it was too late, had an abortion performed. A contraceptive remedy mentioned twice in the Hippocratic writings seems very problematical: it consisted of a potion containing *misy*, a copper salt, of which an amount 'the size of a bean' was dissolved in water. Moreover, it was supposed to protect the woman for a whole year.[40] If it had been effective, the Greeks would have discovered the ideal contraceptive for all times to come. Mechanical devices, wool, salves, and resins introduced into the vagina before intercourse were more effective.

The problem of abortion is a very interesting one. Strongly condemned in many civilizations including our own, abortion was accepted in ancient Greece.[41] The only objection that could be raised was that abortion without consent of the father might deprive him of a desired heir. This is probably the meaning of a passage in Galen where he says that both Lycurgus and Solon forbade the practice of abortion.[42] If they ever did, and this is not at all certain, they did so to protect the father's rights. At any rate, abortion was not only legitimate but even recommended in the fifth and fourth centuries B.C. It is mentioned repeatedly in the Hippocratic writings. Prostitutes who for obvious reasons were not particularly anxious to have children had frequent recourse to abortion.[43] A highly prized singing girl, who much to her dismay became pregnant, was advised by the Hippocratic doctor to jump so that her heels would hit her buttocks. When she had done this seven times, 'the semen fell to the ground with a plop.'[44] It looked like a raw egg without the shell, round, transparent, with blood clots—undoubtedly a blood mole.[45] Abortive drugs were given as potions or pessaries, but as they had no effect whatever there is no point in listing them here.[46] More effective were certain manipulations, such as the puncture of the ovum.[47]

Plato and Aristotle both recommended abortion as a means of controlling the growth of the population. In his inquiry about the ideal state Plato suggested that women after the age of forty should be allowed to have intercourse, but should not give birth to children;

in other words, should have abortions.[48] And Aristotle thought that abortion should be practiced before the embryo had 'sensation and life.' [49] Now, we know that the Hippocratic Oath forbids the physician to 'give to a woman an abortive pessary.' How can we reconcile this prohibition with the fact that abortion was generally practiced, not only by midwives but also by Hippocratic and other physicians; that it was accepted by society and even recommended by the greatest philosophers of the period? The average Greek had not the deep respect for life that the Indian had. Weak and crippled infants were destroyed, not only in Sparta but in Athens also; and once one is prepared to kill born children, why should there be any hesitation to destroy what is a mere embryo, provided it can be done without endangering the mother? There were, however, religious groups in Greek society, notably the Orphics and Pythagoreans, who perhaps under Indian influence, had profound respect for life. We shall see later that the so-called Hippocratic Oath actually was a Pythagorean document, which, therefore, did not represent the general view of the period but was rather a reform program, a manifesto of a relatively small religious group.

It was known that the child was born at the end of a period of about 280 days—that is, of ten moon months or nine months of thirty days each, with ten additional days. Some doctors believed that a child born in the seventh month survived, while one born in the eighth month usually died.[50] The arguments they brought forth for such a theory were purely speculative and not based on facts. The number seven played an important part in the thinking of various schools, and the Hippocratic collection contains a special treatise on the subject.[51] Similar views are reflected in other writings of the same collection. It was believed that life unfolded according to a certain rhythm. Woman menstruated at intervals of four times seven days, the child was born after seven times forty days, and so the number seven appeared to be deeply rooted in nature. As it also played an important part in the thinking of the Babylonians and Assyrians, an Eastern influence on Greece by way of Asia Minor is well conceivable.

When the ten months of pregnancy are over, 'the nourishment and the material for growth that descend from the mother are no longer sufficient for the child . . . for it absorbs the sweetest part of the blood and also gets a little food from the milk. But whenever these sources become inadequate for it and the child is full-grown, it craves more nourishment than actually is available, and so strikes out and bursts the membranes . . . .' [52] When all the membranes have burst, the embryo is freed from its attachment and comes wriggling out. In other words, it was believed that it was the child that initiated labor, a view held until the beginning of the seventeenth century, when Fabricius and Harvey observed and correctly evaluated the contractile powers of the uterus. Vertex presentation was considered the normal and best presentation, as indeed it is. In case of breech presentation no special action was required, while transverse presentation had to be corrected. This was done through manipulations intended to change it to a cephalic presentation, or the child was killed to save the mother. The Greeks had no clear view about the anatomy of the pelvis and its significance in the process of childbirth, and sometimes believed that the hip bones gave way under pressure of the child's head, as they do in the case of certain animals.[53]

The woman probably gave birth in a squatting position, as the Egyptians did. She possibly also used some kind of parturition chair. A midwife assisted her and the doctor was called only in abnormal cases when something went wrong. Conditions, in other words, were very similar to what they are today all over the East. Socrates was the son of a midwife, and he sometimes alludes to that profession.[54] He tells us that midwives were elderly women who had passed the age of pregnancy and childbirth, but had experienced what it meant to have a child. Better than anyone else they were able to diagnose early pregnancy, and they had drugs and charms to activate labor pains and make them milder at will, to induce labor in a woman who gave birth with difficulty, or to cause miscarriage when the embryo was still young. Yet midwives were also excellent matchmakers, who knew well enough what man and what woman should be brought together so that they would produce the best children. Honest midwives, however, had to be careful in this respect, to avoid the reputation of being procurers.

When the child was born it was bathed—not in wine as in Sparta, but in warm water—anointed with oil, and swaddled with bands of woolen cloth that covered the entire body including arms and head. As a rule, the mother nursed the child, or if she did not have enough milk, a wet nurse took her place, possibly a household slave who happened to have a child at that time. Children were breast-fed for a long time, as everywhere in antiquity. Sudhoff collected interesting documents concerning wet nurses from Ptolemaic and Roman Egypt;[55] contracts of people who turned over their own child or one of their slaves' children to a nurse who agreed to bring it up for a certain length of time, usually two or three years, for which service she was paid in money or kind, or both. Much later, Soranus in his book on gynecology gave detailed instructions about the selection of a wet nurse. She was to be not younger than twenty, nor older than forty years of age, was to have borne children two or three times before, was to be free from disease, of good constitution, well built, and of good complexion. Both breasts should be evenly formed, loose, soft, without wrinkles, and the nipples should be neither too large nor too small, neither too hard nor too porous, and they should let the milk flow out in a steady stream. The nurse, moreover, must be of sound mind, must be kind, not irascible, a Greek, and clean.[56] Soranus then goes on to discuss the quality of mother's milk, the diet and entire mode of living appropriate for a nurse. But we are anticipating by centuries, for Soranus wrote in imperial Rome at a time when many ladies refused to nurse their children. The fact that the Hippocratic writings rarely discuss the wet nurse [57] may not be accidental; it seems very likely that in those early days many more mothers were prepared to nurse their children than in imperial Rome.

When the child was weaned it was given cow's milk or goat's milk, which it drank from bottles with an opening, many of which may be seen in our museums.[58] It was also fed porridge made from

various cereals, and the nurse or mother sometimes chewed more
solid food first and then stuffed it into the child's mouth.[59] Until the
age of six the child remained in the care of the women of the house,
playing with toys very similar to those of our own children, dolls
made of terra cotta with movable arms and legs, dolls' houses, all
kinds of animals made of clay, carts and hoops, and a variety of
other playthings. Then, at the age of six, life began to be more serious
as the child went to school.

Athenian education was very different from that of Sparta. The
training of soldiers was not its primary purpose. All served in the army
and were ready to fight for their country, as did Socrates in the campaign against Potideia.[60] Athenian education was aristocratic in the
beginning and only people of means could afford teachers for their
children, but from the middle of the fifth century on it became increasingly democratic. Every citizen was expected to have at least an
elementary education, and since not every family could afford its own
teachers, educators would teach a group of children. This was the
beginning of the school as an institution of the Western world. It was
a private school; the teachers were paid by the parents not by the
state. A slave, the pedagogue, escorted his master's children to and
from school.

The Ionic ideal, unlike that of the Dorians, was the education of
man as a whole, both physical and mental, the attainment of universal culture—what the Greeks called *paideia*. The perfect Ionian
gentleman was καλοκἀγαθός, good and noble, and also well built,
handsome. This was an educational ideal, to be sure, which also had
great hygienic value: an individual perfectly balanced in body and
mind was the highest result that hygiene could possibly achieve.
Where such a view prevailed, the physician's task was much easier;
general education and health education went hand in hand, and
educator, trainer, and physician were close allies. At all times, success
or failure of health education depended not only on the physician's
knowledge and methods but also—and to a very high degree—on
society's readiness to accept advice. Wherever health was highly
valued, when people accepted a duty to health or when *mens sana*

in corpore sano seemed a desirable goal, people were eager to listen to the doctor and to practice what he taught them.

The Athenian boy went to elementary school from the age of six to fourteen, and was instructed in reading, writing, arithmetic, music, and also—and very much so—in sports. To that end he was placed in the charge of a παιδοτρίβης, a trainer of boys who kept a palaestra, a building with a central courtyard covered with sand, dressing rooms, and baths. There he was instructed in running, jumping, throwing of discus and javelin, wrestling, and boxing. He exercised in the nude after anointing his body with oil as a protection against the sun, just as we use cold cream when we go mountain-climbing or sailing in summer. When the training period was over and the young man sweaty and dirty, he scraped off the sand that stuck to his body with a special instrument, the ξυστήρ, a scraper that we find represented on vase pictures and on the famous statue of an athlete by Lysippus. A bath followed.

The Greeks at that time did not bathe in tubs, as did the Romans and the Cretans, and as we do, nor was their bath a steam bath. In the middle of the room was a large washbasin. A servant filled it with water, hot or cold, according to the season. Vase paintings, good sources for scenes of everyday Greek life, display a variety of bath rooms, men's and women's baths, shower baths where the water poured from spigots shaped like a lion's mouth, low basins for foot baths, and others held on the knees for the daily morning ablutions. They also show us women washing and combing their hair; permanent waves were made with hot sand.[61] The Greeks were very clean, like all peoples who have no taboos on nudity and who dress lightly.

From the age of fourteen to eighteen boys of the richer classes continued their education in a higher school; physical training and the study of literature and music were intensified. At eighteen the Athenian boy acquired the official status of an ephebe. He was trained for the army or navy for one year, and did garrison duty for a second year. Later the total period of military service was reduced to one year. Training ground for ephebes and adults was the

gymnasium, which, as a rule, included a palaestra and also facilities
for horseback riding, and even for cavalry parades. The gymnasium
was a public institution, supported by the community and administered by a special board. Athens had three such gymnasia located
in sacred groves on the outskirts of the city, and one of them, the
Academy,[62] became particularly famous, because Plato conducted his
school there. The gymnasium was not only a training ground but
also a meeting place where you found your friends, and where you
began a love affair with an ephebe. In Plato's *Symposium* Alcibia-
des tells how he tried to seduce Socrates by inviting him to train
with him, since this would give him a chance to display his body in
all its beauty.[63] This cult of the male body, this constant effort to
nurse it, to train it, to make it attractive to other men, seems strange
to us, yet it contained a very sound element. Men did not try to
become attractive by wearing expensive clothes and jewelry and by
adorning themselves with cosmetics, as women do today. It was the
perfect harmony of body and mind that counted, and this could be
developed and preserved only through constant exercise. Very few
of our best dressed and seemingly attractive women could stand the
test of appearing in the nude and remain attractive, even if they
were not expected to say one word, for their so-called 'beauty culture'
is artificial and merely on the surface.

Greek men, young and not so young, trained daily, systematically, and under the supervision of a professional trainer. This
trainer was the health educator of ancient Greece even more so than
the physician. He was in daily touch with the people who frequented
his palaestra or the gymnasium to which he was attached. He advised
them not only in matters of gymnastics but also in regard to their
diet; and the Greek word for diet had a much broader meaning
than we give it today. By diet the Greeks meant a man's entire mode
of living, the relation between sleep and being awake, between
exercise and rest, and, of course, also, the choice of food, the quantity
to be consumed, evacuations, and all other factors that constitute a
man's life and must be under control if the individual is to be not
only healthy but also strong and beautiful. Hence these trainers were

great experts in matters of hygiene. Perhaps they did not have a philosophical explanation for all their precepts as had physicians, but they had experience, the experience of a century-old tradition. The Olympic games were founded in the eighth century B.C. Athletes were trained in the pentathlon: five exercises which they had to master equally well—running, jumping, throwing of discus and javelin, and wrestling. The purpose of the pentathlon was to develop not record-breakers in one field but all-round athletes, strong, skillful, agile, graceful, and beautiful.[64] The statues of Olympic victors have created a canon of beauty for all times. How different they are from Roman gladiators or modern boxers, whose muscles are quite unevenly developed and whose entire habitus reflects nothing but brute force!

We found one source of Greek medicine in the teachings of the pre-Socratic philosophers. They provided the physician with methods of thought and reasoning. Another source is Greek gymnastics. Like the philosophers the trainers taught the physician a great deal, and again like the philosophers in turn learned much from him. As a matter of fact, there never was any antagonism between the two; rather, there seems to have been a very close co-operation between them. The Hippocratic writings, particularly those on diet, mention gymnastics frequently. Thus we read in the treatise *On Diet* [65] that food and exercise have opposite effects but that together they contribute to the maintenance of health. By exercising we spend energy and substance, but food and drink restore both. Hence the art consists of knowing accurately the effect of exercises on the body, as well as the effect of food, and to prescribe both in the right proportion. In doing so we must take into account the constitution of the individual, since no two persons are alike; we must also consider his age, the seasons, the winds that happen to be blowing, the locality in which an individual lives, and the general condition of the year. These are very correct observations, for we all know that children, adults, and old people require different food, that we crave different foods in summer from those we desire in winter. We know well enough the effects of such winds as *sirocco*, *föhn,* or *mistral.* We are aware of the importance of climate for an individual's well-being, and of the fact that the years differ. All these factors must be considered very carefully in order to keep a person fit and in good health throughout the year, and to this end physician and trainer should work hand in hand.

We possess a very interesting document which describes what the physicians considered a day spent hygienically. It is a fragment from a book of Diocles of Carystus, a famous physician who lived at Athens toward the end of the fourth century B.C. He was later than the Hippocratic doctors, but the views on hygiene and hygienic life had hardly changed during the century. The fragment is too long to be quoted in full and verbatim, and the following is an abstract and paraphrase: [66]

The cultivation of health begins with the moment a man wakes up. This should as a rule be when the food he ate the previous day has already moved from the stomach to the bowels. A young or middle-aged individual should take a walk of about 10 stadia [67] just before sunrise, in summer however he should walk only 5, and older men will take a shorter walk in winter as well as in summer. After awakening one should not arise at once but should wait until the heaviness and torpor of sleep have gone. After arising one should rub one's neck and head thoroughly in order to overcome the stiffness caused by the pillow. Then rub the whole body with some oil. Those who are not accustomed to empty their bowels immediately after arising should perform this rubbing before the evacuation, while others will do it after evacuation but before undertaking anything else. ... Thereafter one shall every day wash face and eyes with the hands using pure water. One shall rub the gums in order to strengthen the teeth or shall simply rub the teeth inside and outside with the fingers using some fine peppermint powder and cleaning the teeth of remnants of food. One shall anoint nose and ears inside, preferably with well-perfumed oil. ... The head is a part that requires a great deal of care, such as rubbing, unction, washing, combing, and close shaving. One shall rub and anoint the head every day but wash it and comb it only at intervals. ... After such a morning toilet people who are obliged or choose to work will do so, but people of leisure will first take a walk. Long walks before meals evacuate the body, prepare it for receiving food, and give it more power for digesting it. Moderate and slow walks after meals mix foods, drinks, and gases contained in the body. . . . After the walk it is good to sit down and to attend to private affairs until the time arrives when one has to think of caring for the body. Young people and those who are accustomed to exercise or who need it should go to the gymnasium. For older and weaker people it is better to go to the bath or to some other warm place to be anointed. For people of that age if they have a gymnasium exclusively for their own use a moderate rubbing and light exercise are sufficient. . . . After such physical exercise it is time for the mid-day meal, which in summer should consist of white barley groats with aromatic white wine well mixed with some honey and water—or some other gruel that does not produce flatulence, is nourishing and easy to digest. Those who do not care for such foods shall take cold bread. In addition to that, one shall eat some boiled vegetable such as gourds or cucumber, prepared simply. One shall drink white wine and water until the thirst is quenched, but before eating one should drink water in large quantity if one is thirsty, otherwise less. Soon after eating one should go to sleep in a shady or cool place well protected from wind. After the siesta one can attend to private affairs, take another walk, and go to the gymnasium. After exercising and being covered with dust it is good for strong young people to have a cold bath. Older and weaker people, on the other hand, shall be anointed and rubbed gently and shall then have a hot bath. A general rule is that one should never or only rarely wash the head with hot water. . . . The chief meal is to be taken when the body is empty and does not contain any badly digested residue of food. Dinner should be taken in summer soon before sunset and consist of bread, vegetables, and barley cake. Dinner begins with raw vegetables, with the exception of cucumber and horseradish, for these are vegetables that should be eaten toward the end of the meal. Boiled vegetables are eaten in the beginning of the meal. Other dishes are cooked fish and meats; kid or lamb meat shall be preferably from very young animals, pork from middle-aged pig, and as far as birds are concerned one shall eat chicken, partridge, or pigeon. All must be cooked simply. . . . Before dinner one shall drink water and continue to drink it some time afterwards. Lean people shall drink dark and thick wine and after the meal white wine. Fat people shall drink white wine all the time, and they all shall drink their wine with water. Fruits from trees are of little use, but if one takes them in moderate quantities before the meals they do relatively little harm. ... After dinner lean and flatulent people who do not digest well should go to sleep at once while others will take a short and slow walk before going to sleep. It is good for everybody to lie on the left side first as long as the food is still in the region of the stomach, but when the abdomen has become soft one should turn to the right. It is not good for anybody to sleep on the back.

This was a very elaborate personal hygiene that required time and leisure. It was the hygienic way of life that could be led only by a citizen whose sole occupation was politics and service to the state in general. The metics, freedmen, traders, artisans, farm laborers and other slaves obviously could not afford to lead such a life. The Hippocratic book *On Diet* has advice for 'the mass of people who drink and eat what they happen to get, and who are obliged to work, and to travel by land and sea in order to make a living, who are exposed to unwholesome heat and unwholesome cold, and who otherwise lead an irregular life.' [68] All they can do is consider the season in which they happen to be and try to adapt their meals, exercise, and sex life to it as best they can. It is little enough but they are people who 'by necessity must lead a haphazard life and who cannot, neglecting all, take care of their health.' This was particularly true of the slaves, who had no control over their hours of work and rest or over their food. Their well-being was protected only by the fact that their owners were materially interested in keeping them fit and in good health.

Our science of nutrition is based on physiology and biochemistry. The latter is a very young science which could develop only after Lavoisier's revolution of chemistry had taken place and had paved the way for the development of organic chemistry, and thus had made possible the investigation of the chemistry of the human body. In antiquity, experience alone revealed the action of a given food on the organism, and in the fifth and fourth centuries an enormous amount of observation was devoted to ascertaining the effect of

innumerable foods, solid and liquid, raw and cooked, on the human
body in health and disease. The Hippocratic treatise *On Diet* was
by no means the first of its kind, for the writer criticizes his pre-
decessors in this subject, but it is the best early treatise on diet preserved. It begins with statements which are as true today as they
were in the past, namely that in order to be able to write a good
treatise on diet the physician must know the nature of man in
general, and must know how to diagnose the individual's nature.
He must also know what constitutes the human body originally and
what parts have the faculty to influence it or to gain power over it,
because this is exactly what we aim at when we prescribe a special
diet. To that end we must also be familiar with the faculties of the
various foods and drinks. Thus Book I of the treatise *On Diet* discusses the nature of man, that he is constituted of two elements, fire
and water, which have the elementary qualities of hot and dry, cold
and moist. Book II then treats of the qualities of the various foods,
those they have by nature and those that may be developed in them
by cooking, boiling, roasting, and similar processes. We eat few foods
raw, as nature supplies them; they are made palatable in the kitchen
and the preparation largely determines their dietetic effect. Centuries
later Galen wrote a treatise in three volumes *On the Faculties of
Foods* in which he gave detailed instructions on the effects and uses
of practically everything we eat and drink.

The Hippocratic collection contains another treatise on diet,
Περὶ διαίτης ὑγιεινῆς, *On Sound Diet*. It is only a few pages
long but is full of interesting observations and reveals the way of
life of the Greek upper class. It does not discuss the general effect
of individual foods—this was done in other books—but begins with
a chapter on how you should live during the various seasons. Thus
in winter you should eat much and drink little. Drink your wine
as pure as possible, eat bread, roast your meats, and eat few vegetables. In the summer, however, eat barley porridge instead of bread,
eat vegetables, raw and cooked, boil the meat, and drink plenty of
well-diluted wine. This was sound common sense, but there was
also a theory behind it. The seasons affect man's constitution as we

all know, and the diet was meant to offset evil seasonal effects by keeping the body hot and dry in winter, cool and moist in summer. We shall have to say more about these and similar theories.

The treatise then goes on to discuss a man's mode of living according to his constitution and age. A fat individual must live differently from a lean one, and what is good for an old person is not good for a young one. The many people who are trying to reduce today may wish to hear what the Hippocratic doctor recommended:

Fat people and all those who wish to reduce must do all hard work on an empty stomach, and then begin eating while they are still out of breath from exertion and without having refreshed themselves, having had only some diluted and not very cold wine. Their food should be prepared with sesame, sweet spices, and similar substances, and should be rich, for thus they will feel satiated with a minimum of food. Furthermore one should have only one meal a day, should not bathe, and should sleep on a hard couch. One should walk nude as much as possible. Those who wish to gain weight should do the contrary.[69]

The book also has a chapter on vomiting and the taking of enemas as a matter of hygiene. For more than two thousand years people evacuated the body by way of the stomach and bowels to liberate it from superfluities. This was a Greek heritage, the result of Greek physiological and pathological theories as we find them first expressed in the Hippocratic writings. Vomiting was recommended during the six winter months, because at that time phlegm dominated in the upper parts of the body. During the summer heat, however, enemas were indicated, because the body then became bilious, with heaviness in the lumbar region and knees. Prescriptions were given for the diet of children and women. Small children should have long hot baths. Wine was given to them as a matter of course, but it was to be well diluted and only such wine as does not cause flatulence. The women's diet must be essentially dry: such a diet was considered becoming to the softness of the female flesh. This did not mean that the diet was to be of dry materials but rather of dry quality. A long chapter is devoted to athletes, whose exercises and diet must be adapted to the seasons and whose individual constitution must be taken into consideration. In the manuscripts this short treatise ends with an aphorism which occurs also in another Hippocratic book:

An intelligent man must understand that health is the people's most valuable possession and must know how to help himself by his own thought in case of illness.[70]

Many of the Hippocratic treatises were written for physicians and laymen alike. Every educated person was supposed to have some knowledge of health and disease, and medicine was not yet the specialized science it became in Alexandria.

Higher education evolved greatly from the second half of the fifth century on.[71] The teachers were the sophists, some of the most prominent of whom are well known to us from Plato's dialogues. Their task was παιδεύειν ἀνθρώπους, to educate people, namely for statesmanship. A sophist would take over the education of a young man or of a group of young men for a period of three to four years, and the fee charged was sometimes quite considerable. In this higher education the chief accent was no longer on gymnastics but on intellectual pursuits. The young man was instructed in all the subjects that a statesman, a leader of people needed: first of all philosophy and rhetoric, but also mathematics, science, and medicine. This higher education was to be as universal as possible and was to lead the young man on the road to success. The sophists were itinerant teachers who, like the physicians, remained in a place so long as they found work there remunerative. In the course of time they acquired a bad reputation, and the word 'sophistry' is anything but complimentary. It is certainly correct that they were not primarily seekers of truth, that they worked for money, that many were cynical and not too scrupulous in selecting the road to success. On the other hand, it must be admitted that among the earlier sophists there were men of high character, and that they contributed a great deal to the spread of knowledge, including medical learning. Their profession had much in common with that of the physician.

In this chapter we have discussed private life in the Greek city-states in the fifth and fourth centuries B.C. In doing so we consulted a number of medical books which indeed proved to be a first-rate source for our knowledge of small details of daily life. Herodotus visited Egypt in the fifth century B.C. and gave us a graphic account of the customs and general way of life he observed. But no Egyptian or other foreigner wrote a book on Greek customs at that time. Philosophers, historians, and tragic poets do not write about such trivial matters as daily meals or the swaddling of infants. In the comedies of Aristophanes, however, we find many interesting details, since the comic writer is allowed to be trivial and no one objects to his presenting even crude physiological matters on the stage. But it is the books of the physicians who entered all homes and were forced to inquire into most intimate affairs that remain one of our chief sources, one which, it seems to me, has not been fully exploited as yet.

We talked about diet and saw that physicians greatly emphasized its importance for the people's health. We saw that Greek meals were frugal as a rule. Two meals a day, with the chief meal in the evening before sunset, were enough even for people of wealth. Flat loaves of bread baked from wheat flour or barley porridge were staple food in every household. Fruit and vegetables were plentiful during the good season, and onions and garlic were eaten throughout the year. Fish was consumed by rich and poor, and salted or smoked, could be preserved or even imported from afar. Meat and poultry frequently mentioned in the physicians' writings were not cheap and appeared only occasionally on the poor man's table. Like all Eastern peoples, the Greeks loved sweets, and the famous Attic honey was used in the preparation of a great variety of sweetmeats.[72] It was not only the Spartans who led a simple life; the Athenians of the classical period were moderate in eating and drinking, too. There obviously was room for feasting also. Men had their banquets, and a Greek symposium was not a mere academic discussion, with the papers presented to be published as a book. There was discussion, and sometimes of a very high order, as we know from

Plato's immortal dialogue. But social drinking went with the discussion, as the word implies, and all this took place after a hearty meal. In the periphery of Greece, in Asia Minor where Greeks lived in close touch with Asiatics, or in Sicily where brilliant courts were flourishing, luxury was displayed at an earlier time than on the mainland. Athenian daily life remained simple in its external manifestations throughout the Golden Age, as long as the people were able to create great artistic and spiritual values. Luxury is usually a sign of a decadent culture, which under an apparently brilliant surface tries to conceal the hollowness of the ruling class.

Greek dress at that time was also simple. Its basic elements were the same as in the early days, consisting of a tunic and a cloak. The tunic or *chiton*—sometimes short, sometimes long, particularly on formal occasions—was made of wool in the Dorian style and pinned up on the shoulders, or made of linen and sewn in the Ionian way. It was sleeveless or had short sleeves, was sometimes pleated, sometimes not, and was held in at the waist with a belt. It was an undergarment, the only dress of people at work, and the one worn at home. Outside of the house a cloak, the *himation*, was worn over the tunic, a piece of material, light in summer, warm in winter, gracefully draped so that it covered the whole body, sometimes even the head. At home people went barefoot, but in the street they wore sandals; not always though, for Socrates was known to walk about barefoot even outside the house.

The woman's dress was basically the same, except that she wore a *strophion*, a band to hold the breasts up. It had no straps as do our present brassières, so it had to be worn rather tightly. Otherwise women wore tunic and cloak like men, made of the same materials, and a woman leaving the house could put on her husband's cloak without becoming conspicuous, or vice versa. People riding on horseback or engaged in some violent occupation would have felt handicapped wearing the cloak and therefore adopted a Thessalian garment, the *chlamys*, a light cape also frequently worn by ephebes. Hats were rarely used by either men or women, unless there was some compelling reason such as particularly strong exposure to the sun, when a parasol served the purpose equally well. But it was simpler to protect the head by drawing the cloak over it.

We often think of the Greeks as being dressed in white garments, because their marble statues in our museums are white today. Yet they used to be colored in antiquity, and as a matter of fact costumes were made in all conceivable colors and color combinations. The Greek dress was very hygienic: it did not deform the body and did not hinder the free movement of the limbs; it was light enough to permit the body to perspire freely when it was hot, and could be made and worn in such a way as to provide warmth in winter. It was, moreover, an extremely graceful costume. The cloak could be draped in a variety of ways, thus permitting individual taste to manifest itself. The well-known statue of Sophocles in the Lateran Museum shows the dignity of a man well wrapped in the *himation,* and the charming Tanagra statuettes reveal how women could dress with an infinite grace, to be found today only in India where the *sari* is worn very much as Greek women used to wear their *himation.*[73]

The house in the classical period was also simple. At a time when temples, theaters, and other public buildings were built of the most beautiful marble, in exquisite style and grandiose proportions, the Athenian lived in unpretentious houses, simply furnished. The Athenian citizen led an outdoor life and was at home only for meals and for the night. The house followed the Mediterranean pattern, opening into a courtyard, the *aule.* It had one or two stories above the ground floor. The women's quarters were usually on the upper floors. The foundation of the houses was of stone, the rest of bricks or of timber. This is why hardly any Athenian house of that period has been preserved, and why we have to rely mostly on literary sources. In the Hellenistic period courtyards became larger and were frequently ornamented with pillars. Rooms opened on loggias, and walls were decorated with paintings; but this was a later development when life had become more luxurious. In the fifth century B.C. in Athens and other Greek cities of the mainland, living conditions even of the wealthier citizens were very modest, and the poor population lived in tenements which were probably not very different from what we can see in the East today.

Most Greek cities developed haphazardly at first, with the market place as center, houses being built irregularly with no apparent city plan. There were exceptions, however. The city of Olynthus on the Chalcidic peninsula, excavated by D. M. Robinson on numerous expeditions,[74] reveals planning. The houses were built opening onto long straight streets, following a plan which reminds us of that of certain Egyptian towns. The chance to rebuild Greek cities more hygienically came after the Persian Wars, during which so many were destroyed. Thus the Piraeus had to be rebuilt around the middle of the fifth century B.C. This was done following a plan of Hippodamus of Miletus, an architect and town planner, who is usually credited with having introduced the 'gridiron' system into continental Greece and Italy—that is, a system of squares with avenues and streets cutting one another at right angles. It was very much the same system that William Penn applied when he outlined the city of Philadelphia. Town planning became the rule in the Hellenistic period, and the excavation of such cities as Priene, Miletus, Pergamum, Corinth, or Selinus in Sicily shows how clever and sound these plans were, making the best use of the geographic features of the site.[75]

A special treatise of the Hippocratic collection is devoted to *Airs, Waters, Places*. It clearly shows what great attention was paid by physicians to the location of a dwelling place, the winds to which it was exposed, the nearness of the sea, rivers, or swamps, and the quality of water available to the population. Centuries later a Roman architect and engineer, Vitruvius Pollio, who lived at the time of Augustus, wrote a famous treatise *On Architecture*. Since it is the only ancient book of its kind that has come down to us, it became a classic and was reprinted frequently from 1486 on. Vitruvius was concerned not only with building materials, machines, and technical problems of the building of public and domestic structures, but also with questions of public hygiene. A whole book of his work is devoted to the problem of water supply. We shall have more to say about him in our chapter on Rome, and this will give us an opportunity to discuss public health in Graeco-Roman antiquity in greater detail.

NOTES

1. See *Oxford Classical Dictionary*, 'Slaves'; also A. W. Gomme, *The Population of Athens in the Fifth and Fourth Centuries B.C.*, Oxford, 1933; and still useful K. J. Beloch, *Die Bevölkerung der griechisch-römischen Welt*, Leipzig, 1886.
2. About the Greek *polis* see N. M. Fustel de Coulanges, *La Cité antique*, a classic book first published in 1864 and reprinted ever since; Jakob Burckhardt, *Griechische Kulturgeschichte*, Berlin, 1898, vol. I; Gustave Glotz, *The Greek City and Its Institutions*, London, 1929; E. Howald, *Griechische Kulturgeschichte*, Zurich, 1948; W. Jaeger, *Paideia*, New York, 1945, vol. I.
3. See, e. g., R. M. Dawkins, 'The Sanctuary of Artemis Orthia at Sparta,' *J. Hell. Stud.*, Suppl. Paper 5, London, 1929.
4. *Pelop. War*, II, 6.
5. On Sparta in general see H. Berve, *Sparta*, Leipzig, 1939; T. Meier, 'Wesen der spartanischen Staatsordnung,' *Klio*, Beiheft 42, 1939; P. Roussel, *Sparte*, Paris, 1939.
6. See *Webster's New International Dictionary*.
7. The classical sources on Spartan education are Xenophon, *Polity of the Lacedaemonians*, 2; Plutarch, *Lycurgus*, 16–17; Plato, *Laws*, I, 633 A-C. About Greek education in general see H. I. Marrou, *Histoire de l'éducation dans l'antiquité*, Paris, 1948.
8. Plutarch, *Lyc.*, 15.
9. Ibid. 16.
10. Ibid. 25.
11. Ibid. 27.
12. Ibid. 22.
13. Ibid. 14.
14. See the very pertinent discussion of this point by H. I. Marrou, op. cit. p. 51ff.
15. W. Jaeger, *Paideia*, vol. III, p. 171.
16. A rich collection of source materials is in L. R. de Pogey-Castries, *Histoire de l'amour grec dans l'antiquité par M. H. E. Meier, augmenté d'un choix de documents originaux et de plusieurs dissertations complémentaires*, Paris, 1930; E. Bethe, 'Die dorische Knabenliebe, ihre Ethik, ihre Idee,' *Rhein. Mus.*, 1907, 42:438–75; H. Hoessli, *Eros, die Männerliebe der Griechen*, Munster-Berlin, 1924; D. M. Robinson and E. J. Fluck, *A Study of Greek Love-Names, including a Discussion of Paederasty*, Baltimore, 1937.
17. Plutarch, *Lyc.*, 18.

18. In fascist Italy this development was counteracted by the influence of the Catholic Church.

19. Plutarch, *Lyc.*, 18.

20. Herondas, *Mime*, VI.

21. See *Cambridge Ancient History*, vol. V, p. 28.

22. Citizens who could not afford to buy the equipment of a hoplite or heavy infantryman could serve in the light infantry or in the navy.

23. See H. Wallon, *Histoire de l'esclavage dans l'antiquité*, Paris, 1879, 3 vols.; E. Meyer, 'Die Sklaverei im Altertum,' *Kleine Schriften*, Halle, 1924, vol. I, pp. 169–212.

24. *Cambr. Anc. Hist.*, vol. V, p. 8.

25. Ibid. p. 15.

26. About the mines see E. Ardaillon, *Les Mines du Laurion*, Paris, 1897; G. Glotz, *Ancient Greece at Work*, New York, 1926; G. Rosen, *The History of Miners' Diseases*, New York, 1943.

27. About four cents.

28. For details see Xenophon's Περὶ πόρων, *Ways and Means*, namely, to improve the Athenian finances.

29. Thucydides, VII, 27.

30. The temples also owned land which they leased to tenants.

31. See Xenophon, *Oeconomicus*, 16, 12ff.

32. See *Cambr. Anc. Hist.*, vol. V, p. 13f.

33. Prescriptions for its preparation are given in Galen's treatise on *Hygiene*, Kühn, VI, 271ff.

34. *Cambr. Anc. Hist.*, vol. V, p. 21f. A drachma had 6 obols, a mna 100 drachmas or 600 obols, and a talent 60 mnas.

35. On Greek life in general see I. von Müller and A. Bauer, 'Die griechischen Privat- und Kriegsaltertümer,' *Handbuch der klassischen Altertumswissenschaft*, Munich, 1893, vol. IV, pt. 1, 2; H. Blümner, *Leben und Sitten der Griechen*, Leipzig, Prag, 1887; British Museum, *A Guide to the Exhibition Illustrating Greek and Roman Life*, 2nd ed., London, 1920.

36. See the Hippocratic treatise Περὶ ἀφόρων, *On Sterile Women*, Littré, VIII, 408ff. The classic book on Hippocratic gynecology and obstetrics is H. Fasbender, *Entwicklungslehre, Geburtshülfe und Gynäkologie in den hippokratischen Schriften*, Stuttgart, 1897. Recent books on ancient gynecology are I. Fischer, 'Geschichte der Gynäkologie,' *Biologie und Pathologie des Weibes*, Berlin and Vienna, 1924, vol. I, pp. 1–202; P. Diepgen, *Geschichte der Frauenheilkunde*, I. 'Die Frauenheilkunde der Alten Welt,' *Handbuch der Gynäkologie*, ed. by W. Stoeckel, 3rd ed., Munich, 1937, vol. 12, part I.

37. Hippocrates, L. VIII, 416.

38. Ibid. L. VIII, 486.

39. Ibid. L. VIII, 408ff.

40. Ibid. L. VII, 414; L. VIII, 170.

41. René Monpin, *L'Avortement provoqué dans l'antiquité*, Paris, 1918.

42. Galen, XIX, 179.

43. Hippocrates, L. VIII, 610.

44. Ibid. L. VII, 490. See also *Hippocrates on Intercourse and Pregnancy,* An English translation of *On Semen* and *On the Development of the Child,* by Tage U. H. Ellinger, with introduction (and notes) by Alan F. Guttmacher, New York, 1952.

45. See Guttmacher, op. cit. note 5.

46. See, e. g., Hippocrates, L. VIII, 170ff.

47. Ibid. L. VIII, 220.

48. Plato, *Republic,* 461C.

49. Aristotle, *Politica,* VII, 16.

50. See the Hippocratic treatises Περὶ ἑπταμήνου and Περὶ ὀκταμήνου, *On the Seven-Months Embryo* and *On the Eight-Months Embryo,* L. VII, 436–61. See also the passage, VIII, 612.

51. There is a special edition of this treatise by W. H. Roscher, *Die hippokratische Schrift von der Siebenzahl in ihrer vierfachen Ueberlieferung,* Paderborn, 1913.

52. Hippocrates, L. VII, 530f., Engl. trans. by Ellinger, op. cit.

53. Hippocrates, L. VII, 538.

54. Plato, *Theaetetus,* 149.

55. Karl Sudhoff, *Aerztliches aus griechischen Papyrus-Urkunden,* Leipzig, 1909, p. 150ff. On wet nurses in general see also W. Braams, *Zur Geschichte des Ammenwesens im Altertum,* Jena, 1913.

56. Soranus, *Gynaecia,* II, 12.

57. She is mentioned, e. g. L. V, 323.

58. See our illustration p. XXX.

59. Aristophanes, *Thesmophoriazusae,* 692. The comedies of Aristophanes are a rich source for such details of daily life.

60. Plato, *Symposium,* 219Ef.

61. See K. Sudhoff, *Aus dem antiken Badewesen,* Berlin, 1910, 2 vols.

62. The gymnasium was named after the hero Academus, or Hecademus. The word 'academy' has assumed very different meanings in the course of time.

63. Plato, *Symposium,* 217C.

64. E. N. Gardiner, *Athletics of the Ancient World,* Oxford, 1930.

65. Hippocrates, *On Diet,* L. VI, 470.

66. The fragment is preserved in the works of Oribasius (ed. U. C. Bussemaker and C. Daremberg, Paris, 1858, vol. III, p. 168ff.). See also M. Wellmann, *Die Fragmente der sikelischen Aerzte,* Berlin, 1901, p. 177ff.

67. A stadium was 600 feet or 200 yards.

68. *On Diet,* L. VI, 594ff.

69. Ibid. 76f.

70. Ibid. 86.

71. See Marrou, op. cit. p. 84.

72. About food in ancient Greece see J. Burckhardt, 'Über die Kochkunst der späteren Griechen,' in *Vorträge 1844–87,* Basle, 1918, p. 103ff.

73. About Greek dress see Lady Evans, *Chapters on Greek Dress,* London, 1893;

E. B. Abrahams, *Greek Dress,* London, 1908; M. Bieber, *Griechische Klei-dung,* Berlin, 1928.

74. On housing and town planning see the numerous archaeological works, notably the publication by D. M. Robinson and J. W. Graham, *Excavations at Olynthus. Part VIII. The Hellenic House,* Baltimore, 1938.

75. See A. von Gerkan, *Griechische Städteanlagen,* Berlin, 1924.

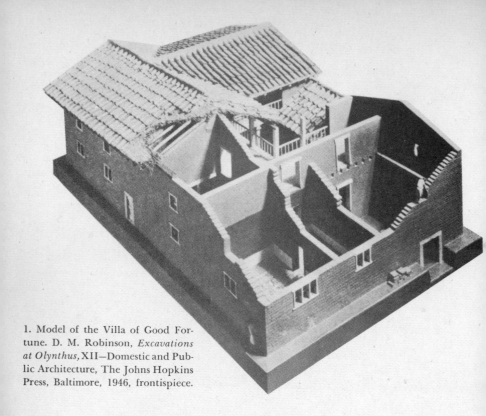

1. Model of the Villa of Good Fortune. D. M. Robinson, *Excavations at Olynthus,* XII—Domestic and Public Architecture, The Johns Hopkins Press, Baltimore, 1946, frontispiece.

2. Andron of the Villa from the South. D. M. Robinson and J. W. Graham, *Excavations at Olynthus,* VIII—The Hellenic House, The Johns Hopkins Press, Baltimore, 1938, pl. 17, 2.

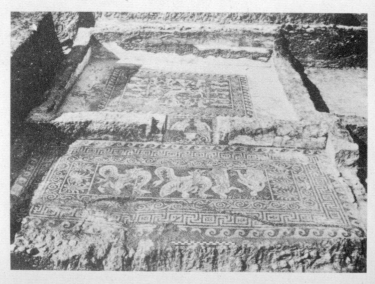

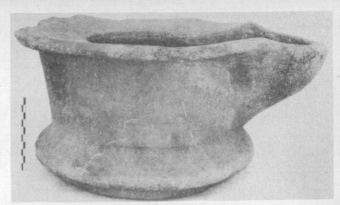

3. Terra-cotta toilet seat. Ibid. pl. 55, 1 a.

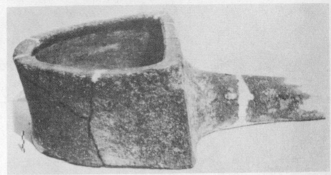

4. Terra-cotta vessel. Ibid. pl. 55, 2.

5. Bathtub. Ibid. pl. 53, 2.

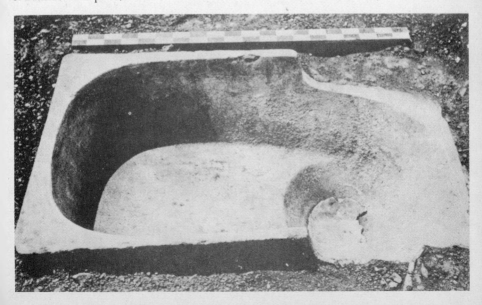

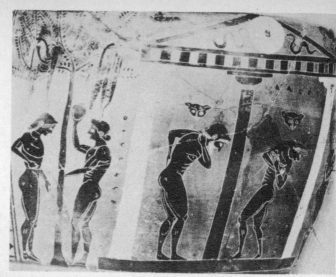

6. Shower in bathhouse. From Bruno Schröder, *Der Sport im Altertum*, Hans Schoetz,
Berlin, 1927, pl. 99.

7. Vase in black. From Karl Sudhoff, *Aus dem
antiken Badewesen*, Allgemeine Medizinische
Verlagsanstalt, Berlin, 1910, p. 52, fig. 41.

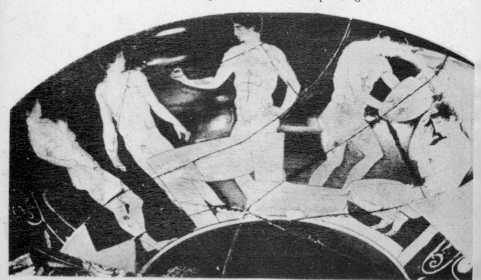

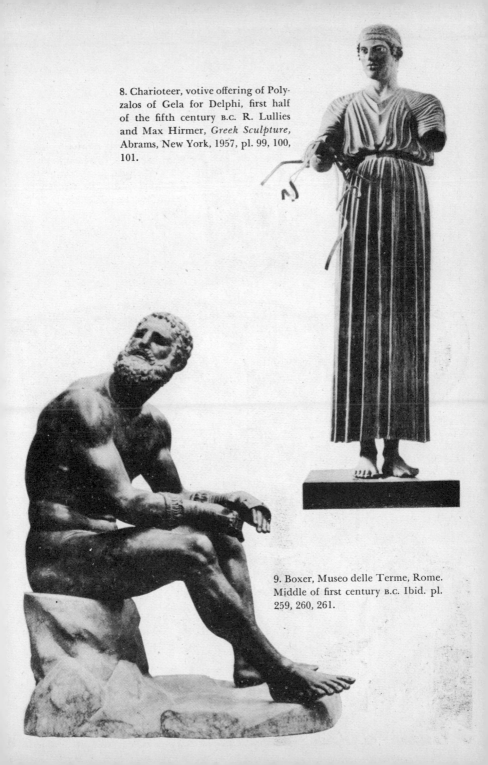

8. Charioteer, votive offering of Poly-
zalos of Gela for Delphi, first half
of the fifth century B.C. R. Lullies
and Max Hirmer, *Greek Sculpture,*
Abrams, New York, 1957, pl. 99, 100,
101.

9. Boxer, Museo delle Terme, Rome.
Middle of first century B.C. Ibid. pl.
259, 260, 261.

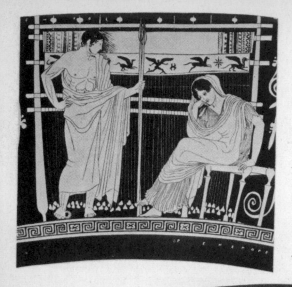

10. Loom of Penelope, from a vase in Bologna. (Furtwängler-Reichhold, *Vasenmalerei*, pl. 142.) M. Bieber, *Griechische Kleidung*, Walter de Gruyter, Berlin and Leipzig, 1928, p. 2, illustration 3.

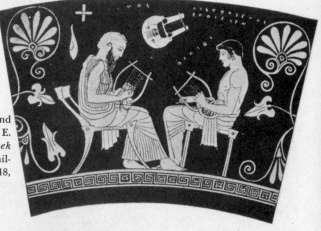

11. Music lesson: Iphikles and Linos. Kotyle from Caere. E. Pfuhl, *Masterpieces of Greek Drawing and Painting*, Macmillan, New York, 1926, pl. 48, fig. 67.

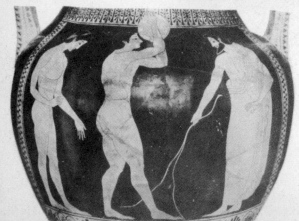

12. Discus thrower. From an amphora by the painter Euthymides, end of the sixth century B.C. Ibid. pl. 25, fig. 40.

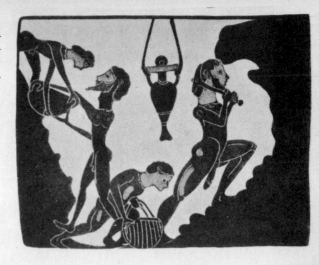

13. Corinthian clay tablet (dedications), sixth century B.C. Poseidon, Amphitrite and Hermes: Copper-mine. Ibid. pl. 10, fig. 17.

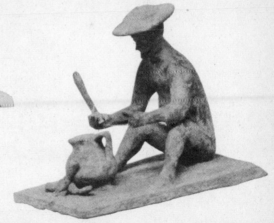

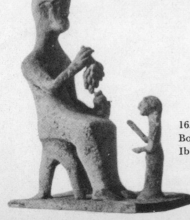

14. Barber, terra cotta. Seventh-sixth century B.C. (?). Boston Museum of Fine Arts. *Festschrift für James Loeb*, F. Bruckmann, München, 1930, p. 47.

15. Man cooking, terra cotta. Boston Museum of Fine Arts. Ibid. p. 47.

16. Old man and girl, terra cotta. Boston Museum of Fine Arts. Ibid. p. 47.

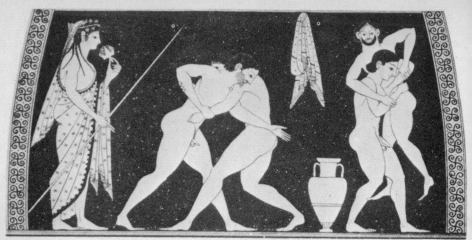

17. Wrestlers. Bruno Schröder,
op. cit. pl. 61.

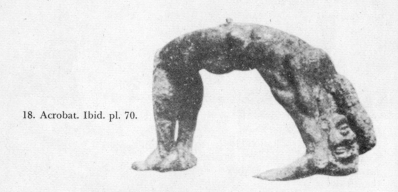

18. Acrobat. Ibid. pl. 70.

19. Jumping. Ibid. pl. 54.

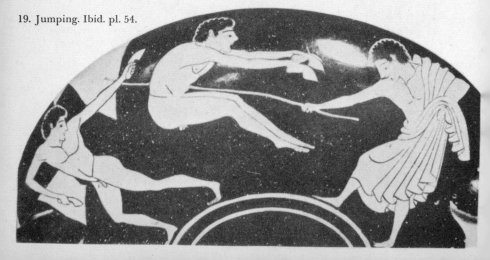

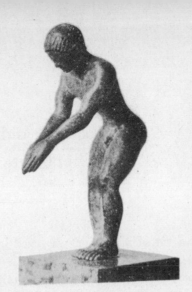

21. Satyr swinging girl at the spring festival. Bowl, middle of the fifth century B.C. From E. Pfuhl, *Masterpieces of Greek Drawing and Painting*, pl. 70, fig. 101. ·

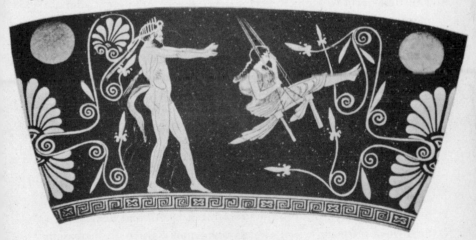

22. Swimmer. From Bruno Schröder, op. cit. pl. 39.

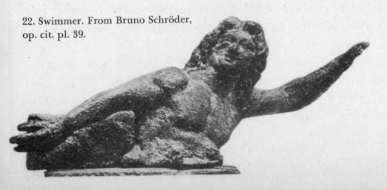

2. Hippocrates and the Collection of Hippocratic Writings

No physician's fame was ever greater than that of Hippocrates. The magic of his name for the Western medical world can be compared only to Charaka's for India. To be called a second Hippocrates or the Hippocrates of his time was the highest title of honor that could possibly be bestowed on a Western physician, and whenever something went wrong in medicine, when theory and practice did not harmonize, or when fantastic theories came up and began to dominate the field, the cry 'Back to Hippocrates,' was heard. The Hippocratic Oath was sworn by young physicians for many centuries, either in its original wording or with modifications, and is still sworn in some countries and in medical fraternities. In our very days, journals are named after him, and so is a medical publishing firm. Before World War II a movement arose which was called neo-Hippocratic; it emphasized the value of clinical observation at a moment when physicians were relying more and more on laboratory findings. To the Western world Hippocrates was the ideal physician, and Hippocratic medicine, although obviously dated in details, seemed to embody the right approach to the problems of health and disease. At a time when medicine was no longer anonymous, when an increasing number of doctors were known by name as teachers and practitioners, Hippocrates became the dominating personality, the 'Father' of European medicine. Who was Hippocrates?

A disappointment awaits us, for we actually know very little about him. The only contemporary references are in two dialogues of Plato. In the *Protagoras* a young man by the name of Hippocrates—a not uncommon name in Greece—wants to study with the sophist Protagoras who has lately arrived in Athens. He requests Socrates to make the necessary arrangements, whereupon Socrates, in order to test him, asks him a few questions:

Tell me, Hippocrates, you now wish to approach Protagoras and pay him tuition for your instruction, what do you expect to find in him and what do you intend to become? Let us assume you were thinking of going to your namesake, Hippocrates of Cos, the Asclepiad, and of paying him tuition for your instruction—if someone asked you, 'Tell me, Hippocrates, in what quality do you intend to pay Hippocrates tuition? What would you answer?' 'I should say, in his quality as a physician.'—'And what then would you wish to become yourself?'— 'A physician.' [1]

Socrates then goes on to ask the same questions with respect to the sculptors Polycletus and Phidias, and finally comes back to Protagoras, who is a sophist; but with him the answer is that one attends a sophist's teaching not to become a sophist—that is, a paid teacher— but to improve his general education.

From this passage we learn that the Asclepiad Hippocrates, a native of the island of Cos, was a teacher of medicine who accepted students upon payment of a tuition fee. And we also learn that he was so well-known a physician that you could refer to him as you referred to the sculptors Polycletus and Phidias and be sure that everyone knew whom you meant.

The other passage is even more important. In the dialogue *Phaedrus* Socrates compares rhetoric with medicine [2] and says that in both one must know nature: the nature of the human body in medicine, and the nature of the human soul in rhetoric. Without such knowledge, physician and orator can act only with the help of tricks or empirically. But if the physician knows nature he can give health and strength to the human body skillfully with drugs and foods, and if the orator knows nature he can impress his conviction and virtue upon the human soul with arguments and examples. To the question whether it is possible to recognize the nature of the human soul without knowledge of the nature of the whole, Phaedrus answers:

If we may trust Hippocrates the Asclepiad, it is impossible without this method to have any knowledge of the human body either.

Socrates—that is, Plato—then goes on expounding the method of Hippocrates, according to which we are first to ask 'whether that which we wish to learn and to teach is a simple or multiform thing, and if simple, then to inquire what power it has of acting or being acted upon in relation to other things; and if multiform, then to number the forms; and see first in the case of one of them, and then in the case of all of them, what is that power of acting or being acted upon which makes each and all of them be what they are.' [3]

This is not too clear and gives us little, but it provides more than the previous passage. It tells us not only that Hippocrates was a famous physician and medical teacher, but also that he had a philosophical approach to medicine which was basically dialectic. In the words of Edelstein, 'Hippocrates considered the body an organism; medical practice he based on the knowledge resulting from the comprehension of the scattered particulars into one concept and the division of the whole in turn into its natural species.' [4]

This is not too clear either and cannot be, as Plato's is merely a short general statement. More specific was a student of Aristotle, Meno, who compiled a doxographical compendium of early Greek medicine, parts of which have been found in a papyrus of the British Museum, the so-called *Anonymus Londinensis*.[5] The papyrus contains three different texts which may be quite unconnected: (1) definitions (I-IV, 25), (2) the etiology of diseases according to various authorities (IV, 26-XXI, 9), and (3) the development of physiology after 300 B.C., from Herophilus to Alexander Philalethes. We are here concerned only with the second part, which states the views of twenty medical authorities, among whom is Hippocrates. Since the passage is very important it may be quoted here in full: [6]

Hippocrates says that breaths (φῦσαι) are causes of disease, as Aristotle has said in his account of him. For Hippocrates says that diseases are brought about in the following fashion. Either because of the quantity of things taken, or through their diversity, or because the things taken happen to be strong and difficult of digestion, residues are thereby produced, and when the things that have been taken are too many, the heat that produces digestion is overpowered by the multitude of foods and does not effect digestion. And because digestion is hindered residues are formed. And when the things that have been taken are of many kinds, they quarrel with one another in the belly, and because of the quarrel there is a change into residues. When, however, they are very coarse and hard to digest, there occurs hindrance of digestion because they are hard to assimilate, and so a change to residues takes place. From the residues rise gases, which having arisen bring on diseases. What moved Hippocrates to adopt these views was the following conviction. Breath (πνεῦμα), he holds, is the most necessary and the supreme component in us, since health is the result of its free, and disease of its impeded passage. We in fact present a likeness to plants. For as they are rooted in the earth, so we too are rooted in the air by our nostrils and by our whole body. At least we are, he says, like those plants that are called 'soldiers.' For just as they, rooted in the moisture, are carried now to this moisture and now to that, even so we also, being as it were plants, are rooted in the air, and are in motion, changing our position now hither now thither. If this be so, it is clear that breath (πνεῦμα) is the supreme component. On this theory, when residues occur, they give rise to breaths, which rising as vapour cause diseases. The variations in the breaths cause the various diseases. If the breaths are violent [many], they produce disease, as they also do if they are very light [few]. The changes too of breaths give rise to diseases. These changes take place in two directions, towards excessive heat or towards excessive cold. The nature of the change determines the character of the disease. This is Aristotle's view of Hippocrates.

But what Hippocrates himself says is that diseases are caused by the differences in the elemental components of the human organism ... that these diseases arise in us through inflammation. For these things apart from ... of excessive fatigue, chill or heat. And it is because of the chilling or heating of bile and phlegm that diseases result. But as a matter of fact Hippocrates goes on to say that diseases have their origin in either the air (πνεύματος) or regimen, and the outline of these matters he thinks fit to set out thus. Whenever, he says, many are attacked at one and the same time by the same disease, the cause must be attributed to the air. For if the air produce a disease, it will be the same one. When, however, many different forms of diseases occur, we must attribute them to errors of regimen, he says, employing an unsound method of argument. For there are times when many different diseases have one and the same cause. For surely fever, pleurisy and epilepsy may be the result of a surfeit, which produces diseases corresponding to the constitution of the body that takes it in. For certainly one and the same cause does not bring one and the same disease to every body, but, as we have said, many and various forms. On the other hand, sometimes different causes produce the same affection. For diarrhoea is caused through surfeit, as well as through acridness if there be any untoward flow of bile. From these facts it is manifest that Hippocrates is mistaken in this matter, as we shall show in the course of our narrative. Yet it must be said that what Aristotle tells us about him does not tally with Hippocrates' own statements about the origin of diseases.

This is all we find on Hippocrates in contemporary sources or such as were written one generation later. We may add a passage from the *Politics* of Aristotle which implies that Hippocrates was great as a physician but small of stature.[7]

In other words, we know very little about the historical Hippocrates, his teaching or his life. We know his birthplace, know that he was a famous physician and teacher of medicine, and that is all. As to his theories and method the only authentic sources are those we just quoted, and we have no guarantee that Plato and Meno reported his views correctly. They certainly would not explain the fame of Hippocrates. But then we possess the *Corpus Hippocraticum,* a collection of medical writings which have been transmitted through the ages with the label Hippocrates attached to them. If all or at least some of them are his work, then we certainly must know more about his medicine.

Again we are disappointed, for the books of the collection are obviously the work of different authors belonging to different schools. Some are Coan and even designated as such,[8] others are undoubtedly

Cnidian, while still others reflect views of the Sicilian philosophers and physicians. They are also totally different in character and style. There have been attempts even in our days to prove that all the writings were the work of one man, Hippocrates himself,[9] but in order to explain the contradictions one had to assume that Hippocrates had changed his theories every few years, a very naïve assumption.

Now, if the Hippocratic method and theory of disease reported by Plato and Meno are authentic, we should expect to find them, and in more detail, in the Hippocratic collection. But this it not the case. There is not a single treatise which would present Hippocrates in such a light, although elements of the theory may be traced here and there. The view that residues of undigested food produce air or breath ($\pi\nu\epsilon\tilde{\upsilon}\mu\alpha$) and that this air, invading the body, causes illness, may be found in a very inferior treatise of the collection, the treatise *On Breaths* ($\pi\epsilon\rho\grave{\iota}$ $\varphi\upsilon\sigma\tilde{\omega}\nu$), a dissertation which clearly betrays its sophistic origin. Does that mean that the historical Hippocrates was a medical sophist who traveled about making speeches, teaching young people, and also, of course, curing patients, and that the best writings of the collection were somebody else's work? This is possible, but it is also possible that Plato and Aristotle were wrong. At any rate, there is not one treatise in the entire *Corpus Hippocraticum* that could be ascribed to Hippocrates with any degree of certainty. Dozens of volumes have been written in an attempt to find the 'genuine' works of Hippocrates,[10] and every editor, translator, and commentator of the Hippocratic collection had his own list of 'genuine' and 'spurious' works. It was observed in antiquity that not all books could have been written by the same man, and it was also noticed that certain books could be grouped together. They were written in the same style [11] and reflected the same basic attitude toward health and disease. Physicians at all times were inclined to consider those books 'genuine' which were medically the best—that is, revealed a high degree of accurate observation and sound reasoning. Philologists, on the other hand, worked with the passage from the *Phaedrus,* and from 1893 on with the fragment from Meno. But both passages are so vague that no convincing conclusions can be drawn from them.

Personally I incline to the belief that the *Corpus Hippocraticum* does contain books written by the master himself, although I cannot prove it and cannot tell which books must be his work. But it would be difficult to understand why the whole collection should have been named after him rather than after Herodicus, Euryphon, or any other physician, unless his own writings were a part of it.

According to Edelstein the process by which this entire literature was attributed to Hippocrates was the following: [12] To his contemporaries Hippocrates was not a particularly outstanding figure, a famous physician and teacher but one among many. As a matter of fact, Plato refers to a number of other doctors whom he implies to be as well known as Hippocrates, and in the fragment of Meno Hippocrates is one of twenty famous physicians.

The early Alexandrian doctors became interested in the history of medicine. In an important document of that time [13] it is said that dietetics was inaugurated by Herodicus and brought to perfection by Hippocrates, Praxagoras, and Chrysippus. Herophilus, the great Alexandrian physician, was a student of Praxagoras of Cos, and his equally famous fellow doctor Erasistratus was a student of Chrysippus of Cnidus. Hippocrates, Praxagoras, and Chrysippus were mentioned together as the three leading men in the field of dietetics in which medicine had achieved its greatest progress. Hippocrates, however, was the senior of the three.

The Alexandrian library possessed a certain amount of fifth- and fourth-century medical books which must have been anonymous when they were brought to Alexandria.[14] As soon as interest in Hippocrates was aroused, Alexandrian physicians and philologists endeavored to ascertain which of these anonymous books could be the work of Hippocrates. In this way a nucleus of Hippocratic writings was formed. As time went on, the fame of Hippocrates increased. To Celsus, whose work reproduces late Alexandrian knowledge, he appears as the oldest medical writer—*vetustissimus auctor*—as the first worthy of being remembered.[15] It is obvious that more and more anonymous medical treatises were now ascribed to him. This process continued as Hippocrates became more famous. To imperial Rome the fifth century B.C. was the Golden Age of Greece, the time of the great writers, and Hippocrates was one of them. Erotian, who lived at the time of Nero and wrote a glossary on Hippocrates, considered him a writer ranking with Homer. He was Galen's ideal of a physician,[16] was now the 'Father of Medicine,' and the entire extant medical literature of the Golden Age was naturally attributed to him, although Galen and other critical minds had their doubts as to the genuineness of some of the treatises. Hippocrates was not deified as was Imhotep, but he was heroized particularly on his native island. It is quite possible that this was the process by which the *Corpus Hippocraticum* was formed, and I find Edelstein's hypothesis very convincing, but there can be no certainty where the source material is so scanty. Every generation of philologists and every school will develop its own theories.

Although we know very little about the historical Hippocrates, yet there is one more source that we may consult, although with great caution: namely, the traditions about his life, legendary as they probably are. Still, most legends contain an element of truth. As soon as Hippocrates had assumed a prominent position in the history of Greek medicine, people were anxious to know more about his personality and life. Biographies were written in order to satisfy this demand, just as many biographies of Christian martyrs were written in the fifth century of our era. And just as the biographies of the *Acta Sanctorum* are a mixture of historical facts and reminiscences with legendary traits and miracle stories, so the biographies of Hippocrates are a combination of fact and fancy. It would be a mistake, however, to consider them nothing but fairy tales. After all many people must have known him, many must have been his disciples, since it is established that he was a famous teacher, and these students must have had stories to tell about the master which they passed on to their own students. If we had no contemporary written records about William Osler's life, we could still reconstruct it from traditions and reminiscences, not only today but even centuries later. The picture obviously becomes less accurate the later it is drawn after the event, and ancient historians were in the habit of lending color to their narrative by inventing characteristic episodes and by writing speeches their heroes might have made.

We have four biographies of Hippocrates. One is by Tzetzes, a Byzantine writer of the twelfth century A.D.[17] who based his story on an earlier source, a *Vita* attributed to Soranus. The Greek lexicon of Suidas, compiled toward the end of the tenth century, has an article on Hippocrates [18] which follows a somewhat different tradition. A Latin manuscript of the Royal Library in Brussels, written in the twelfth century but containing much earlier texts, has a short treatise entitled *Yppocratis genus, vita, dogma;* [19] in other words, it discusses the ancestry, life and doctrine of the master. And finally we have the *Life of Hippocrates* by Soranus, which probably is the best known of all such biographies. It is supposed to be a chapter of a book, *Lives of Physicians,* which supposedly was written by Soranus of Ephesus.[20] The authorship, however, is uncertain.[21] To this material we must add the pseudo-Hippocratic *Letters* in which the legend is also developed.

What do these biographies tell us? On the whole they agree that Hippocrates was a Coan by birth, an Asclepiad, that he practiced medicine as an itinerant physician, that he died in Thessaly and was buried between Gyrton and Larissa. These data are in all probability correct but were not sufficient to satisfy people's curiosity. Why was he an itinerant? Why did he leave his native island? At the time of these biographies most doctors were settled and did not take to the road. According to one source, he was librarian at Cos and burned the old medical books and archives, whereupon he was forced to flee to the Greek mainland. According to another source, it was not the archives of Cos but those of the rival medical center of Cnidus that he burned, and still another source says that he was ordered by a dream to go to Thessaly.

According to Soranus' biography, Hippocrates was the son of the physician Heraclides and his wife Phaenarete. He traced his ancestry back to Heracles and Asclepius. He studied first with his own father, then with Herodicus; according to some writers, he also studied with the sophist Gorgias and with the philosopher Democritus. The year of his birth was the first year of the eightieth Olympiad, which corresponds to our year 460-459 B.C. After he had left the island of his birth, he traveled all over Greece and amazed the world with the success of his cures. When Perdiccas, King of Macedonia, was sick and was believed to suffer from phthisis, Hippocrates and Euryphon were called to his sickbed; the former recognized that the disease was not phthisis but had psychological causes, whereupon the Abderites invited him to their city to cure the raving Democritus. Several of the pseudo-Hippocratic *Letters* are supposed to be a correspondence between the philosopher and his physician.

When pestilence invaded the lands, the Illyrians and Paeonians called Hippocrates to relieve them from the plague, but being a Greek patriot he felt that his first duty was toward his Greek fellow men, declined the invitation of the barbarian kings, and went to Attica instead, realizing that the pestilence would invade that region too. His very patriotism compelled him also to refuse a call to the court of Artaxerxes, Great King of Persia, to a position that would have been highly remunerative. But he did not care for money, and his self-respect forbade him to serve the enemy of his country. In gratitude the Athenians admitted him to the Eleusinian mysteries. The pseudo-Hippocratic letters contain a decree which may be quoted in full as an illustration of the Hippocratic legend: [22]

It has been decreed by the Council and the People of Athens: Whereas Hippocrates of Cos, a physician and descendant of Asclepius, has shown great goodwill and helpfulness toward the Greeks by sending his disciples to various places when the plague coming from the lands of the barbarians invaded Greece; has prescribed what treatments must be applied to escape safely from the incoming plague, thus demonstrating how the healing art of Apollo transmitted to the Greeks saves those among them who are sick—
whereas he has unselfishly published medical books in his desire to see many physicians prepared to save the people—
whereas, when the king of Persia called him and offered him honors

equal to his own and all the gifts he Hippocrates might ask for, he turned down the offers of the barbarians, hated common enemy of the Greeks—

therefore the People of Athens, desirous of showing their regard for the common welfare of Greece and of giving adequate reward to Hippocrates for his services, decrees: to initiate him at government expense into the great mysteries, like Hercules, son of Jupiter—

to crown him with a wreath of gold of the value of one thousand gold coins—

to announce the crowning publicly at the time of the great Panathenaea, during the gymnastic contest—

to allow all children of Coans to have the ephebes' training in Athens with the same rights as Athenian children, since their homeland has produced such a man—

finally, to give Hippocrates Athenian citizenship and grant him sustenance in the town-hall for life.

Thus, the legend says, Hippocrates was greatly honored, and not only by the Athenians. He was held in high esteem in Cos, Thessaly, and Argos. Free of jealousy, he taught his art to any student who wanted to learn it, after he had sworn the prescribed oath. At the age of ninety he died in Thessaly. A beehive on his tomb had honey with curative properties. He continued to exert his beneficial influence long after his death. His sons, Thessalus and Dracon, and his numerous disciples practiced the art as he had taught them.

I have dealt at such length with this document to give an example of the legend of Hippocrates as it probably began to develop in the third century B.C., that is, when the *Corpus Hippocraticum* began to take shape and Cos was famous for its physicians and its temple of Asclepius. The other biographies differ from that of Soranus in many details and particularly in one basic point. Soranus and, following him, Tzetzes, picture Hippocrates as a Greek patriot who despised Persian gold and devoted all his life to the welfare of his fellow Greeks. Suidas mentions the invitation to the Persian court but does not say that Hippocrates declined it, while the biography of the Brussels manuscript explicitly states that Hippocrates was at the court

of Artaxerxes, that he also went to Egypt and brought books home
from Memphis. In other words, there was a tradition which pictured
Hippocrates as a disciple of the Orient.

There can be no doubt that all these biographies are legendary.
They were written many centuries after the events, based on traditions which had crystallized much later. In every legend episodes are
invented to illustrate a particular trait that people assigned to their
hero. A Christian saint performed miracles and died the death of a
martyr. A heroized physician performed famous cures and had all
the qualities expected of an ideal physician. Some groups in Greece
looked upon Egypt as the source of all wisdom. Hence Hippocrates
went to Memphis, and bought medical books there from which he
derived his knowledge; since he was a student of the East he had no
hesitation to work at the court of the Great King. Other groups had
a deep hatred of Persia, and their Hippocrates could not be anything
but a philhellene, a friend of the Greeks, and hence an enemy of
Persia. But legends are not always pure fiction; they may contain
grains of truth. There is no doubt that a number of writings of the
Hippocratic collection have been influenced from the East, Egypt
and Mesopotamia, and probably much more than we can assess at
the moment. Other incidents related in the legend may also be true.
It may well be that Hippocrates went to Athens in the course of
his peregrinations. The Greek physicians were great travelers, and
distances were short. But we have no means of distinguishing fact
from fiction, and we must admit that we know very little about the
life of Hippocrates.

Since we know so little and since people in antiquity apparently
also knew very little about his life, we cannot expect to have many
authentic portraits of him. We think we know what Pericles, Sophocles, Socrates, Plato, Aristotle and many other great Greeks looked
like, because, at least at some time or other, they all lived in Athens,
the home of great sculptors who made their portrait statues. We do
not know of any authentic old statue of Hippocrates. And yet, when
long after his death he had become the 'Father of Medicine,' people
wanted to know what his physical appearance had been. Physicians

wished to have his statue in their workshop or courtyard. We know from literary sources that this was actually the case. In the second century A.D. the physician Antigonus had a bronze statue of the master which he worshiped as that of a hero.[23] The biographies we just discussed tell that Hippocrates was usually pictured with his head covered with his cloak, which points to the story of his having been initiated into the mysteries of Eleusis.[24] The biography of Soranus mentions that 'on the majority of pictures he was represented with the head covered, according to some with a felt cap as a sign of noble birth like Odysseus, according to others with the cloak.' [25]

We have nothing that corresponds to these descriptions, but we do have several heads and busts which are commonly supposed to be portraits of Hippocrates. How can one possibly decide which one among the large mass of anonymous busts preserved must or may represent Hippocrates rather than some philosopher or poet? Luck has it that the city of Cos issued coins with the head of Hippocrates on them. The name is on the coin so that there can be no doubt whose head is represented. We have four such coins preserved.[26] They are all late, mostly from the first century A.D. It may be that the portraits are the product of some late designer's imagination. On the other hand, they have strong individual features, so that they may go back to some much earlier pictures or statues. If the designer had invented the portrait, he undoubtedly would have idealized it, picturing Hippocrates as a worthy old gentleman, looking like one of the great philosophers or poets, if not like Asclepius himself. Instead, we have the head of a thick-set man who was anything but handsome, with a bald head, a rather thick nose, and short beard.

If among the anonymous busts we find some that correspond to these characteristic features we may assume they represent Hippocrates, and as a matter of fact, there are such busts, two types of them, one showing the master old and wrinkled, with deep-set eyes and a serious expression,[27] and another showing him not quite so old and tired, but rather lively.[28] A new bust found at Ostia in the 1940's is supposed to represent Hippocrates, and that is quite possible.[29] All these portraits are late copies of Hellenistic busts, and we must bear in mind that their identification rests on the rather flimsy resemblance to late Coan coins.

Now that we have written a good many pages on Hippocrates, we must admit that we still know extremely little about the man, his life, and his work. Yet circumstances made him the most influential Western physician. He appeared as the founder of scientific medicine, who excluded the transcendental and based his actions on observation and reasoning. Theories of the Hippocratic writings were attributed to him which, when systematized by Galen and even further by Avicenna, were the dominating theories of the West until very recently, and are still preponderant in large sections of the East.

Hippocrates also appeared as the ideal physician, the good doctor who embodied all the qualities that patients expect to find in their physician. Every period has an ideal physician in mind, indeed, must have one; it is this ideal which determines the physician's ethics. If his actions are in accordance with the medical ideal, his conscience will tell him that he acted correctly and did his duty, while it will censure him in the reverse case. The medical ideal of a period also determines its system of medical education, for its purpose is to train a physician according to a certain educational ideal which in turn is the medical ideal of the time. The Hellenistic ideal obviously had to be a physician of the Golden Age of Greece, and all the qualities that this society wished to find in its physicians, and probably missed in many of them, were attributed to Hippocrates. Not to Asclepius, for Asclepius was a god, while physicians were human beings like their own patients. Thus Hippocrates came to personify the ideal physician and lived endowed with all the features legend had given him. He embodied the eternal values of the medical profession: readiness to help, purity of life, kindness, patriotism, skillfulness, and the like. Every profession needs founding fathers, ancestors, heroes to whom it can look up and of whom it can be proud. In Hippocrates the Western medical profession found its Father.

Once Hippocrates, originally one good doctor among many, had assumed his unique position, once the legend had crystallized and busts of him were being made, once an increasing number of writings were attributed to him, he began to exert a wide influence which is still felt in the West today. His fate may be compared to that of certain Christian saints who were colorless, almost anonymous martyrs in the beginning but, once their legend had been created and given literary form, became extraordinarily influential. And just as Alexander the Great will continue to create great generals and statesmen, and Brutus liberators from tyranny, so will Hippocrates continue to create good doctors.

Before studying the contents of the Hippocratic writings we must briefly survey the collection as a whole. The so-called *Corpus Hippocraticum* is a collection of medical writings which, with few exceptions,[30] are pre-Aristotelian, that is, date from the fifth and fourth centuries B.C. It probably contains all the medical literature of the period that the Alexandrians could find. There has been much speculation on the number of treatises included in the collection, but this is a vain speculation, for, unlike the Hermetic books of Egypt, the *Corpus Hippocraticum* was never firmly constituted, never divided into a set number of books, never rigidly fixed. One source of confusion is that some writers refer to titles while others mean books. Thus the *Epidemics* has seven books and may be counted as one by some, as seven by others. The first commentators who wrote glossaries on these texts—Bacchius of Tanagra and Euphorion, who worked at the end of the third century B.C.—knew books that went under the name of Hippocrates, but do not mention how many there were. Another commentator, Erotian, in the first century A.D. lists the Hippocratic writings known to him. He mentions twenty-nine titles or thirty-eight books. The number of books indicated by the biographers varies from fifty-three to seventy-two. There is no doubt that some books included in the collection in antiquity are lost today, while others were added in the Middle Ages. Diels' list of the manuscripts of ancient physicians contains 130 Hippocratic writings,[31] many of which, however, are trans-

lations or medieval treatises with no connection whatsoever with the
Corpus Hippocraticum. Still, the best Greek manuscripts contain
about sixty books which were transmitted from the fifth and fourth
centuries.

These sixty-odd books may be divided into groups from various
points of view. Early editors liked to make the distinction between
'genuine' books of Hippocrates and 'spurious' works. This was particularly the case in England, with the result that many important
books, notably the gynecological works, were never translated into
English. It seems unbelievable, but there is actually no English
translation of the complete *Corpus Hippocraticum.*[32] We shall not
try to divide the collection into genuine and spurious books: we
are convinced that it is impossible to ascribe any one treatise to
Hippocrates with any degree of certainty or without a great display
of philological acrobatics. It is possible, however, to group the
various treatises according to contents. But here again we face a
certain difficulty. If we had to divide modern medical literature
into groups we would feel no hesitation whatsoever to begin with
anatomy, the foundation of our medicine since the sixteenth century, proceed to physiology, the core of all modern medicine, then
to pathology—anatomical, physiological, and experimental—
further to internal medicine and the specialities that branched off
from it—pediatrics, dermatology, neurology, and psychiatry—to
surgery and its specialities—urology, ophthalmology, oto-rhino-
laryngology, dentistry—to hygiene and public health, and so forth.
When we deal with ancient medical literature, the situation is much
more complicated.

In archaic medicine, theory and particularly anatomy come last.
The starting point of all medical action is the sick man and his complaints—that is, the symptoms of disease. Hippocratic medicine is no
longer archaic. Theories play a very important part in it, and when a
physician prescribed a diet or drugs, he was not guided by experience
alone but very often by theoretical considerations, endeavoring to
evacuate a humor or to aid the organism with its natural healing
power. Yet it is still practically impossible to distinguish between phy-

siological and pathological treatises. Whatever theoretical writings we have deal with man's life in health and illness—that is, with physiology and pathology. There is still little anatomy in the Hippocratic writings. Hippocratic medicine was not based on anatomy, as our modern Western medicine is. The school of Cnidus was known for the localizing of disease in greater measure than the school of Cos, but even there anatomy was in the background. Human bodies were not dissected systematically before the Hellenistic period, and the knowledge of organs was chiefly the result of analogy drawn from animal dissections, although human cadavers may have been opened at times.

The anatomical writings preserved in the Hippocratic collection are very scanty. The treatise *On Anatomy* (Περὶ ἀνατομῆς) is a one-page fragment which merely lists some internal organs. The treatise *On the Heart* (Περὶ καρδίης) [33] is slightly longer. It describes the heart as a muscle with two ventricles and two auricles wrapped in the pericardium. The writer undoubtedly dissected animal hearts carefully. Concerning the function of the heart, the author believes that the right ventricle feeds the lungs with blood and receives air in exchange. The left ventricle contains no blood but merely air, and is the seat of the innate heat and of the intelligence that controls the soul. A third anatomical treatise, transmitted under the misleading title *On the Nature of the Bones* (Περὶ φύσιος ὀστέων), actually deals primarily with blood vessels. The treatise is rather confused and obviously consists of various fragments put together.[34] The heart is pictured as the center of the vascular system, and some writers claim that Hippocrates was familiar with or at least had a vague idea of the circulation of the blood, a view which in my opinion cannot be substantiated. A scientific concept of the circulation of the blood could not be formulated before physicians thought in quantitative terms, and many centuries were to elapse before this was the case.[35] The longer treatise *On Flesh* (Περὶ σαρκῶν) also bears a wrong title; it is not a dissertation on muscles but a speculation on the formation of organs. The number seven plays an important part in it, as it does in several other books of the collection, and it seems probable that this treatise was also influenced from the East. And finally we have a short treatise *On Glands* (Περὶ ἀδένων) in which liver, pancreas, testicles, ovaries, and salivary glands are not mentioned, while the brain is described as the most important gland which draws superfluous humidity from the head into the whole body.

It is still primitive and in a way speculative anatomy that we find described in these treatises, knowledge gained in the kitchen, on the sacrificial altar, but also in the systematic dissection of animals. It must be admitted, however, that some descriptions are correct. The keen sense of observation that these doctors showed at the bedside of patients did not fail them when they looked at organs. Anatomical data are scattered all through the Hippocratic collection, and the surgical treatises obviously presuppose anatomical knowledge. Surgery, however, requires familiarity with topographical anatomy, and an ancient surgeon might have known the shoulder in every detail without having the faintest idea of the pancreas in its relation to the intestinal tract. Still, the ancients knew more anatomy than we commonly assume. In a seminar course we once made a study of the ancient physician's knowledge of the liver and were astonished to find that the Alexandrian anatomists and Galen added very little to what the Hippocratic doctors knew about this organ. Anatomy remained in the background because the entire structure of Greek medicine was different from ours.

The Hippocratic collection also contains a considerable number of theoretical writings. They are as different as possible in character and content. We shall of course discuss later in detail the theories they expound, since they determined or at least influenced the thoughts of generations of physicians. Here we can only list and briefly describe them.

The treatise *On Ancient Medicine* (Περὶ ἀρχαίης ἰητρικῆς) has been the subject of three recent studies;[36] justly so, as it is a beautiful piece of work, addressed not only to physicians but to the general educated public as well. It is philosophical and shows sophistic influence, although it begins by protesting against the

intrusion of philosophy into medicine. Medicine is an art of its own
which originated empirically when it was found that certain foods
and diets improved the condition of sick people. The author mini-
mizes the importance of a limited number of opposites, such as heat
and cold, and emphasizes the part played by humors and qualities.
The treatise *On Breaths* (Περὶ φυσῶν) [37] is usually considered one
of the poorer theoretical books, since it is highly dogmatic, tracing
the origin of all diseases to one agent, breaths or airs or winds,
whichever way we translate the Greek word φῦσαι.[38] Since the
discovery of the Meno Papyrus, however, it has been given increased attention, as it comes closest to the theory attributed to
Hippocrates by Meno. The treatise *On the Nature of Man* (Περὶ
φύσιος ἀνθρώπου) seems to be one of the later writings of the
collection. Its importance lies in the fact that it describes the theory
of the four humors which was to dominate medicine for many
centuries in both East and West.

A considerable number of other books are clinical rather than
theoretical. They all presuppose an underlying theory, and many
have theoretical introductions. They vary in their basic concepts of
health and disease, but their chief accent is not on physiology and
general pathology; their purpose is rather to describe diseases, their
etiology, their course, outcome, complications, and usually also their
treatment. Such are *On Diseases*, Books I-III (Περὶ νούσων),
while Book IV consists of fragments on the humors of the body
and their origin. Such is the book *On Ailments* (Περὶ παθῶν), a
popular book addressed mainly to laymen, telling them what to do in
the case of the more common diseases; or the very detailed book *On
Internal Ailments* (Περὶ τῶν ἐντὸς παθῶν) which gives some excellent
descriptions of diseases.

The short treatise *On Humors* (Περὶ χυμῶν) is clinical also,
in spite of its title, which would rather point to a physiological dissertation. It deals with the effect of the seasons on the constitution of
the human body, and the body's disposition toward disease at
various periods, and gives in a rather sketchy way—it is not an
elaborate book—a description of symptoms and indications of treat-

ments. In its comparisons it sometimes reminds me of Paracelsus: for example when it says, 'What the earth is to trees, the stomach is to animals; it nourishes, warms, and cools; when empty it cools, when full it warms. A manured earth is warm in winter and so is the belly.' [39] Littré pointed out that this treatise was close to *Epidemics*, which is one of the finest books of the whole collection. Books I and III of *Epidemics* belong together.[40] They were written by a physician who worked on the island of Thasos, keeping a record of the patients who went through his office. He endeavored to correlate the diseases he saw to the *katastasis*—that is, to the general weather conditions prevalent at the time. The observations are superb, and we shall have more to say about them. Books II, IV, and VI constitute another group, with various histories of cases observed in Crannon, Perinthus, and other places. The writer was not the same as the author of Books I and III, but he wrote in the same spirit. He too kept diaries and wrote up the case histories of his patients. Books V and VII seem to be later but also contain some very interesting observations. These seven books—and not only I and III—are among the great medical classics of world literature. Another classic writing, one of the early monographs on a single disease, is a treatise on epilepsy, *On the Sacred Disease* (Περὶ ἱερῆς νούσου). This is the name by which it was commonly called, but the author states emphatically that this disease is no more of divine origin than any other.

Clinical monographs of another kind are those *On Crises* (Περὶ κρισίων) and *On Critical Days* (Περὶ κρισίμων). In a region in which malaria was endemic, nothing struck the medical observer's imagination more forcibly than the iron rhythm that the disease followed, with attacks of fever and remissions that could be predicted to the very hour. It was soon found that other diseases such as relapsing fever, pneumonia, and the like also had a certain rhythm, taking a turn for the better or the worse on definite days. This opened the door to speculation with numbers, particularly in a country that was subject to Babylonian influences and where, on the other hand, the Pythagoreans had considered number the essence of all things. Thus the *Corpus Hippocraticum* contains not only treatises on the critical days but also a very puzzling one *On Periods of Seven Days* (Περὶ ἑβδομάδων), transmitted partly in Greek and partly in three different Latin versions.[41] We mentioned in another connection the treatises *On the Seven-Months Embryo* (Περὶ ἑπταμήνου) and *On the Eight-Months Embryo* (Περὶ ὀκταμήνου) in which speculation on numbers also plays an important part. A rather strange treatise which, however, deserves closer examination, bears the title *On Places in Man* (Περὶ τόπων τῶν κατ' ἄνθρωπον). It opens with the statement that the human body is like a circle, having no beginning and no end, and that diseases similarly begin anywhere in the body. Anatomical remarks follow, particularly about the blood vessels. These are believed to originate in the head whence fluxes arise.

A treatise of a very special kind, which has attracted much attention lately and has been the subject of various studies, is *Airs, Waters, Places* (Περὶ ἀέρων, ὑδάτων, τόπων).[42] It is one of the most brilliant books of the collection and the earliest classic of medical geography. The treatise is not homogeneous but consists of at least two different parts. One part, chapters 12-24, is a very fascinating comparative anthropology of Asia and Europe. Asiatics and Europeans differ in constitution and character. Why? Because the geography of their countries, the climate, the entire physical environment are different. Man is conditioned by his environment, physically and mentally. The environment largely determines his constitution, his health, and the diseases to which he may fall prey. These are modern ideas. We know that man is born with hereditary raw materials, but what he makes of them is principally the result of environmental factors. We know furthermore that heredity is not rigid, that genes may be affected by chemical factors, resulting in mutations.[43] Thus the Hippocratic anthropology is a grandiose anticipation of modern ideas.

The first part of the book has a totally different character. Chapters 1-11 are basically a prognostic treatise. In our next chapter we shall discuss why prognosis was so important in Hippocratic medicine. The first part of *Airs, Waters, Places* aimed to instruct the physician who came to a region previously unknown to him, how to observe the surroundings and draw conclusions from them on the nature of the diseases prevailing in such a place, so that he might be able to judge about a patient without even asking questions. The physician who comes to a town must consider not only the season, the winds, the water that people use, and the geographic location of the place, but also the mode of living of the people: whether they drink much wine, eat well, and rest much, or whether they are hard-working, exercise a great deal, eat much, and drink little.[44] Edelstein thinks that chapters 7-9 are interpolated from an otherwise lost treatise *On Waters* (Περὶ ὑδάτων);[45] though this is possible it is not necessarily true. We must not expect more logic in ancient treatises than in modern textbooks.

The treatise on *Airs, Waters, Places* leads us to a brief discussion of the other prognostic books of the collection. One of them, which has the simple title *Prognostic* (Προγνωστικόν), is one of the finest books of the entire *Corpus*. It reveals a power of observation on the part of the physician and a wealth of clinical experience that command greatest admiration. The second chapter gives the description of the face of a moribund patient for which the technical term *facies hippocratica* was coined and is still used today. The brief chapter is a good example of this kind of literature.[46]

In acute diseases the physician must make his observations in the following way. He must first look at the face of the patient and see whether it is like that of people in good health, and particulary whether it is like its usual self, for this is the best of all; whereas the most opposite to it is the worst, such as the following: nose sharp, eyes hollow, temples sunken, ears cold and contracted and their lobes turned out, the skin about the face dry, tense, and parched, the color of the face as a whole being yellow or black, livid or lead-colored. If at the beginning of the disease the face is such and if the other symptoms do not yet permit making a prognosis, one must inquire whether the patient has been sleepless, whether he had strong diarrhea, or whether he has suffered from hunger. If any of these causes be admitted, the condition may be considered less threatening. The crisis will come in the course of a day and a night if the condition of the face was due to any such cause. But if the patient does not tell of any such cause, and if the condition does not clear up within that period, you must know that this is a sign of imminent death. If the disease has lasted more than three days after the face showed these signs, ask the same questions as I recommended before and observe the other symptoms, those of the whole body and also those of the eyes. For if they shun the light or weep involuntarily, or squint, or if the one be less than the other, or if the white of them be red, livid, or have black veins in it, or if rheum appear around the eyeballs, or if they be restless, protruding or are become very sunken; if the color of the whole face be changed—all these symptoms must be considered bad, even fatal. One must also observe what can be seen of the eyes during sleep. For if some of the white of the eyes can be seen while the eyelids are closed and the patient is not suffering from diarrhea, has not taken any purgative, and is not in the habit of so sleeping, then it is a bad and very fatal symptom. If in addition to these symptoms the eyelids or lips or nose be contracted, livid, or pale, one may know for certain that death is close at hand. It is also a fatal symptom when the lips are loose, hanging, cold, and very white.

The book *Prognostic* is a veritable mine of information on the Hippocratic knowledge of disease symptoms and groups of symptoms, and of their prognostic evaluation. The treatise that comes next to it in quality is Book II of the *Predictions* (Προρρητικόν β′), while Book I consists mostly of an abstract from the *Prognostic*. A fourth treatise entitled *Coan Prognoses* (Κωακαὶ προγνώσεις) points to Cos as its place of origin and therefore had much authority. It contains over six hundred brief aphoristic prognoses, some of which are quite correct, but the treatise as a whole is mostly an abstract from other books of the collection.

Treatment in Hippocratic medicine was primarily dietetic. Diets were reinforced with drugs and only as a last resort was the knife used. Hence we expect to find in the collection books specially devoted to therapeutics. It goes without saying that all clinical books, whether they be dietetic, pharmacological, or surgical, discuss treatments; we have, however, special monographs on these subjects, such as the one *On Diet in Acute Diseases* (Περὶ διαίτης ὀξέων), a treatise which for a long time was supposed to be of Coan origin, for it criticizes a now lost Cnidian treatise, *Cnidian Sentences* (Κνιδίαι γνῶμαι). It was also believed to consist of two quite heterogeneous parts, but Edelstein has shown convincingly that the treatise is Cnidian, since it follows the pattern of Cnidian pathology, and also that the second part is not a separate book but belongs to the first, since references may be found in the one to the other.[47] The book, as the title indicates, discusses chiefly the diet that must be prescribed in the treatment of acute diseases 'which are fatal to most people,' [48] such as pleurisy, pneumonia, and other fever diseases. But it is by no means limited to therapeutics; it gives, notably in the second part, excellent descriptions of disease. The books *On Diet* I-III (Περὶ διαίτης α'–γ') have been mentioned before, for they also discuss the regimen for people in health. The second book, containing a disquisition on the virtues of the various foods, was an important reference book not only for the physician but also for the educated layman. Book IV is a treatise of a special kind in that it deals with dreams and their interpretation. The author distinguishes two kinds of dreams. Some are sent by the gods and are omens which presage good or bad luck to individuals or towns. Their interpretation is not the physician's business but that of diviners, who explain such dreams following well-established rules. But then there is another kind of dream of physical origin, in which the soul announces ailments of the body, excessive repletion or evacuation, or some similar process. When the diviner is consulted in such a case he prescribes prayers. Prayers undoubtedly are a very good thing, but while praying to the gods one must help oneself,[49] and there can be no doubt that this kind of dream must be interpreted medically. This is an interesting attempt at rationalizing old folklore.

The short book *On the Use of Liquids* (Περὶ ὑγρῶν χρήσιος) is not a real treatise but merely a collection of notes on the medicinal use of fresh water, sea water, vinegar, and wine, hot or cold.

Drugs are mentioned in a great many books, wherever treatments are discussed, but in its present form the *Corpus Hippocraticum* contains no pharmacological book. A herbal listing the various drugs and describing their preparation and medical indications would have been very useful, as would also have been a collection of recipes such as we find in Egyptian papyri. Actually there are references to a lost book on drugs (Φαρμακῖτις),[50] and some early printed editions have a short treatise of only a page and a half *On Drugs* (Περὶ φαρμάκων) which deals with purgative remedies and must be a late interpolation, for it is never mentioned in antiquity. Pharmacological therapy does not play an important part in Hippocratic medicine. Its drugs were mostly house remedies, the kind of plants that the *rhizotomoi* and *pharmacopolai* gathered and kept for sale.

While we possess no pharmacological treatises we have a whole group of surgical works which are among the best books of the entire collection. They were for a long time attributed to Hippocrates himself,[51] and there can be no doubt that medicine and surgery in those days were not separate crafts and certainly not hostile brothers. A group of three books deals with fractures and dislocations, and the two books *On Fractures* (Περὶ ἀγμῶν) and *On Joints* (Περὶ ἄρθρων) must have been written by the same man. The third book of this group, *Instruments of Reduction* (Μοχλικόν), is mostly an abstract from the other two, and in the course of the centuries the text of the three books became somewhat disarranged, so that at present their order is not always logical, and both fractures and dislocations are discussed in all of them. In the first century B.C. an Alexandrian physician, Apollonius of Citium, wrote a commentary on the book *On Joints,* the chief interest of which lies in the fact that it was illustrated. The need for medical illustrations was felt as much in antiquity as it is felt today; it was recognized that a picture sometimes tells more than many words could do. The earliest Greek medical illustrations that have come down to us can be traced back to the first century B.C. They are pictures of medicinal plants; the pictures illustrating methods of reducing dislocated joints are a fine specimen of early bookcraft. Of course, we do not have the originals, only copies of copies; however, even in the manuscript of the ninth century A.D. preserved in the Laurentian Library of Florence the pictures in their Byzantine frames are impressive.[52]

The books on fractures and dislocations imply observations in the palaestra and gymnasium, where such accidents must have been frequent and the physician had an ideal opportunity to gain experience. The book of *On Wounds in the Head* (Περὶ τῶν ἐν κεφαλῇ τρωμάτων), on the other hand, points to the battlefield. It too is a remarkable treatise, full of splendid observations describing the wounds, the clinical symptoms they produce, complications that may be expected, and finally the treatment. Wound treatment in general is discussed in a special short treatise *On Wounds* (Περὶ ἑλκων), and we have two other short dissertations on ailments commonly treated by the surgeon, *On Hemorrhoids* (Περὶ αἱμορροΐδων) and *On Fistulae* (Περὶ συρίγγων). The surgical books, finally, include a treatise or rather the sketchy outline of one entitled *In the Surgery* (Κατ' ἰητρεῖον). It consists of loose notes about the surgeon's workshop and what it should include by way of instruments, apparatus, and bandages. It discusses some general principles of surgery and particularly the use of various bandages and dressings.

Men and women have many diseases in common, but women, as a result of their sex, have diseases of their own, or ailments common to both take a different course with women. The physician has a difficult task, because women hesitate to call him and consult with another woman or a midwife first. When the doctor has been called, he often finds that the patient in her ignorance cannot tell what ails her or is ashamed to reveal the origin of her disease. The doctor, on the other hand, frequently makes the mistake of treating sick women as if they were men and neglects to ascertain the cause of their illness at the very start.[53] So it is necessary as well for physicians to know the maladies peculiar to women, and the Hippocratic collection has a number of treatises on the subject, notably the two books *On Women's Diseases* (Περὶ γυναιχείων α'–β'). We quoted from them in a previous chapter. The two books cover the whole wide field of gynecology and obstetrics, mixing sound observations, well-described case histories, and good reasoning with traditional superstitions. In no field of medicine do we encounter more old folklore, which in an age of reason becomes superstition, than in that concerning women and children. In the *gyneceum* and in the nursery, old beliefs persist through the ages in antiquity, just as they still do in harems today and wherever women are uneducated.

The collection also contains a number of shorter treatises on gynecological ailments. One, *On Sterile Women* (Περὶ ἀφόρων), immediately follows the textbook just mentioned and was probably meant to be Book III. It undoubtedly was written by the same author. The rather long book *On the Nature of Woman* (Περὶ γυναιχείης φύσιος) is a mere abstract of the major textbook. Such abstracts were probably the work of students who could not obtain a complete copy of a book. They were sometimes carelessly made, as in the present case, with mistakes and repetitions.

The treatises *On Generation* (Περὶ γονῆς) and *On the Nature of the Child* (Περὶ φύσιος παιδίου) have been mentioned in the previous chapter. They belong together, and Littré is probably right when he assumes that Book IV of the treatise *On Diseases* (Περὶ νούσων δ') is their sequel, and that the whole constitutes a considerable textbook which presents the formation and development of the human body and the genesis of disease.

A few short treatises dealing with embryology and obstetrics have also been mentioned before, such as those that discuss the chances of survival of a child born in the seventh month and of that born in the eighth month. Two other treatises, the very short one *On Superfetation* (Περὶ ἐπικυήσιος) and the longer one *On the Excision of the Embryo* (Περὶ ἐγκατατομῆς ἐμβρύου), are on the whole mostly abstracts from the main textbook. Finally, there are two more treatises that might be mentioned in this connection, a short collection of aphorisms *On Teething* (Περὶ ὀδοντοφυίης) and the ailments that children have at that age, and an equally short fragment *On the*

Diseases of Maidens (Περὶ παρθενίων). This undoubtedly is merely a fragment, for the author of the main textbook on gynecology refers twice to a book which he had written on the diseases of maidens. Short as the fragment is it is not without interest, for it apparently considers the heart the seat of all mental functions, not the brain, as the author of the treatise *On the Sacred Disease* does, following Alcmaeon. When a young girl begins to menstruate and the blood cannot flow out freely, it reverts to the heart and diaphragm and causes mental symptoms, anxieties, delirium, and even the desire to commit suicide. The remedy consists in having such girls marry as soon as possible.

A last group of treatises remains to be mentioned: namely, those on medical ethics and etiquette. Since their content will be analyzed and the subject discussed in detail in our next chapter, we shall only list them here without further comment. Foremost in the influence it exerted in later centuries stands the *Oath* (Ὅρκος). Next we may mention the *Law* (Νόμος), which deals with the study of medicine. *Decorum* (Περὶ εὐσχημοσύνης) is the title of another piece which gives valuable information on conditions of practice. *Precepts* (Παραγγελίαι) is one of the older treatises of this group; it discusses questions of etiquette and other important problems. The short treatise *The Physician* (Περὶ ἰητροῦ)[54] like most of these deontological books is addressed to beginners. The first chapter indicates the physical and mental qualities required of the physician, and the book then goes on to picture the workshop, the *iatreion,* in which the apprentice-student receives his training. General medical and particularly surgical principles are discussed, and the final chapter is devoted to remarks about military medicine. It is recommended that students who wish to become proficient surgeons attach themselves to mercenary troops fighting in foreign lands, since this will give them the best opportunity to practice surgery.

Although it is not deontological, we may mention here another general treatise which has attracted much attention, *The Art* (Περὶ τέχνης), an apology for medicine,[55] the oration of a sophist. Gomperz thought that the author was Protagoras, others that it might have been Hippias.[56] There is no doubt that the author was not a physician but a philosopher who developed the subject in the manner of the sophists. Medicine was attacked then as it was at all times, and usually with the same arguments. It was pointed out that patients recovered spontaneously, without medical care, that cures were due to sheer luck, that patients died in spite of all treatments, and that physicians refused to handle hopeless cases. The author refuted every point, very cleverly and very eloquently, as we would expect of a sophist.

And finally I must mention the Hippocratic work which became the most famous of all, was printed early, was reprinted in the original Greek and in the Latin translation innumerable times, and was translated into many vernacular languages, the work that seemed to synthesize the entire wisdom of Hippocratic medicine and was studied, quoted, and assimilated by endless generations of physicians, the *Aphorisms* ('Αφορισμοί), in seven books, to which an eighth book was added much later. The initial sentence of the first aphorism is known far beyond the narrow circle of the medical profession, for it applies to all other branches of knowledge as well: 'Life is short, the art is long; the opportunity is elusive, experience is fallacious, judgment is difficult.' In a vein more strictly medical though not without far-reaching application, the aphorism goes on to state: 'It is not enough for the physician to do what is necessary, but the patient and the attendants must cooperate as well and circumstances must be favorable.' [57] The first section of the *Aphorisms* deals primarily with evacuations and nutrition; the second is a regular hodge-podge of medical precepts; while the third is more systematic and discusses the influence of the seasons, winds, and atmospheric constitutions on the genesis and course of diseases. The fourth section deals again with evacuations, and moreover with fever diseases and their complications. Book V is mainly devoted to spastic diseases, diseases of the chest, the examination of various treatments, ailments of women, and wounds. Book VI evaluates which symptoms are favorable or not; it is in other words chiefly prognostic, at least in the beginning, while the later parts are purely symptomatic or give thera-

peutic prescriptions. Book VII finally repeats some of the preceding
statements and adds a number of symptomatic, prognostic, and therapeutic observations and recommendations. The *Aphorisms* is a very
remarkable book and we can well understand its popularity through
the ages. Numerous commentaries were written on it, for every
single aphorism might be used as a starting point of an entire dissertation. Littré was perfectly right when in 1844 he wrote of the book:
'Aujourd'hui comme jadis, il excite la méditation et fortifie la
pensée, genre de service que tous les livres ne rendent pas.' [58]

We listed the major Hippocratic writings, dividing them roughly
into groups according to subjects, and found that in spite of gaps
they covered a very wide field. We might also have grouped them
from other points of view, according to form and style. Some books
are regular textbooks, addressed to physicians, written for instruction
and constant reference; others, as we saw, are abstracts from these
textbooks made by some doctor or student. Before the invention of
printing the text of a medical book was never rigid, because such
books served a practical purpose and were in constant use. Therefore the doctor who owned a few medical books [59] added his own
observations to them, or added recipes that he had found effective,
or cancelled others that he did not like, and later copyists frequently
incorporated such changes into the original text.[60] This also explains
why at the end of some Hippocratic treatises we often find a number
of uncorrelated notes.

Some books, such as *Epidemics* I and III are a doctor's day-by-
day notes and case histories; still others are addressed to a lay
audience. A number of treatises were written for young men just
entering the profession. Some treatises are well-rounded monographs,
such as the book *On the Sacred Disease,* while others consist of rough
notes which were never meant to be 'published,' that is, to be copied
and circulated for centuries.

A much more interesting division of the books would be according
to schools. In fact, the books represent views not only of individuals

but of schools. There can be no doubt that the majority of the books preserved originated in the schools of Cos and Cnidus. They were the two leading medical centers in the second half of the fifth century and the first half of the fourth century B.C., but the other schools in southern Italy, Sicily, and North Africa were still active, and the influence of Alcmaeon and of the Sicilian school can be traced unmistakably in a number of Hippocratic writings. It would be most pleasing if we could attach a label to every book, designating it as Coan, Cnidian, Sicilian, or whatever its school of origin may have been, but unfortunately this cannot be done with any degree of certainty except in a limited number of cases, and there is much disagreement among philologists.[61]

Our knowledge of the Cnidian school derives from what later writers such as Galen tell us, and from the criticism of the *Cnidian Sentences,* one of the major works of the school, as we find it in the introduction of the treatise *On Diet in Acute Diseases.* The heads of the school were Herodicus and Euryphon, both outstanding physicians beyond any doubt. Both are mentioned in the Meno Papyrus along with Hippocrates.[62] Cnidus was a town on a peninsula of the mainland. Although not very distant from Cos and despite the fact that both had originally been Dorian colonies, Cnidus was infinitely closer to the civilizations of Asia and particularly of Mesopotamia.

The authors of the *Cnidian Sentences* were criticized for describing accurately what the patients experienced in every illness and what the outcome of the various diseases was, a matter that a layman could do as well, if he took the trouble to inquire carefully into what the sick felt. They neglected observation of symptoms, paid too little attention to making a correct prognosis, and their treatment was wrong in that they did not use a sufficient number of remedies. They were also criticized for their system of diseases, which seemed too artificial, for their disease entities would be almost innumerable if every symptom experienced by patients were held to constitute a disease and receive a different name.[63] The critic admits that the second edition of the *Cnidian Sentences* was much improved, but Cnidus remained known for its tendency to subdivide diseases. Galen,

in his commentary on the treatise *On Diet in Acute Diseases,* says
that the Cnidians described seven diseases of the bile, twelve of the
bladder, four of the kidneys, twelve kinds of strangury, four of
tetany, four of jaundice, and three of phthisis.[64] This tendency to list
symptoms, diseases, and treatments reminds us of the Mesopotamian
medical literature, which shows the same tendency to a very marked
degree, and it is quite possible that there was a direct influence. When
a book of the Hippocratic collection reveals this characteristic
approach to the problems of disease, we are obviously inclined to
attribute it to the Cnidian school. This applies to *On Diseases* Book
II, *On Internal Diseases,* and the numerous gynecological writings;
and we mentioned before that Edelstein even attributes *On Diet in
Acute Diseases* to the Cnidian school, an assumption which, if
correct, would prove that there were dissenting opinions and criticism
within the schools.

On the other hand, there is another group of writings which undoubtedly are related in character, style, and general outlook. They
are the books commonly considered the 'genuine' works of Hippocrates, and although we cannot attribute any one of them to the master
or any other definite individual, we are justified in assuming that they
were the works of the Coan school. They include such books as *Prognostic, Epidemics* I and III, *Airs, Waters, Places, On the Sacred
Disease,* and most of the surgical books. It is impossible today to determine the origin of many treatises with anything like certainty, and
there is no agreement among philologists even in regard to the two
major schools. For us who are primarily interested in the medical
content of these books, it is not so important to know on what island
or what part of the mainland a book was written, nor is it so important for us to establish in every case which philosopher influenced the writer of a given treatise. We must be grateful that so many
excellent books of the period have survived the vicissitudes of the
centuries, and we study them to find out what diseases the physicians
had to struggle with, how they treated them, whether treatments
were effective, and of course what ideas were guiding the doctors in
their actions.

NOTES

1. Plato, *Protagoras*, 311 B-C.
2. Plato, *Phaedrus*, 270 B-D.
3. Translation by B. Jowett, Oxford, 1892.
4. L. Edelstein, 'Hippocrates,' *The Oxford Classical Dictionary.*
5. *Anonymi Londinensis ex Aristotelis Menoniis et aliis medicis eclogae,* cd. H. Diels, Supplementum Aristotelicum iii. I (1893), v. 35f. A German translation by H. Beckh and F. Spät was published in Berlin, 1896, *Anonymus Londinensis, Auszüge eines Unbekannten aus Aristoteles-Menons Handbuch der Medizin.* An excellent English translation has been published with a reprint of the Greek text, *The Medical Writings of Anonymus Londinensis,* by W. H. S. Jones, Cambridge, 1947.
6. Reprinted here with the kind permission of W. H. S. Jones and the Cambridge University Press.
7. 1326 a 15f.
8. E. g. the *Coan Prognoses,* L. V, 588ff.
9. So Georg Sticker in the introduction to his German translation of Books I and III of the *Epidemics,* Klassiker der Medizin, Leipzig, 1923, vol. 28; and Gaston Baisette in his *Hippocrate,* Paris, 1931.
10. Three recent attempts are K. Deichgräber, 'Die Epidemien und das Corpus Hippocraticum,' *Abhdl. Preuss. Akad. Wiss.,* 1933, Phil.-Hist. Kl. No. 3; M. Pohlenz, *Hippokrates und die Begründung der wissenschaftlichen Medizin,* Berlin, 1938; W. Nestle, 'Hippocratica,' *Hermes,* 1938, 73:1ff. See L. Edelstein's discussion and refutation of the arguments, 'The Genuine Works of Hippocrates,' *Bull. Hist. Med.,* 1939, 7:236–48.
11. The analysis of the style of various writings is a promising method; see Margit Gutmann, *Die Nebensätze in ausgewählten Schriften des hippokratischen Corpus und ihre Bedeutung für die Verfasserfrage,* Thesis, Munich, 1929.
12. L. Edelstein, Περὶ ἀέρων *und die Sammlung der hippokratischen Schriften,* Berlin, 1931, p. 116ff.
13. Scholion on *Iliad,* 11, 515.
14. We know the names of the first editors, see M. Wellmann, 'Hippokrates-Glossare,' *Quellen u. Stud. Gesch. Naturwiss. Med.,* Berlin, 1931, vol. 2.
15. *Primus ex omnibus memoria dignis,* Celsus, I, 18, 12–13.
16. See E. Wenkebach, 'Der hippokratische Arzt als das Ideal Galens, Neue Textgestaltung seiner Schrift, "Ὅτι ὁ ἄριστος ἰατρὸς καὶ φιλόσοφος,' *Quellen u. Stud. Gesch. Naturwiss. Med.,* Berlin, 1933, vol. 3. Se also H. Diller, 'Zur Hippokratesauffassung des Galen,' *Hermes,* 1933, 68:167–81.
17. Tzetzes, *Chiliades,* VII, 944–89.
18. The lexicon is arranged alphabetically.
19. Codex Bruxellensis 1342–50. The biography of Hippocrates was published by H. Schöne, 'Bruchstücke einer neuen Hippocrates-vita,' *Rhein. Mus.,* N. F., 1904, 58; pp. 56–66.

20. The latest edition of this biography is that by J. Ilberg in *Corpus Medicorum Graecorum*, vol. IV, Leipzig and Berlin, 1927, p. 173ff.

21. For a critical discussion of the various biographies see L. Edelstein in *Pauly-Wissowa*, suppl. VI, col. 1290ff.

22. L. IX, 400ff. (All translations of Hippocrates are made from the Greek text; I have, of course, compared and used the available translations. See note 32, below.)

23. Lucian, *Philopseudes*, 21.

24. See L. Edelstein in *Pauly-Wissowa*, op. cit. col. 1306f.

25. Ed. Ilberg, p. 177, 10–12.

26. O. Bernhard, *Griechische und römische Münzbilder in ihren Beziehungen zur Geschichte der Medizin*, Zurich, 1926, plate IX, figs. 205, 206; J. J. Bernoulli, *Griechische Ikonographie*, Munich, 1901, Münztafel II, 8; *Catalogue of Greek Coins of Caria, Cos etc.*, 1897, plate XXXIII, fig. 7, p. 216.

27. Galleria Geographica Vaticana no. 113 and six replicas.

28. Villa Albani no. 1036, no replicas known.

29. G. Becatti, *Rend. Pont. Acc. Archeol.*, 1945–46, 21:123ff.

30. Such as the book *On Nourishment* and Book VII of the *Epidemics*.

31. H. Diels, *Die Handschriften der antiken Aerzte, I. Hippokrates und Galenos*, Berlin, 1905, pp. 3–57, and *Nachtrag*, 1908, pp. 25–9.

32. The Loeb Classical Library (Hippocrates, vol. I–IV, 1923ff.) missed a great opportunity to provide the English-speaking medical profession with a complete translation of the Hippocratic collection; France and Germany have excellent translations.

33. Περὶ καρδίης, *Libei Hippocraticus De Corde*, ed. F. C. Unger, Leiden, 1923, with text and Latin translation.

34. The fragments have been rearranged so that they make much more sense in R. Kapferer (with A. Fingerle and F. Lommer), *Die anatomischen Schriften, Die Anatomie, Das Herz, Die Adern in der hippokratischen Sammlung*, Stuttgart, 1951.

35. R. Kapferer, who made the most thorough study of Hippocratic anatomy, believes that Hippocratic physicians had some notion of a circulatory motion of the blood (op. cit. p. 29). P. Diepgen, on the other hand, came to opposite conclusions, 'Haben die Hippokratiker den Blutkreislauf gekannt?,' *Klin. Wschr.*, 1937, p. 1826; 'Die Hippokratiker und die Lehre vom Blutkreislauf,' *Münch. med. Wschr.*, 1939, p. 299.

36. H. Wanner, *Studien zu Περὶ ἀρχαίης ἰητρικῆς*, Thesis, Zurich, 1939; W. H. S. Jones, *Philosophy and Medicine in Ancient Greece, with an Edition of Περὶ ἀρχαίης ἰητρικῆς*, Baltimore, 1946; Hippocrate, *L'Ancienne Médecine*, Introduction, traduction et commentaire, par A.-J. Festugière, Paris, 1948.

37. Axel Nelson, *Die hippokratische Schrift Περὶ φυσῶν, Text und Studien*, Uppsala, 1909.

38. L. VI, 94: Πνεύματα δὲ τὰ μὲν ἐν τοῖσι σώμασι φῦσαι καλέονται, τὰ δὲ ἔξω τῶν σωμάτων ἀήρ.

39. L. V, 490.

40. See the German translation and commentary by G. Sticker, Hippokrates, *Der Volkskrankheiten erstes und drittes Buch,* Klassiker der Medizin, Leipzig, 1923, vol. 28.

41. W. H. Roscher, *Die hippokratische Schrift von der Siebenzahl in ihrer vierfachen Ueberlieferung,* Paderborn, 1913.

42. L. Edelstein, Περὶ ἀέρων *und die Sammlung der hippokratischen Schriften,* Berlin, 1931; H. Diller, 'Die Ueberlieferung der hippokratischen Schrift Περὶ ἀέρων, ὑδάτων, τόπων,' *Philologus,* Suppl. XXIII, 3, 1932; L. von Brunn, 'Hippokrates und die meteorologische Medizin,' *Gesnerus,* 1946, 3:151–73, 1947, 4:1–18, 65–85. See also Gerhard Jacoby, *Geographische Beobachtungen und Anschauungen im Corpus Hippocraticum,* Thesis, Jena, 1928.

43. B. Peyer, 'Das Problem der Vererbung von Reizwirkungen,' *Vierteljahrsschr. naturf. Ges.,* 1952, 97:65–81.

44. L. II, 10.

45. L. Edelstein, op. cit. p. 25ff.

46. *Prognostic,* L. II, 112.

47. L. Edelstein, op. cit. p. 154ff.

48. L. II, 232.

49. L. VI, 642.

50. Ermerins, *Hippocratis ... reliquiae,* II, LXVII.

51. Galen reports that Ctesias of Cos, a kinsman of Hippocrates, and later several others, condemned Hippocrates' reduction of the hip joint, a subject discussed at length in the book *On Joints.* See the discussion of E. T. Withington in the Loeb edition of Hippocrates, vol. III, p. 84.

52. H. Schöne published the text and illustrations of Codex Laurentianus LXXIV, 7 in: *Apollonius von Kitium, Illustrierter Kommentar zu der hippokratischen Schrift* Περὶ ἄρθρων, Leipzig, 1896.

53. L. VIII, 126.

54. Edited and discussed by J. F. Bensel in *Philologus,* 1922, 78:88–130.

55. T. Gomperz, *Die Apologie der Heilkunst, eine griechische Sophistenrede des fünften vorchristlichen Jahrhunderts,* Leipzig, 1910.

56. See the discussion of W. H. S. Jones in the Loeb Hippocrates, vol. II, p. 187f.

57. Even in recent times commentaries have been written on the first aphorisms, see, e. g., R. Koch, 'Auslegung des ersten hippokratischen Aphorismus,' *Festgabe Georg Sticker,* Berlin, 1930, pp. 1–10; 'Auslegung des zweiten hippokratischen Aphorismus,' *Festschrift Max Neuburger gewidmet,* Vienna, 1928, pp. 209–18; 'Auslegung des dritten hippokratischen Aphorismus,' *Sudhoffs Arch. Gesch. Med.,* 1933, 26:281–8. See also by the same author, 'Warum kamen die hippokratischen Aphorismen zu klassischer Bedeutung?,' *Münch. med. Wschr.,* 1933, 80:189–91.

58. L. IV, 440.

59. The number of books owned by a physician cannot have been large in

antiquity. Cf. the relief showing a doctor's library consisting of about eight papyri in E. Holländer, *Plastik und Medizin,* Stuttgart, 1912, p. 451, fig. 336.

60. Once books were printed doctors made marginal notes, as we find them in many old medical books. But these notes never became part of the text.

61. E. g. *On Diet in Acute Diseases,* usually considered Coan and in opposition to Cnidian views, is now looked upon as representing younger Cnidian views in opposition to those of the older generation; see note 47, above.

62. W. H. S. Jones, *The Medical Writings of Anonymus Londinensis,* Cambridge, 1947, p. 32ff.

63. *On Diet in Acute Diseases,* L. II, 224ff.

64. Galen, XV, 427f.

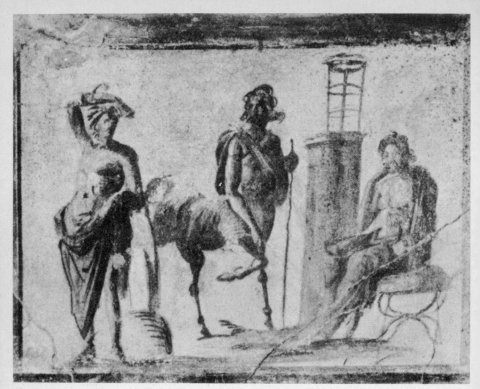

1. Wall portrait of Hippocrates from Casa d'Anonide. Naples, Museo Nationale. From L. Curtius, "Miscellen zur Geschichte der griechischen Porträts," *Archaeologisches Institut des Deutschen Reichs, Römische Mitteilungen,* 1944, vol. 59, p. 27.

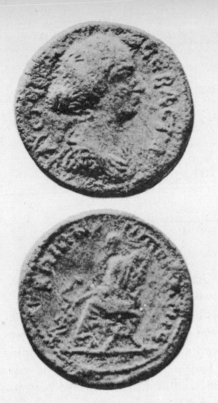

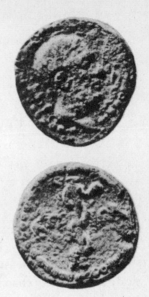

3. Coin of Cos. First century A.D.
Ibid. pl. 9, fig. 205.

2. Coin of Cos. Second century A.D. From
Oskar Bernhard, *Griechische und römische
Münzbilder*, pl. 9, fig. 206.

*

3. Patient and Physician

What did illness mean to the Greek patient of the Golden Age, and what was the physician like who advised and treated him?

We saw in the first volume of this history that the position of the sick man in society changed a great deal in the course of time. Some primitive tribes simply abandoned the sick, so that he was dead socially before his physical life had been ended. In others he was considered a victim of evil spirits, and as a man who had been in touch with the transcendental world he was looked upon with awe and sometimes great respect. In all archaic civilizations, including those of Greece and India, we encountered the view that disease was a punishment for sin sent by the deity, but in no literature was this more strongly expressed than in that of Mesopotamia and in the Old Testament. The patient of these early Semitic civilizations was burdened with the odium of sinfulness. He suffered, but justly so, in atonement for sin, his own sins, those of his parents, or of his clan.

The time of Hippocrates was an age of reason. It was by no means irreligious. The theatrical festivals in Athens were deeply religious experiences, and the author of *On the Sacred Disease* does not deny that there is θεῖόν τι, a divine element in the genesis of disease. His contention is merely that epilepsy is no more 'sacred' than any other disease but has a natural cause.[1] It was a rational age which would not have been satisfied with ascribing disease to the wrath of the gods. But the Greek patient was burdened with an odium also, that of inferiority. The Greek world of the classical age was a world of the healthy and the sound. Health was not only a treasured possession but an ideal. Jaeger, very justly, even goes so far as to say 'that the Greek ideal of culture was the ideal of health,' [2] because equality and harmony are the very essence of health. Physical culture as practiced by the Greek gentlemen 'imposed one supreme standard upon men—the duty of preserving a noble and healthy balance between their physical powers.' [3] Without health there could be no beauty, and as long as the Platonic ideal of *kalokagathia,* of perfect physical and mental balance in man, prevailed, health was of necessity valued very highly and illness was considered a great curse. Illness renders man inferior. It reveals to all that a man's harmony has been disturbed; it not only upsets the rhythm of his life but also disfigures him. The sick, the cripple, the weakling are inferior people and may count on society's attention only if their condition is likely to be improved. This is why weak infants were destroyed, and not only in Sparta. There never was any organized care for cripples or the blind. The sick man had to recover his health in order to be restored to his full status in society. But if his condition was hopeless, his disease incurable, the physician would not touch him. Treatment would have been senseless, since the goal, the restoration of health, was unattainable.[4] Thus the Greek patient was burdened with odium also, one from which he was freed by Christianity.

The Stoics attempted to overcome this point of view by declaring health and disease to be *adiaphora,* indifferent matters. Virtue is the only good, wickedness the only evil. However, in the later development of their philosophy, the Stoics made concessions to the needs of everyday life by admitting differences of value in the *adiaphora.* Health became a desirable *adiaphoron,* illness one to be rejected. Chrysippus, one of the leading Stoic philosophers, declared it insane not to desire health, wealth, and freedom from pain. An incurable disease seemed a sufficient justification for suicide, and Zeno is said to have hanged himself because of a broken finger.[5]

Health remained a highly desirable end throughout the classical

period, and this attitude obviously had deep repercussions in medicine and largely determined the physician's position in society. As a
man who worked for money, who sold his services on the open
market, who practiced a *techne,* a craft, much of which was manual,
the Greek doctor would not have held a very high social position.
Greek society at that time despised manual labor and the making of
money. However the service sold was considered extremely important, since it helped people to remain normal individuals or to regain
a normal status; the physician, therefore, among all craftsmen was
the most highly esteemed. Medicine, moreover, was a *techne,* a
craft—or an art, as we like to translate the word—of a special kind
in that it had a philosophy. There is no philosophy of shoemaking or
of baking. They are arts and crafts, too, important to the well-being
of man and even to the maintenance of health, but the baker makes
his bread without inquiring into the physiology of digestion or meta-
bolism. The physician, however, when he prescribes a diet or drugs
or performs an operation, is guided—at this stage of medical history
—not only by experience but also by ideas, by theories, by philosophy.
Indeed, educated people engaged in medical studies without ever
intending to practice the art.

The young man who wanted to study medicine, not in order to
broaden his philosophic outlook but to exercise the profession, became
apprenticed to a physician. He paid him a fee and worked with him
for a number of years, seeing patients with him, assisting him in
preparing remedies and in performing operations, keeping his surgery
in order and listening to the oral instruction of the master, making
notes of what he saw and heard.[6] If the student could afford it, he
went to a famous physician, an Asclepiad such as Hippocrates was.
Not all physicians were called Asclepiads, 'sons of Asclepius,' although
there may have been a time when the word was synonymous with
iatros—that is, 'physician.' I am inclined to believe that at the time
of Hippocrates the Asclepiads who were not priests but practicing
doctors represented an aristocracy among the profession, that they
were members of families in which medicine had been practiced for
generations.

The biographies of Hippocrates relate that he accepted students upon payment of a fee and after they had sworn an oath. It was long assumed that this was the Oath preserved in the Hippocratic collection, but recent investigation has shown that the document is probably late and has no connection with the school of Cos.[7] Since it has played such an important part in the history of medical ethics, we must discuss it in greater detail. The text reads, in the translation of Edelstein:

I swear by Apollo Physician and Asclepius and Hygieia and Panaceia and all the gods and goddesses, making them my witnesses, that I will fulfil according to my ability and judgment this oath and this covenant:

To hold him who has taught me this art as equal to my parents and to live my life in partnership with him, and if he is in need of money to give him a share of mine, and to regard his offspring as equal to my brothers in male lineage and to teach them this art—if they desire to learn it—without fee and covenant; to give a share of precepts and oral instruction and all the other learning to my sons and to the sons of him who has instructed me and to pupils who have signed the covenant and have taken an oath according to the medical law, but to no one else.

I will apply dietetic measures for the benefit of the sick according to my ability and judgment; I will keep them from harm and injustice.

I will neither give a deadly drug to anybody if asked for it, nor will I make a suggestion to this effect.

Similarly I will not give to a woman an abortive remedy.

In purity and holiness I will guard my life and my art.

I will not use the knife, not even on sufferers from stone, but will withdraw in favor of such men as are engaged in this work.

Whatever houses I may visit, I will come for the benefit of the sick, remaining free of all intentional injustice, of all mischief and in particular of sexual relations with both female and male persons, be they free or slaves.

What I may see or hear in the course of the treatment or even outside of the treatment in regard to the life of men, which on no account one must spread abroad, I will keep to myself holding such things shameful to be spoken about.

If I fulfil this oath and do not violate it, may it be granted to me to enjoy life and art, being honored with fame among all men for all time to come; if I transgress it and swear falsely, may the opposite of all this be my lot.

This is a beautiful document and at the same time one which presents a number of puzzles. Like every oath it begins with the invocation of the gods, who in a medical oath are first of all the healing deities: Apollo, Asclepius, and some of his children. Then follows a very interesting covenant, a kind of contract between teacher and student. The student is adopted into the teacher's family and shares the rights and obligations of the teacher's own children. Medicine, although not a secret lore, is not to be taught except to members of the family or to such outsiders as have joined the family by swearing to such a covenant.

The main part of the Oath concerns the duty of the physician to his patients. It is constructed quite symmetrically. In the center is the sentence, 'In purity and holiness I will guard my life and my art,' the only positive pledge of the whole Oath. It is preceded by three prohibitions, not to do harm or injustice to the sick, not to give a deadly drug to anybody, and not to give abortive remedies to women. And it is followed by three more prohibitions, not to practice surgery, not to have sexual intercourse with any member of the patient's household, male or female, and not to divulge secrets heard in the course of practice. Finally, the last paragraph indicates that the reward for fulfilling the Oath will be fame and good reputation, breaking the Oath will result in loss of face.

It is puzzling that in Hippocratic medicine abortion was in no way frowned upon but was considered a perfectly legitimate method of regulating the population, as we discussed in a previous chapter. Suicide, particularly under the influence of Stoic philosophy, was generally accepted, in Greece as well as in Rome, and we know of many cases in which poison was supplied by physicians. The Hippocratic doctor was physician as well as surgeon, and the surgical writings of the *Corpus Hippocraticum* are among the best of the whole collection and were frequently attributed to the master himself. Hence there was no reason why the physician should not 'use the knife'—that is, not practice surgery.

The explanation of all these contradictions is simply that the Oath originated in an environment which was totally different from that of Cos or Cnidus: namely, in a philosophical environment, among the Pythagoreans, as Edelstein has convincingly demonstrated. There it was considered unethical for the physician to lend a hand to any action that might lead to the destruction of life in any form. There the shedding of blood in operations and the risk of having a patient die under the knife was left to the surgeon. It is not at all certain that the Oath was ever sworn in antiquity. It is never mentioned in the pre-Christian era.[8] Pythagorean physicians may have drawn it up as a reform program and possibly even as a protest against current practices.

This theory of the origin of the Oath is confirmed still further by a document to which Charles Singer has drawn the attention of the medical historians.[9] The goddess Agdistis had a private shrine at Philadelphia in Lydia around 100 B.C., on which an inscription was found which required worshipers coming to the shrine to swear the following oath:

Let men and women, slave and free, when coming into this shrine swear by all the gods that they will not deliberately plan any evil guile, or baneful poison against any man or woman; that they will neither know nor use harmful spells; that they will neither turn to nor recommend to others nor have a hand in love-charms, abortives, contraceptives, or doing robbery or murder; that they will steal nothing but will be well-disposed to this house, and if any man does or purposes any of these things they will not keep silence but will reveal it and avenge. A man is not to have relations with the wife of another, whether a free woman or a married slave, or with a boy, or with a virgin, or to counsel this to another. . . . Let not woman or man who do the aforementioned acts come into this shrine; for in it are enthroned mighty deities, and they observe such offences, and will not tolerate those who transgress their commands. . . . These commands were set up by the rule of Agdistis, the most holy guardian and mistress of this shrine. May she put good intentions in men and women, free and slave alike, that they may abide by what is here inscribed; and may all men and women who are confident of their uprightness touch this writing, which gives the commandments of the god, at the monthly and the annual (?) sacrifices in order that it may be clear who abides by them and who does not. O Saviour Zeus, hear our words, and give us a good requital, health, deliverance, peace, safety on land and sea.

I do not think that there is any direct relation between this oath and the Hippocratic Oath, but the document is very important nonetheless, for it shows what ethical rules prevailed in certain religious circles. It also suggests how the Hippocratic Oath became so popular in the Christian world. A Christian, of course, could not swear by Apollo and Asclepius, but the beginning could be changed to 'Blessed be God, the Father of Our Lord Jesus Christ who is blessed for ever and ever; I lie not,' as we find in several manuscripts.[10] It is interesting that the Christian version omits the clause which forbids the physician to perform operations: and it also omits the covenant which makes the doctor a member of a restricted group. I fully agree with Jones that aristocratic exclusiveness was in sharp contrast with the Christian idea of universal brotherhood.[11]

One final point concerning the Oath must be mentioned here, since it illustrates conditions of practice. The aim of the Oath was to win for him who fulfilled it and did not violate it, *doxa*—that is, a good reputation and even fame. To have a good reputation is important for every doctor at all times, but to the itinerant Greek doctor *doxa* meant even more. There was no license to practice medicine granted by the state or any other organization, as we have had in the West since the Middle Ages. Nobody guaranteed that an individual who treated patients for a fee had any medical knowledge at all. There were quacks, and there must have been many of them.

In the *Precepts* we read of such charlatans who are 'at the bottom of ignorance of the Art,' who had no medical education, are a disgrace, yet manage 'to get credit for having been lucky in the treatment of some rich people.' [12] They are the fellows who endeavor to impress the people by displaying undue luxury in clothing, using rare perfumes,[13] and displaying showy instruments. Medicine, we read in the *Law,* the most distinguished of all the arts, is by far the least esteemed by the public, because there are so many ignorant practitioners, and the chief reasons for this condition is that medicine is the only art not subject to penalty in the city-states except dishonor, and this does not hurt the quacks.[14] Hence *doxa,* a good reputation, was the only credential a physician had, and this he acquired through his learning, skill, conscientiousness, correct prognoses, by finding out things that the patient does not tell him,[15] and in a general way by leading a worthy and dignified life.[16]

The short deontological writings of the *Corpus Hippocraticum* are addressed primarily to students and young doctors. What qualities must a young man possess who wishes to enter the profession? The *Law* gives an answer to this question:

Whoever is to acquire a competent knowledge of medicine ought to possess the following advantages: a natural ability, instruction, a favorable place for study, tuition from childhood, love of labor, time. First of all, a natural ability is required, for if nature is opposed, all efforts are in vain. But when nature leads the way to what is best, then the instruction of the art begins which the student must try to appropriate to himself by reflection, becoming an early pupil in a place favorable for learning. Moreover, he must labor for a long time so that learning may take root and bring forth proper and abundant fruits.[17]

The text then goes on to compare the learning of medicine to the growth of a plant. The student's natural aptitude is the soil on which the teacher sows the seeds at the right season—that is, early in life. In a proper environment the plant grows, until with time it reaches maturity. The first chapter of the treatise on the *Physician* tells us what qualities were expected of a good doctor.[18] He was to look healthy, and appear to be fit and in good physical condition: the common people are only too ready to assume that a doctor who cannot take care of himself is unable to help others successfully. He was expected to be very clean, decently dressed, and anointed with sweet-smelling unguents. He was to be silent, lead a morally irreproachable life, be grave and kind to all, serious without being harsh.

Doctors who made jokes and laughed immoderately in the presence of the sick, were frowned upon. The physician was to be fair in every respect and never lose his self-control, for the relationship between doctor and patient is a very intimate one: the sick man puts himself into the doctor's hands. The doctor is constantly in touch with women and girls, close to precious possessions, so that he must at all times remain bodily and spiritually clean. These are golden words, as true today as they were when a Greek teacher told them to his students.

At that time most physicians practiced as itinerants,[19] traveling from one city to another, offering their services as did other craftsmen, or artists, or sophists. In their youth they traveled with the master, assisting him. Later, themselves masters, they took young people along. A doctor needed assistance, particularly when he also practiced surgery, and it was advisable to leave a disciple at the bedside of patients who needed special attention, to carry out instructions and administer the treatment. Greece had no professional nurses as we do, and the young assistant physicians seem to have taken their place, at least in the case of patients of means. Doctors did not like to have laymen carrying out their instructions, because if anything went wrong, the blame fell on the physician.[20] A young assistant at the bedside of a patient, moreover, was able to act independently, if necessary, and could observe symptoms in the interval between visits of the master.

When a physician came to a town and found that there was sufficient work for him there, he settled down for a while, rented a shop or an entire house in some good location, perhaps in the market place. His assistants unpacked the surgical instruments, appliances, knives, drugs, and whatever a doctor needed in everyday practice. It was recommended that the doctor should always have a second physician's case handy when on a journey,[21] and that he should have a good supply of drugs prepared in advance, 'emollients classified according to their various uses,' draughts, purgative remedies 'taken from suitable localities, prepared in the proper manner.' [22] In a short while the house, which may have been a craftsman's workshop before, was turned into an *iatreion,* a physician's surgery, and the doctor was ready to see patients. People came, bringing their sick relatives for examination and treatment, and whoever has been in eastern Europe can well imagine the scene. The relation between physician and patient was intimate if the patient was rich and could afford to have the physician come to his home; otherwise, there was probably little privacy in the doctor's surgery. Relatives and neighbors would stand around, giving advice and all talking at the same time. Dislocated joints were reduced, broken extremities splinted, and other operations performed, more or less in public.

We know what such a surgery looked like, because two Hippocratic writings discuss the requirements it had to fulfill.[23] It was to be easy of access, like the workshop of other craftsmen—that is, it probably had a direct entrance from the street—but it was not to be drafty or glary. Too much light did not disturb the doctor but was unpleasant to the patient. The physician, as a rule, worked in daylight, but he undoubtedly also saw patients in the evening, and emergency operations might have been performed at night. This required artificial lighting. It was to be direct light, with the brightest spot turned on the part to be operated upon. Another important requirement was that plenty of pure water be available in the doctor's office, drinking water for the patient as well as water needed for various treatments. Chairs were to be of equal height, so that the patient and the examining physician would be on the same level. Lints and sponges used to wipe the eyes or wounds were to be clean and soft, and all instruments easy to handle. Detailed instructions were given for the preparation of the room for major operations. We shall come back to this point when we discuss Hippocratic surgery.

The question has been raised whether physicians took patients for general treatment or post-operative treatment into their houses, so that the *iatreion* would have been not only the doctor's office but some kind of private nursing home and as such the precursor of the ancient Western hospital.[24] There is no documentary evidence to support such an assumption, but on the other hand it seems only logical that after a serious operation patients, particularly out-of-town patients, were kept for a while at the doctor's house, where they could be nursed by the physician's assistants or slaves, be under constant observation, and be sure of immediate attention in the case of complications. Every Greek house had guest rooms (ξενῶνες), and it is quite possible that patients were kept in such rooms for a period of time.

Patients of means did not seek the doctor's office but were examined and treated in their homes. Operations were performed in private houses, as was the case in some European countries until the end of the nineteenth century. The book on *Epidemics,* a doctor's diary and case book, frequently gives the patients' addresses, which means that the doctor went to see them in their homes. The many instructions about bedside manners given in the deontological writings apply mostly to this private practice which was the doctor's *praxis aurea.*

On entering [the sickroom] remember the manner of sitting down, reserve, arrangement of dress, authoritative demeanor, brevity of speech, perfect composure, assiduous attention, care, replies to objections, calm self-control to meet the troubles that occur, severity to rebuke disturbance, goodwill to do what has to be done. ... Make frequent visits, examine carefully ... thus you will know the case more easily and at the same time you will be more at ease. ... Watch also the faults of the patients, many of whom often lie about the taking of things prescribed. For by not taking disagreeable drinks, purgative or other, they sometimes die. The fact is never admitted but the blame is thrown upon the physician. The bed also must be considered. The season and the kind of illness make a difference. Some patients are put into breezy spots,[25] others into covered places or underground. Consider also noises and smells, particularly the smell of wine. This is very bad and you must shun it or change it. Perform all these things quietly, skilfully, and conceal from the patient most of what you are doing. Give necessary orders cheerfully and with serenity, turn his attention away from what is being done to him; sometimes you have to reprimand him sharply and severely, and sometimes you must comfort him with attention and solicitude.[26]

This was good advice, as valid today as it was then. The controversial question whether the patient should be informed about his condition was not evaded. The writer of *Decorum* was very outspoken on the subject and urged the physician not to reveal anything to the patient, either about his present condition or about the prognosis, at least—this must have been understood—if it was not favorable, for many patients have been brought close to death for having been told the truth.[27] Another delicate question was also discussed: namely, consultation with a colleague.[28] The doctor was strongly advised not to hesitate to call in other physicians, if the case was not clear or if he had not sufficient experience. But the physicians who attend a patient together must never quarrel or ridicule one another, 'for I swear that no physician should envy a colleague's reasoning; this would reveal the weakness of his own thought.'

There are many golden words in these short deontological treatises. They have been quoted for centuries, since the profession found them to be true. In the sixteenth century, Paracelsus said, 'Der höchste grund der arznei ist die liebe'[29] (Love is the foundation of medicine), and two thousand years earlier the author of *Precepts* said, 'Where there is love of man, there is also love of the art.'[30] And *Decorum* postulates that wisdom be transplanted into medicine and medicine into wisdom, for a physician who is a *philosophos* —that is, a lover of wisdom—is god-like.[31] Medicine has all the noble qualities of philosophy and they are similar in purpose. The physician, furthermore, must be humble, realizing that many sick people recover spontaneously. In the sixteenth century, the great French surgeon Ambroise Paré used to say, 'Ie le pensay . . . et Dieu le guarist' (I dressed the wounded man . . . and God cured him), and similarly the Hippocratic writer said, 'The gods are the real physicians, though people do not think so.'[32]

Physicians were paid for their services but not for every individual service, as happens in many countries today. When the doctor took over a case, a certain fee, a lump sum, was agreed upon for the entire treatment. And the physician could be urged to visit his patient frequently, as we mentioned before, since this did not increase the cost of the treatment. The treatise *Precepts* has some pertinent remarks on the subject of fees.³³ The doctor is advised not to be too greedy and to take the economic status of his patient into consideration, even to be prepared to give free services occasionally, either because he has some obligation toward an individual or for the sake of his reputation. This is especially desirable in the case of some poor foreigner who has fallen ill far away from home, without the possibility of obtaining the funds necessary for treatment. The agreement in advance upon payment of a certain fee was not without advantages, for the patient knew where he stood and had a certain guarantee that the physician would do all that was in his power and would not abandon him. On the other hand, the doctor was urged not to raise the question of fees in the beginning in certain cases, particularly with patients suffering from acute diseases. Such patients should not be worried with financial matters, for their condition would be unfavorably affected. The physician, of course, runs the risk of not being paid at all, but glory is better than gain, and it is better to be forced to scold people whose lives you saved than to exploit patients who are in danger.

Greek society was strictly divided into social classes—citizens, metics, and slaves—and there was a class distinction not only of patients but correspondingly also of physicians. In the *Laws* and the *Republic* Plato gives us a picture of conditions as they existed in Athens in the fourth century B.C.³⁴ The free gentleman-physician treated people of his own class. He treated them for money, to be sure, but still they were people of similar education with whom he could discuss problems of health and disease, and of philosophy at large. The sick slave and other patients of moderate means were treated by the physician's assistants or even by his slaves. A carpenter and other craftsmen who had to make a living had no time for elaborate cures. The doctor gave them a vomitive or purgative, cauterized or cut them without further explanation, and many who could not afford the expense went without any treatment at all, or sought healing in the temples of Asclepius.

Most doctors were itinerant physicians, but larger communities were obviously anxious to have a permanent physician who was a resident of their town. In order to attract a doctor they liked, they appointed him municipal physician and paid him an annual salary, the amount of which was raised through a special tax. The salaried physician therefore is not a new institution but one that has a very old tradition. We mentioned before that Democedes of Croton was municipal doctor in Aegina, and there can be no doubt that from the sixth century B.C. on most larger Greek cities had their publicly appointed doctor, who in addition to his salary was allowed to accept fees from patients of means.[35]

Today we have a whole army of auxiliary medical personnel— nurses, public health nurses, midwives, highly specialized laboratory technicians, optometrists, pharmacists, and many others. Ancient Greece had midwives, as we mentioned before, but otherwise the physician and his assistants working as a team did practically all the work. They compounded the remedies they prescribed, yet some of the drugs they may not have collected themselves but may have bought from the *rhizotomoi,* 'root cutters,' people who knew medicinal plants and knew where to find them and when they should be cut.[36]

NOTES

1. *On the Sacred Disease,* L. VI, 352. See also L. Edelstein, 'Greek Medicine in Its Relation to Religion and Magic,' *Bull. Inst. Hist. Med.,* 1937, 5: 201–46.
2. W. Jaeger, *Paideia,* New York, 1944, vol. III, p. 45.
3. Ibid.
4. Plato, *Republic,* III, 408.
5. The sources of this subject may be found in E. Zeller, *Die Philosophie der Griechen in ihrer geschichtlichen Entwicklung,* 5th ed., Leipzig, 1923, vol. III, pt. I, in the chapter on the Stoics.
6. See T. Puschmann, *Geschichte des medizinischen Unterrichts,* Leipzig, 1889.
7. L. Edelstein, *The Hippocratic Oath,* Baltimore, 1943. On the Oath in general, see W. H. S. Jones, *The Doctor's Oath,* Cambridge, 1924; J. Hirschberg, *Vorlesungen über Hippokratische Heilkunde,* Leipzig, 1922, p. 26ff.

8. The earliest ancient reference to the Oath dates from the first century A.D. and is to be found in the preface to the *Compositiones* of Scribonius Largus.

9. Charles Singer, 'An Early Parallel to the Hippocratic Oath,' *Gesnerus*, 1951, 8:177–80. The text is given in W. Dittenberger's *Sylloge Inscriptionum Graecarum*, 3rd ed., no. 985. The English translation is from A. D. Nock, *Conversion: The Old and the New in Religion from Alexander the Great to Augustine of Hippo*, Oxford, 1933, p. 216.

10. See W. H. S. Jones, op. cit. p. 23.

11. Ibid. p. 54.

12. *Precepts*, L. IX, 258ff.

13. Ibid. L. IX, 266.

14. *Law*, L. IV, 638.

15. *On Diet in Acute Diseases*, L. II, 224.

16. *Decorum*, L. IX, 227; *Physician*, L. IX, 204.

17. *Law*, L. IV, 638ff.

18. *Physician*, L. IX, 204ff.

19. *Law*, L. IV, 640.

20. *Decorum*, L. IX, 242.

21. Ibid. p. 236.

22. Ibid. p. 238.

23. *Physician*, L. IX, 206ff. and *The Surgery*, L. III, 272ff. The details are from these two works.

24. The chief publication on the subject is T. Meyer-Steineg, *Kranken-Anstalten im griechisch-römischen Altertum*, Jena, 1912.

25. The reading of Ermerins εὐπνόους adopted by Jones gives better sense than the ὑψηλούς of Littré.

26. *Decorum*, L. IX, 238ff.

27. Ibid. p. 242.

28. *Precepts*, L. IX, 262ff.

29. Theophrast von Hohenheim gen. Paracelsus *Sämtliche Werke*, herausgegeben von Karl Sudhoff, I. Abteilung, siebenter Band, Munich, 1923, p. 369.

30. *Precepts*, L. IX, 258, ἢν γὰρ παρῇ φιλανθρωπίη, πάρεστι καὶ φιλοτεχνίη.

31. *Decorum*, L. IX, 232.

32. Ibid. p. 234. The text of this chapter is very corrupt, but there can be no doubt of its general meaning. I follow the interpretation of W. H. S. Jones. Paré, *Apologie, et traité contenant les voyages faits en divers lieux*. Oeuvres complètes d'Ambroise Paré revues etc. par J. F. Malgaigne, Paris, 1841, vol. III, p. 698.

33. *Precepts*, L. IX, 254ff. The text is very corrupt.

34. See T. A. Sinclair, 'Class-Distinction in Medical Practice: A Piece of Ancient Evidence,' *Bull. Hist. Med.*, 1951, 25:386–7. The crucial passages are *Laws*, IV, 720; IX, 857, and *Republic*, III, 406ff.

35. See R. Pohl, *De Graecorum Medicis Publicis*, Berlin, 1905.

36. Root cutters were first mentioned by Theophrastus, *Historia Plantarum*, 9.1.7; 9.8.1.

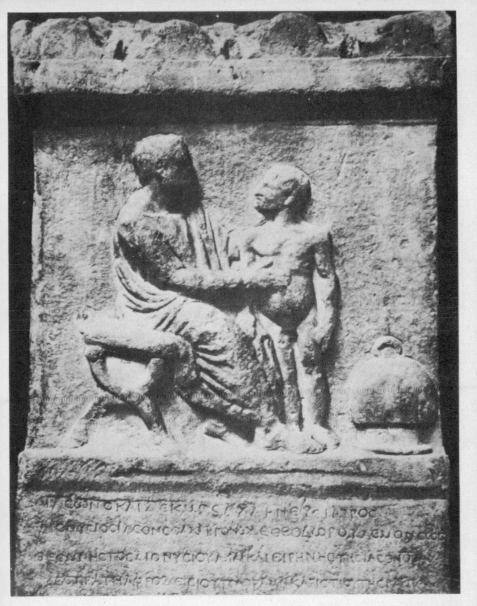

1. The physician Jason palpating the liver of a patient, funeral stele found in Athens, British Museum. From *Histoire générale de la médecine,* published under the direction of Laignel-Lavastine, Albin Michel, Paris, 1936, vol. I, p. 275.

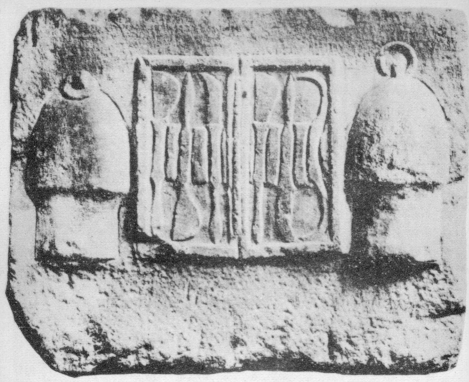

2. Instrument case, found in Asclepieion, Athens, in Athens Museum. Ibid. p. 285.

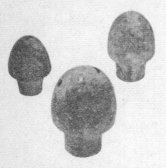

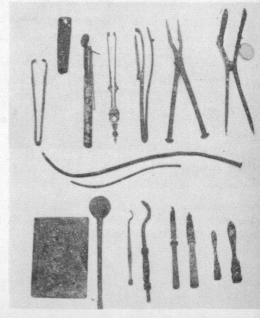

3. Bleeding cups. Found at Colothon. From the collection owned by The John Hopkins University and deposited in The Institute of the History of Medicine, Baltimore.

4. Surgical instruments. Found at Colothon. The Institute of the History of Medicine, Baltimore.

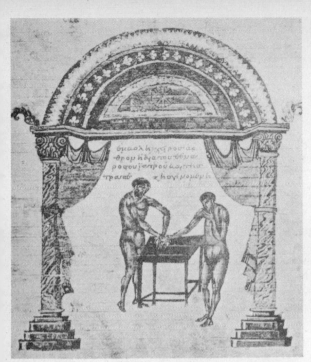

5. Resetting of a dislocated hand. From *Apollonius von Kitium, illustrierter Kommentar zu der hippokrateischen Schrift.* Περὶ ἄρθρων, ed. Hermann Schöne, B.G. Teubner, Leipzig, 1896, pl. 25.

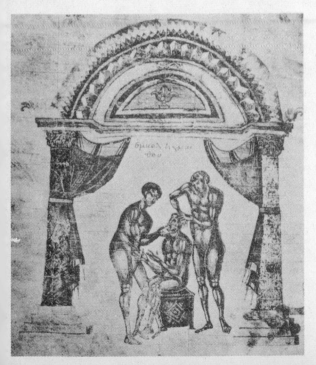

6. Resetting of a dislocated lower jaw. Ibid. pl. 14.

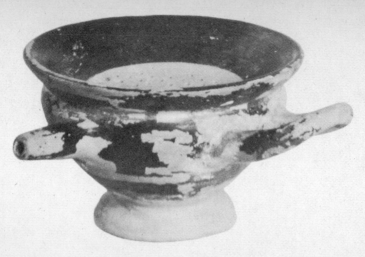

7. Feeding cup. Cleveland Museum of Art. Courtesy of Dr. Howard Dittrick, Cleveland Heights, Ohio.

8. Relief showing birth. Photograph from Dr. F. Merke, Basel, after correspondence with Professor Ludwig Curtius.

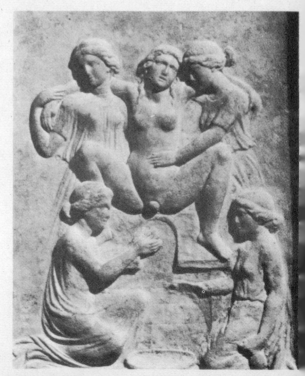

4. Medical Theories

What is health, what is disease? When is a man healthy, when is he sick, and what makes him so? If we have answers to these questions and if we know what factors are responsible for an individual's condition we obviously can act more purposefully than otherwise. Every period thinks, must necessarily think, in the categories of thought available at the time, and in every epoch these categories are limited. There are always individuals who are ahead of their time and think in completely different terms but they usually find no response. The Alexandrian Aristarchus outlined the heliocentric system, but the geocentric system of Ptolemy was considered correct up to the time of Copernicus.

The Hippocratic physicians were obviously influenced by the philosophy of nature and the scientific outlook of the pre-Socratics, and particularly by the Pythagoreans and Sicilians. Plato was a younger contemporary of Hippocrates, and Aristotle was yet to come. Hence to most Hippocratic writers health appeared as a condition of perfect equilibrium, while illness resulted when this balance was disturbed for some reason or other. This was a perfectly scientific view which excluded all transcendent forces. And it was a correct view and one that we still hold today. To us, too, health is a condition of perfect equilibrium. We differ from the Greeks when it comes to analyzing what constitutes the elements of the

human body. An equilibrium is impossible in a vacuum; it requires
a material substratum. After twenty-five hundred years of experience we know that the organism consists of cells and intercellular
substances which are kept alive and functioning by chemical and
physical forces. Some of these we can measure and reproduce ex-
perimentally, some we cannot. Our theory, in other words, has
highly speculative elements too.

The Greeks obviously did not possess our knowledge of chemistry
and physics, but like us they knew that elementary forces or qualities
(δυνάμεις) such as heat, cold, dry, moist, sweet, bitter are active
in the human body and that the perfect balance of these qualities,
whose number is not limited, constitutes health.[1] Force and
quality, however, were rather vague concepts, and we understand
that the physicians looked for more tangible substances which could
explain the phenomena of health and disease. Such a substance
necessary to life is air, and it seemed possible that too much or
not enough or contaminated air or air of wrong composition is
the determining factor in the genesis of disease.[2] But then there are
also humors in the human body as everybody knew: blood which
is found everywhere, phlegm that runs out of the nose and keeps
the mucous mer..branes moist, bile whose bitterness is sometimes
felt in the mouth, all the moistures which escape the body with
feces and urine. These humors seemed to explain health and disease
better than anything else, and we find several such humoral theories
developed in the Hippocratic writings.

The treatise *On Ancient Medicine* assumes that an unlimited
number of humors are found in the human body. They have elementary qualities. When their blend is perfect, man is in perfect
health. However, if wrong nutrition or some other mistake upsets
the balance, or if for some reason or other a certain humor is drained
from the body, then of necessity disease will result.[3] Another Hippocratic treatise holds that undigested food produces a humor which
ascends to the head and from there may invade any part of the
body. In such a case heat or cold may produce a flux which may
affect any organ.[4] Gradually we find the tendency to limit the

number of humors to four. Two pairs of humors with opposite qualities come to constitute the ideal balance. In the treatise *On Diseases* IV the humors are phlegm, blood, bile, and water.[5] They enter the semen, male and female, from which the embryo is formed. This explains why children have the same humors as their parents, healthy as well as vitiated humors. Each humor has a source, an organ of origin. Thus blood comes from the heart, phlegm from the head, water from the spleen, and bile from the gall bladder. And just as plants draw from the soil the substances appropriate to their nature, the humors are constantly renewed from the food and drink we absorb. Nutrition, therefore, is all-important. If the humors cannot find what they need in the intestinal tract they will take it from their sources of origin, thus drawing from the substance of the body. A surplus or a deficiency of any one of these humors may be the cause of disease. Similarly fever develops when the body has a surplus of digested food, when the individual has no evacuation and new food is being taken. In such a case the body, filled with old and new humors becomes inflamed and the result is fever. Plethora, in other words, or the accumulation of humors is one and probably the main pathogenic process. Other diseases are caused by violence, such as a fall, a wound, a blow, or fatigue. And a third pathogenic principle is to be sought in atmospheric conditions. All these factors act on the humors, make them coagulate, liquefy, or change in some other way. The vitiated humor attaches itself to some part of the body and the diseases are usually named after the organ affected.[6]

Why did water not become a cardinal humor equal in importance to blood, phlegm, and bile? The latter three humors could be seen on every occasion. Blood escaped from every wound, phlegm ran through the nose, bile was vomited occasionally. Water, however, was neither vomited nor secreted. Urine was watery, to be sure, but it was urine, not water. Water, moreover, was one of the elements of which the world was constituted, like earth, fire, and air. Was it not logical to look for another more physiological substance in establishing a system of physiology and pathology? Such a substance was black bile.[7] What is black bile, that humor which, for over two thousand years, was to play an extremely important part in people's thinking, and not only in medicine? We know of no such substance today, but I am inclined to believe that in this as in other cases the Greeks based their theories on observations. We know that the stool of patients suffering from bleeding gastric ulcers is black, as sometimes are the substances vomited by patients with carcinoma of the stomach. A form of malaria is still known as 'blackwater fever' because the urine as a result of acute intra-vascular hemolysis suddenly becomes very dark, if not black at least mahogany-colored. Similar observations may have led to the as-sumption that ordinary yellow bile through corruption could become black and that this black bile caused diseases, notably the 'black bile disease,' namely melancholy. In the writings of the fifth century B.C. black bile is not a cardinal humor, but a pathogenic agent. Müri has collected the pre-Aristotelian passages in which black bile occurs and found that it is mentioned not only in medical writings but in the works of Aristophanes, Plato, and Menander.[8] It was held responsible for a great variety of diseases ranging from headache, vertigo, paralysis, spasms, epilepsy, and other mental disturbances, to quartan fever and diseases of the kidneys, liver, and spleen.[9]

In the Hippocratic treatise *The Nature of Man,* one of the latest of the collection and commonly attributed to Polybus, black bile is mentioned as one of the four cardinal humors. In other words, we find it here for the first time not only as a cause of disease but as a normal constituent of the human body. This treatise, short as it is,[10] is most interesting and is the starting point of the theory of the four humors, which dominated medicine for many centuries. Other treatises of the Hippocratic collection have a greater appeal to today's medical reader because of their wealth of observation. They all presuppose an underlying theory, but these theories are usually vague, while this treatise is outspokenly theoretical and attempts to explain health and disease from a few simple principles. Its very simplicity is impressive.

The Eleatic philosopher Melissus, who flourished in the middle of the fifth century B.C., had opposed Empedocles' theory of the four elements and had postulated that all things are one. His views had influenced physicians who tried to explain man from one principle. Some claimed that the human body was made of blood, others that it consisted of bile, and still others looked upon phlegm as the one substance responsible for health and disease. Under the influence of heat and cold the one humor changed in appearance and quality, became sweet, bitter, white, black, and so on. This is wrong, says Polybus, or whoever the author of our treatise was, for if man were one he would never suffer.[11] From what cause would he suffer being one—that is, a simple organism? And if he did suffer disease, there would in such a case be one remedy only. Now we know that there are many remedies, and indeed there are many substances in the human body which by becoming abnormally hot, cold, dry, or moist produce illness—and not only one form of illness but many; this explains why we have many different treatments. But the substances which constitute the human and animal organism do not occur in unlimited numbers, they are four—blood, phlegm, yellow bile, and black bile—and they are responsible for health and disease. Perfect health prevails when these substances are well balanced with regard to temperament,[12] strength, and quantity and when their blend is perfect. Disease results when there is not enough or too much of one of these humors or when one of them separates from the rest. Indeed when one humor isolates itself, goes its own way, and no longer co-operates with the others, then not only the place it left suffers but the one in which it settles becomes congested and pain results. Similarly the abnormal evacuation of a humor be it outside or inside the body will cause pain.

These humors are not fictitious, not mere principles, but are very real. Wound the body anywhere and you will see blood. Give a drug that acts on phlegm and the individual will vomit phlegm, or bile if you give him a cholagogic remedy. Similarly he will evacuate black bile in response to certain drugs. This happens in every season, no matter how old the individual is. The physician must always consider the seasons, since they have a definite influence upon the humors. Phlegm, the coldest of all humors, increases in winter. At that time therefore phlegm diseases are prevalent, and you see people sneezing and blowing their noses. In the spring phlegm still is powerful but the blood increases, for it is moist and hot like spring. Dysenteries, bleeding from the nose, and other hemorrhages are not infrequent at that time. The hot and dry summer sets the bile in motion, and bile dominates until autumn. People vomit bile, their stools are bilious, fevers have a bilious character, and the skin is frequently yellow. Autumn is a dry season, beginning to be cold. At that time the black bile dominates in the body. Thus the four humors are always present in man just as the qualities hot, cold, dry, and moist are always present in nature, but the blend is not always the same, and this explains the different disposition of man toward diseases according to the seasons of the year.[13]

Simple as this theory is it opened up wide horizons. Two pairs of humors with opposite qualities were indeed the ideal carriers of the balance of health. But more than this: the qualities corresponded not only to the seasons but also to the elements which according to Empedocles constituted the universe, earth, water, fire, and air. Thus it was possible to establish a direct relationship between the macrocosm of the universe and the microcosm of the organism and to link them up with the atmospheric changes due to the seasons. The same elementary qualities were found in nature and in man, who thus appeared as an integral part of nature. This relationship also paved the way for further systematizing. Not only the elements, humors, and seasons had elementary qualities but the organs, diseases, and remedies. Once the principle was established that contraries should be cured by contraries [14] and once one had a key to the qualities of the various objects of nature, treatment became mathematical and medicine seemed to have lost its conjectural character. We shall come back to these problems when we discuss the work of Galen. The relation between element, humor, and season is best illustrated by the following figure:

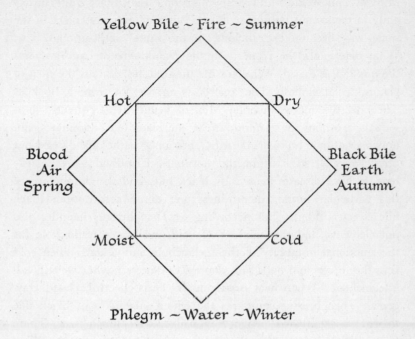

We may anticipate somewhat at this point and draw attention to another possibility that this theory offered. Experience had taught that many diseases had a seasonal character, and, as we just mentioned, this was explained by the assumption that the humor which had the same quality as the season dominated physiologically at such a time and thus created a disposition to certain diseases. Experience taught, furthermore, that individuals differ a great deal from one another. There are tall and short, lean and fat, blonde and brunette, intelligent and stupid, irascible and placid people. It was observed that certain somatic qualities were frequently combined with very definite mental qualities. Fat people are usually benevolent. The devil is pictured as lean; if he is fat he is a good devil. In other words, it was found at an early date that there are what we would call psychosomatic constitutional types of men. Every individual is unique, to be sure; no two have the same fingerprint or handwriting and different people may react quite differently to the same stimulus or lesion. But they may also react in the same way because they belong to the same constitutional type. What determines the type? [15] In the pseudo-Aristotelian *Problems* the question is raised, 'Why are the unusual individuals, the men of genius, melancholics?' The answer is an excerpt from a book of Theophrastus on melancholy. Men of genius are frequently individuals in whom the *melaina chole,* the black bile, dominates, not only in autumn but permanently, not in a pathological way but physiologically, still within the norm. Such individuals obviously tend to have diseases caused by black bile, and the dominance of this particular humor determines their entire constitution. Black bile is cold and dry but according to Theophrastus includes also hot elements, and this mixture of cold and hot is responsible for the emotional instability of the melancholic individual. When cold is in the foreground he is sad, depressed, dejected, what we still call 'melancholic.' When heat predominates he is cheerful, elated, gay, genial. Theophrastus compares the emotional effects of black bile to what is experienced when a man drinks too much wine. There too you have these sudden changes from hilarity to depression. When heat and cold are well-tempered then the melancholic individual may accomplish great feats and this is why so many poets, artists, philosophers, and statesmen were found to belong to this particular constitutional type.[16]

This discovery of Theophrastus was extremely important, for it showed what good use could be made of the theory of the four humors for the interpretation of human constitutions. If there are individuals in whom black bile dominates at all times physiologically, there obviously must also be people in whom one of the other humors—blood, phlegm, or yellow bile—dominates. The Arabs developed and extended this theory, describing the sanguine, phlegmatic, and choleric constitutional types as Theophrastus had pictured the melancholic. Combined with astrological elements the theory was developed and extended still further in the West in the Middle Ages and the Renaissance. And strangely enough, modern psychosomatic studies made by psychiatrists, notably E. Kretsch-mer,[17] have shown that most of these ancient constitutional types are not fictitious, not the result of a desire to systematize vague observations, but are very real, and may be described in scientific terms.

The physiological and pathological theory expounded in *On the Nature of Man*, like other Hippocratic theories, emphasized the humors of the body. They were considered the most important part of the organism, were found everywhere, and were responsible for health and disease. We therefore speak of a 'humoral pathology.' Later in this book we shall discuss other theories in which the solid particles of the body, the atoms, were in the foreground of the doctors' thinking. Humoral considerations, however, dominate Hippocratic medicine even in writings where this is not stated explicitly and the reason is easily conjectured. If health is understood to be a condition of perfect equilibrium, and disease the result of a disturbed balance, then humors certainly provide a better explanation than elements or qualities. Humors are tangible and can be mixed and unmixed; it is much more difficult to conceive a perfect blend of fire and water, or of bitter and sweet. Thus the theory of the four humors was decidedly a great step forward, and its success through the centuries shows how workable it was.

Humors were not enough to explain life in health and disease. A driving force was needed to generate the humors from food, to keep them in motion, to blend them, to drive out superfluities, and to restore a disturbed balance. This driving force was believed to be the *'innate heat,'* ἔμφυτον θερμόν, which had its seat in the left ventricle of the heart.[18] This is why the heart is so hot and has to be cooled by respiration. In newborn children the innate heat is greatest, because in addition to all functions of life their bodies must grow; the heat is lowest in old people. This is why young people need much food, old people very little. And for the same reason fevers are not as acute in old people as in young. In winter and spring, moreover, the bellies are naturally hotter and people sleep longer. In these seasons one has to eat more: the innate heat is more abundant, more food is needed. Young people and athletes are evidence of this.[19]

What is the origin of this interesting concept of an innate heat? We must realize that the Hippocratic physicians distinguished three different kinds of heat. One was what we would call physical heat, the heat of summer, of fever, the heat applied externally in the treatment of certain ailments. Heat, however, was also an inherent quality of elements, humors, foods, and other products of nature. Galen was later to explain that pepper was hot, and the rose cold not ἐνεργείᾳ or ἁπλῶς, not by their inherent nature but ἐπικρατείᾳ, because these qualities dominated in them.[20] This became evident from their action on the human body. Pepper is not hot as fire is, but it burns when we eat it or get it in the eyes. The rose is not cold as ice is, but rose ointments have a cooling effect and were used in the treatment of burns.[21]

Innate heat was totally different, and Lichtenthaeler has suggested, in my opinion very convincingly, that the concept was derived from religion, that the innate heat was to the body what the sacred fire was to the Greek and Roman home.[22] In all Indo-European religions the sacred fire played a very important part.[23] It was kept burning on the altar of every home: it was worshiped as *Agni* in India; it was worshiped in ancient Persia and protected the family against all evils. In the same way the innate heat, sacred fire of the body, was kept burning in the heart, the body's hearth, and protected the individual against evil, keeping him alive and restoring health when it had been lost.

The innate heat is the essential part of a man's *physis*, his nature, and it is nature that heals. 'Nature is the physician of diseases. Nature finds ways and means all by itself, not as a result of thought.' [24] The discovery that there is a *vis medicatrix naturae,* a natural healing power in the human body, a force that tends to restore the lost balance, was one of the greatest discoveries medicine could make. It determined the physician's actions, since it became his main task to understand the intentions of nature, to prescribe a treatment that would support them, and to avoid whatever might antagonize them. 'To be helping or at least not harming' [25] became the basic principle of Hippocratic therapy. People had observed at all times that patients occasionally got well without any medical aid but such an event could be ascribed to the intervention of the deity. The Greek considered nature responsible for it, the individual's *physis,* and they also found that nature could be helped very effectively if the physician had knowledge of nature. Some characteristic examples to illustrate this point will be given in the next chapter.

It was observed that diseases had a natural course. A common cold lasts one week. A patient suffering from pneumonia is very ill for about a week, then in many cases there is a most dramatic crisis, his fever drops, he sweats profusely, falls asleep, and wakes up with a feeling of well-being. A sick man suffering from what we today call typhoid fever is very sick for about three weeks, then the disease ends in recovery or, formerly in 10 per cent of the cases, in death. Ten per cent was also the death rate of pneumonia before the modern era of chemotherapy. What caused these diseases? What determined their course? The Greeks observed that with a common cold we evacuate a great deal of matter through the nose and that this matter changes during the week. It is liquid and light in the beginning, later thickens and changes color, becoming yellow or green, and then the evacuation stops. In the case of pneumonia we cough and the sputum also changes, being liquid and sero-sanguineous in the beginning, becoming rusty or brown, thick and tenacious until the crisis puts an end to our coughing. The typhoid patient has evacuations through the intestinal tract, painful diarrheas at times, and in the case of an intestinal hemorrhage the stools will contain gross blood. How was all this to be understood? The humoral theory as it developed gradually explains this very well. For some reason or other—faulty diet, wrong mode of living in a certain season, exertion, or whatever the cause might have been—one of the humors dominated in an abnormal way, became what was later called a *materia peccans,* and had to be driven out of the body so that the balance might be restored. To that end, however, the faulty matter had to undergo a process which was called *pepsis* or coction. It had to become ripe to be expelled. The body mobilized all its defensive forces and attacked the raw, faulty humor which under the influence of the innate heat became 'cooked,' ripe, and ready to be expelled. 'Sputa are cooked as soon as they have become similar to pus; urines, however, when they have a red sediment like the seed of bitter vetch.' [26] The expulsion was quick and dramatic, in the form of a *crisis;* or slow and gradual—in the latter case we still speak of a *lysis.* The crisis is defined in the treatise *On Diseases* as a condition in which a disease suddenly takes a turn for the worse or for the better or changes its character or ends by being healed.[27] It is the decisive battle between man's nature and the disease.

We mentioned before that the Greeks had observed that the course of many diseases followed a certain rhythm and that the crisis occurred on definite days. This is no wonder in a country where malaria prevailed; few diseases have a more regular rhythm, so that the time when the patient will be shaken by fever can be predicted to the hour. Starting from such observations some physicians assumed that all acute diseases had their critical days, and this opened the door to speculation and a playing with numbers in which the influence of Assyria as well as of the Pythagorean school may be discerned. The author of *Epidemics* I declares:

Those diseases which have their paroxysms on even days have their crises on even days. Those which have their paroxysms on uneven days have their crises on uneven days. The first period of those which have their crises on even days, is the 4th day, then the 6th, 8th, 10th, 14th, 20th, 30th, 40th, 60th, 80th, 100th. The first period of those which have their crises on uneven days, is the 3rd, then the 5th, 7th, 11th, 17th, 21st, 27th, 31st. It should be known that if the crisis take place on any other day than on those described, it indicates that there will be a relapse which may prove fatal. One must pay attention to the crises and know that at such times they decide about life and death or at least indicate changes for the better or worse. Irregular fevers, quartans, quintans, septans, and nonans should be studied in order to find out in what periods their crises take place.[28]

The number four points to the Pythagorean school, the number seven to Mesopotamia. Both numbers played a most important part in all these speculations, which after all are nothing but an attempt to correlate disease with cosmic forces. A very characteristic passage occurs in *Prognostics:*

Fevers come to a crisis on the same days as to number, both those from which men recover and from which they die. For the mildest class of fevers, and those appearing with the most favorable symptoms, cease on the fourth day or earlier; and the most malignant and those setting in with the most dangerous symptoms prove fatal on the fourth day or earlier. The first period of their violence ends thus, the second is protracted to the seventh day, the third to the eleventh, the fourth to the fourteenth, the fifth to the seventeenth, and the sixth to the twentieth. Thus these periods of the most acute disease ascend by fours up to twenty.[29]

The author then very cautiously adds: 'But none of these [periods] can be truly calculated by whole days, for neither the year nor the months can be numbered by whole days.'

Similarly we read in the *Aphorisms*[30] that acute diseases come to a crisis within fourteen days. 'The fourth day is indicative of the seventh; the eighth is the beginning of the second week; and the eleventh, being the fourth of the second week, is also indicative; and again, the seventeenth is indicative, as being the fourth from the fourteenth and the seventh from the eleventh.' There was a strong speculative element in these theories of critical days, to be sure, but they were based on correct observations. Today we know that the rhythm of malaria is determined by the life cycle of its causative agent, the plasmodium. The Greeks did not know the cause but the effect, and from that they attempted to reach general conclusions.

The Hippocratic concept of disease was in many ways different from ours. An example will illustrate this best. The author of *Epidemics* I was a physician who in his practice on the island of Thasos kept a careful record of the patients he saw in his office and also of what the Greeks called *katastasis,* a word which means condition, constitution, and which in later medicine was called *constitutio epidemica* and was to play a great part in the pre-bacterial period of epidemiology. The very correct idea was that there is a direct connection between climate, season, weather, and the occurrence of diseases. Malaria flares up in autumn. We also know that there is more malaria after periods of rain, because the larvae thrive in the numerous puddles and ditches filled with water. The Greeks did not know how malaria was transmitted but were fully aware of its seasonal occurrence, just as we know that epidemics of infantile paralysis subside when cold weather sets in although we do not know why.

Thus the author of *Epidemics* I made careful notes about the weather that prevailed while he was practicing in Thasos. The book begins:

In Thasos during autumn about the time of the equinox and toward the setting of the Pleiads abundant rains, gently continuous, with southerly winds. Winter southerly, light northerly winds, droughts. On the whole the winter was like spring. Spring southerly, cool, with light showers. Summer for the most part cloudy, no rain, Etesian winds [31] few, light, irregular. All atmospheric conditions were southerly with droughts but early in the spring the constitution changed into its opposite, became northerly and a few people were stricken with remittent fevers which, however, were mild, few patients had hemorrhages and no one died. Many had swellings in the region of the ears some on one side but most on both sides, without fever; so that the patients were not confined to bed. Some, however, experienced a slight heat but in all cases the swellings subsided without causing harm; neither did any of them come to suppuration as is common in swellings from other causes. As to their character, they were flabby, large, diffuse, without inflammation or pain, and in all cases disappeared without any sign. They seized youths, young men, and men in their prime, particularly those who frequented palaestra and gymnasiums, but attacked few women. Many had dry coughs without expectoration and their voice became hoarse. In some instances earlier, in others after a while, painful inflammations developed sometimes in one testicle, sometimes in both, some with fever, some without, and causing much suffering to most patients. In other respects the people were free of ailments requiring medical assistance.[32]

This passage is highly significant in many respects. It shows us a Hippocratic physician at work making careful observations of atmospheric conditions and of the symptoms of disease which his patients presented. He gives an excellent description of an epidemic of mumps. Few women are attacked, because they stay at home, while young people who crowd the sports grounds are highly exposed to infection. We miss reference to pain, but the most frequent complication in adult males, the very painful orchitis, is well observed and correlated with the initial disease. The swellings are described very correctly, but it is striking that such a well-characterized disease has no name. The writer speaks in quite general terms of ἐπάρματα παρὰ τὰ ὦτα, of swellings in the region of the ears, and immediately adds that these are different from swellings which suppurate, in other words from abscesses of the parotis. But he does not feel the need to attach a name to this particular disease and this points to a basic difference between the Hippocratic, and especially the Coan, concept of disease and the one we hold. We have names for every disease, to us they are well-characterized entities—abstractions, to be sure, but entities nevertheless. From the Renaissance and more especially from the seventeenth century on we developed an ontological concept of disease.[33] We know that no two individuals have exactly the same disease symptoms because no two individuals are identical,[34] but we also know that frequently patients show very similar, almost identical symptoms, that symptoms occur in well-defined combinations. This was first fully realized in the case of epidemic diseases. The plague attacked large groups of individuals who came down with very much the same symptoms. Some survived, many died, but the plague bubo was an unmistakable sign of the disease. In the Middle Ages physicians spoke of eight contagious diseases all of which were considered well-established entities:

> Febris acuta, ptisis, scabies, pedicon, sacer ignis,
> Anthrax, lippa, lepra nobis contagia praestant.[35]

Epilepsy, which is listed here as *pedicon,* had such striking symptoms that it was looked upon as an entity in itself wherever it occurred, and a special treatise on it preserved in the Hippocratic collection is one of the earliest monographs on a single disease. On the whole, however, the ontological concept developed relatively late. It was strengthened through the findings of pathological anatomy which demonstrated that disease has a seat and explained many symptoms as the result of well-defined anatomical lesions. The concept was strengthened still further through the discoveries of bacteriology. Symptoms, seat, anatomical changes, and causative agent characterized a disease. Tuberculosis of the lungs, of the bones, and of the skin are very different clinically, but since they have the same causative agent they have much in common and may be attacked by similar means. The case is the same with syphilis, also a protean disease.

Thus we were able to establish a system of diseases, by no means as perfect as physicians hoped for in the eighteenth century, but a system which groups disease entities according to various factors, depending upon which factor is in the foreground—etiology, pathological anatomy, or physiology—and our diagnosis is first of all one of the disease. Once we know from what disease a patient is suffering much of our further action is determined. Statistical experience tells us what the prognosis is on an average and also what treatments have the best chances of success. We, of course, must also make a diagnosis of the individual, since different persons react differently to the same lesion; but once an individual is sick, the disease entity dominates the picture.

The Greek approach was different. Diseases obviously were also localized, but roughly. Mumps were swellings in the region of the ears which did not suppurate. Pneumonia was peripleumonia, the disease in the region of the lungs. The malarial fevers with their iron rhythm were obviously well characterized, but the other continuous and ardent fevers were conditions under which the patient was hot and suffered, from which he recovered or died. We know that the term fever covered a great many of our disease entities.

Similarly a pain in the abdomen could be anything from appendicitis, to peritonitis or an intestinal tumor. In every case the disease was due to an upset balance of the constitutional elements of the body, such as for instance the humors, and the humors were everywhere in the body. This explained why in every case of illness the whole individual was sick and not just one of his organs, although the faulty humor frequently attached itself to an organ or a region of the body. Treatment, therefore, was to be not only local but also general, and the importance of the psychological element in every case of illness was not overlooked.

It is usually said that the Cnidian school was much more localistic than that of Cos, and we have already mentioned Galen's comment according to which the Cnidians described seven diseases of the bile, twelve of the bladder, four of the kidneys, and so on. But these were also very rough localizations and, as we pointed out, the listing of diseases according to their approximate seat was probably the result of Mesopotamian influences. The Cnidian concept of disease was as far removed from ours as that of the Coan school. All early Greek medical schools differed in theoretical points, but their basic approach was very similar [36] because they were contemporary and had common origins.

NOTES

1. This theory is developed in *On Ancient Medicine,* L. I, 570ff. See especially L. I, 602.
2. This theory is developed in *On Breaths,* L. VI, 91ff.
3. *On Ancient Medicine,* L. I, 618ff.
4. *On Places in Man,* L. VI, 276 and 290ff.
5. This and the following in L. VII, 542ff.
6. Ibid. p. 580ff.
7. In Greek, μέλαινα χολή, *melaina chole,* hence our 'melancholy,' 'melancholic.' About the early history of black bile see the most enlightening study of Walter Müri 'Melancholie und schwarze Galle,' *Museum Helveticum,* 1953, 10 (facs. 1):21–38.
8. The term, μελαγχολᾶν, 'to suffer from the black bile' must have been commonly used in Attica in the sense of 'to be crazy,' Müri, op. cit. p. 34f.

9. The passages are listed in Müri, op. cit. p. 32.

10. Chapters 9–15 do not belong to the book as Galen rightly remarked (XV, 9f).

11. The following is a paraphrase of chapters 2ff. of the treatise *On the Nature of Man* (L. VI, 35ff), which I felt would be clearer than a literal translation.

12. The Greek word is κρᾶσις, which means not only 'mixing,' 'blending,' but also 'temperature.' When it occurs in medical texts it is usually translated by 'temperament.'

13. Müri (op. cit. p. 28) makes the very fine observation that until the middle of the fifth century B.C. the Greeks spoke of three seasons only. Autumn was considered part of the summer, the part when the fruit ripens. It was only from the middle of the century on that autumn was looked upon as a season of its own, and it may well be that the separation of black bile from bile in general was a similar process. The author of *On the Nature of Man* frequently speaks of blood, phlegm, and bile only and actually has not much to say about black bile, which, however, he needed to match the seasons and to develop his theory in conformity with that of Empedocles. He needed two pairs of humors with opposite qualities, and black bile was better than water.

14. See *On the Nature of Man*, L. VI, 53.

15. On the history of these problems see the classical monograph of E. Panofsky and F. Saxl, *Dürers Melencolia I*, Leipzig, 1923; revised English edition, Princeton, 1948. See also Müri, op. cit.

16. *Problemata*, XXX, 1.

17. E. Kretschmer, *Körperbau und Charakter*, Berlin, 1921 (revised edition 1955); English edition, New York, 1925.

18. *On the Heart*, 6; L. IX, 84.

19. *Aphorisms* I, 14, 15; L. IV, 466.

20. Galen, XI, 542f.

21. Galen, XI, 561.

22. See his preliminary publication in *Actes Soc. Helvet. Sc. Nat.*, Berne, 1952, p. 172.

23. Fustel de Coulanges, *La Cité antique*, Bk. I, Ch. III.

24. Hippocrates, *Epidemics* VI, 5, 1; L. V, 314.

25. ὠφελεῖν ἢ μὴ βλάπτειν L. II, 634f.

26. L. II, 462f.

27. L. VI, 216.

28. L. II, 678ff.

29. L. II, 168ff.

30. Book II, 23–24, L. IV, 476.

31. Periodic winds blowing from the northwest during the summer.

32. L. II, 598.

33. See O. Temkin, 'Die Krankheitsauffassung von Hippokrates und Sydenham in ihren "Epidemien",' *Arch. Gesch. Med.*, 1928, 20:327-52.

34. Even identical twins are not quite identical.

35. Acute fever which may be anything from typhus to plague, tuberculosis, scabies, epilepsy, erysipelas, anthrax, an eye disease, possibly trachoma, leprosy. The verses are in the *Lilium medicinae* of Bernard Gordon, Venice, 1496, fol. 35V. Variations of these verses are discussed by K. Sudhoff, *Arch. Gesch. Med.*, 1913, 6:454f.

36. See O. Temkin, 'Der systematische Zusammenhang im Corpus Hippocraticum,' *Kyklos*, 1928, 1:9–43.

★

Index of Names and Places

HINDU

★

Subject Index

Abaton, 62, 64, 66, 67
Abortion, 201, 230–31, 301, 302
Ague, *see* Malaria
Air, 33, 91, 92, 97, 106, 109, 110, 322
Amulets, 23, 137–8, 140–42, 158, 160
Anatomy, 33, 277, 280, 293 n35
Animals, dissection of, 101, 114 n51
  paintings, 17
Anthropology, Hippocratic, 280
Arrow shooting, 20, 21, 26, 156
  poisoned, 28, 38 n76, 50
  and sudden death, 20–21, 47
Art, works of, as offerings, 72
Artemisiae (plants), 50
Aryans, 121, 122, 137, 141, 144, 152
  diet, 152 3
  migration of, 148, 149, 150, 151
  religion, 150, 153
  social structure, 153
Asclepiads, *see* Index of Names and Places
Asclepieia, 45, 57–73, 270, 310
  architecture, 63–4
  case histories at, 64, 65, 66
  hostels, 73
  patients, 64
  places, *see in* Index of Names and Places: Athens, Carthage, Cos, Epidaurus, Pergamum, Tricca
Asclepius
  Athenian reliefs to, 71
  blameless physician, 30, 52, 56
  coin, 55
  cult of, 29, 44–74, 95, 161; Epidaurian pattern, 45
  deification, 57
  dog of, 54, 62, 65, 69
  Imouthes, 60
  Panhellenic healing god, 61
  Phinaios, 55
  physician or surgeon, 67
  picture on a votive offering, **70–71**

snake of, 54, 58, 65, 67, 71
  temples of, *see* Asclepieia
  see also Index of Names and Places
Asphodel, 86
Astronomy, 88, 89, 90
Athens
  Acropolis of, 11, 58, 213
  Asclepieion in, 58, 63, 70–71
  center of culture, 214, 228
  democracy of, 223, 227
  Ecclesia, 223, 226, 227
  education, 234–5; gymnasium, 235–6
  reliefs to Asclepius, 71
  slaves in, 223–5

Barley, 12, 225
Bathrooms, 19, 143
Beans, taboo, 96
Bedside manners, 308
Bile, 319, 321, 322
  black, 320, 321, 322, 324, **333 n7, 333 n8**
  yellow, 321
Birth, 217, 232, 233
  rate of, in India, 127
Blindness, 65–9, 130, 132, 299
Blood, 102, 319, 321, 322
  circulation of, 106–7, 276, 293 **n35**
  origin in heart, 109
  vessels, 34, 102
Brahmanism, Brahmans, 149, 150, 169, 174, 175, 177, 179, 181
Brain, 99, 102, 108, 277
Bread, 12, 33, 86, 109
Breath, regulation of, 172
Buddhism, Buddhists, 169, 173, 176, 179, 181, 182, 185, 188 n24
  canon, 149
  period of, 148, 185
  pre-Buddhistic thought, 170, 174
Bull-god, 140

The indices have been compiled by Mrs. H. T. Perkins of the Department of the History of Medicine, Yale University.